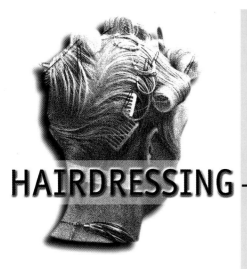

HAIRDRESSING – A Professional Approach

Levels 3, 4 & 5

David Bendell

PEARSON
Longman

Acknowledgements

I would like to thank all those who taught me the craft of hairdressing and all friends and colleagues in hairdressing, education and other spheres for their help and encouragement.

In particular, my sincere thanks to:

Robert Thomson, who is in charge of the scanning electron microscope at Victoria University of Wellington, and his staff for their continued enthusiasm and professionalism in producing the many dozens of interesting micrographs. Dr John Adams, dermatologist, and lecturer in the Department of Medicine, Wellington Clinical School, for supplying the scabie and also for the photographs of the scalp disorders. Dr Reid Basher, Manager, Climate Analysis and Application, NIWA, for his assistance in redrafting the section on New Zealand's ultra-violet radiation.

My hairdressing associates at The Open Polytechnic, and in particular Mary Young, for their advice and comments on a large number of scripts. My colleagues at the Wellington Polytechnic (now Massey University) for their time and professional expertise in checking the science, accounting, electrical, first-aid and computing content. David Sallinger, trichologist. L'Oréal, for permission to use its colour techniques for multi-shading.

Finally, my wife, Marie Wilson, for her advice, suggestions, patience, tolerance and continuing support during the time I spent writing the text.

www.pearsoned.co.nz

Your comments on this book are welcome at
feedback@pearsoned.co.nz

Pearson Education New Zealand
a division of Pearson New Zealand Ltd
67 Apollo Drive, Rosedale,
North Shore 0632,
New Zealand

Associated companies throughout the world

© Pearson Education New Zealand 1999, 2000

Originally published 1988 by GP Publications © David Bendell 1988
Reprinted 1990, 1994
Reprinted by Addison Wesley Longman New Zealand Limited 1999
Second edition published by Pearson Education New Zealand 2000
Reprinted 2004, 2005, 2006, 2007, 2008 (twice), 2009, 2010

ISBN 978-0-582-54259-4

Produced by Pearson Education New Zealand
Printed in Malaysia via Pearson Malaysia, VVP
Typeset in 10.5/12pt Palatino

Contents

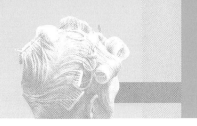

Preface

First, congratulations on completing the Level 1 and Level 2 stages of your training. As the next step in achieving your goal to become a professional hairdresser, this textbook introduces you to Levels 3, 4 and 5.

The time has come to 'move up a notch'. This is the stage in your training when your responsibilities will increase. The expectations will include:

- building up a clientele;
- attending cutting, perming and colouring workshops;
- deciding on your own colour selection;
- choosing the correct solutions and formulas for your clients;
- recommending correct product ranges for clients;
- taking part in competitions;
- assisting junior staff;
- going to seminars and shows;
- learning banking procedures;
- understanding the day-to-day running of a salon;
- completing practical assessments.

Accept these new challenges and show the salon that you are ready for, and willing to, undertake more responsibility. Let your employer know you are keen to learn and acquire more knowledge as part of your development. This book will assist you in developing such knowledge and extra responsibility. Constantly strive to improve: read this text, answer the questions, check the results – and you will reach your ultimate goal of becoming a professional hairdresser. Don't give up, go for it!

Good hairdressing.

David R. Bendell

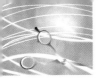

Pathway to National Certificate in Hairdressing
MIND MAP

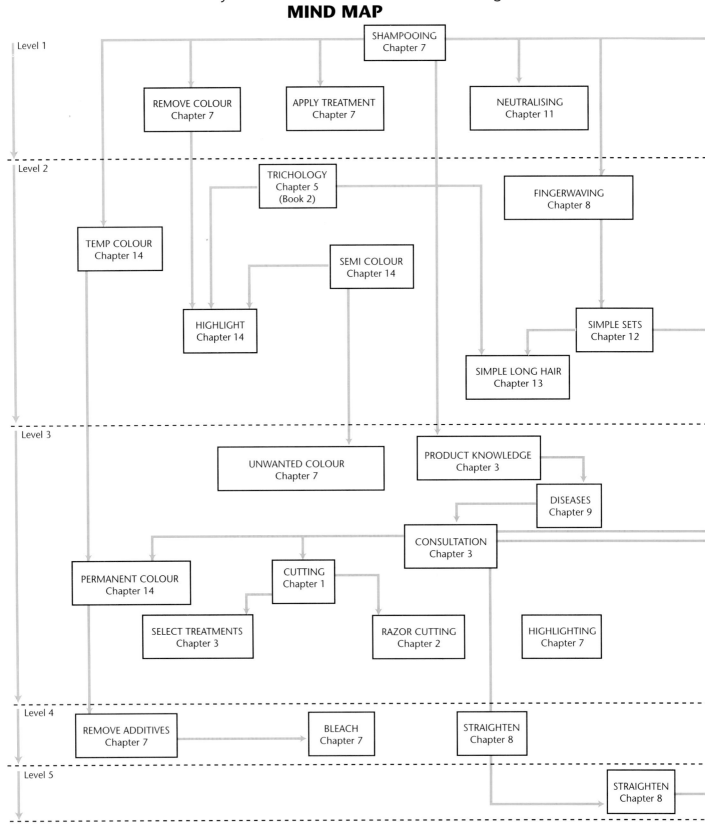

Level 1

SHAMPOOING
Chapter 7

REMOVE COLOUR
Chapter 7

APPLY TREATMENT
Chapter 7

NEUTRALISING
Chapter 11

Level 2

TRICHOLOGY
Chapter 5
(Book 2)

FINGERWAVING
Chapter 8

TEMP COLOUR
Chapter 14

SEMI COLOUR
Chapter 14

HIGHLIGHT
Chapter 14

SIMPLE SETS
Chapter 12

SIMPLE LONG HAIR
Chapter 13

Level 3

UNWANTED COLOUR
Chapter 7

PRODUCT KNOWLEDGE
Chapter 3

DISEASES
Chapter 9

CONSULTATION
Chapter 3

PERMANENT COLOUR
Chapter 14

CUTTING
Chapter 1

SELECT TREATMENTS
Chapter 3

RAZOR CUTTING
Chapter 2

HIGHLIGHTING
Chapter 7

Level 4

REMOVE ADDITIVES
Chapter 7

BLEACH
Chapter 7

STRAIGHTEN
Chapter 8

Level 5

STRAIGHTEN
Chapter 8

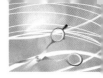

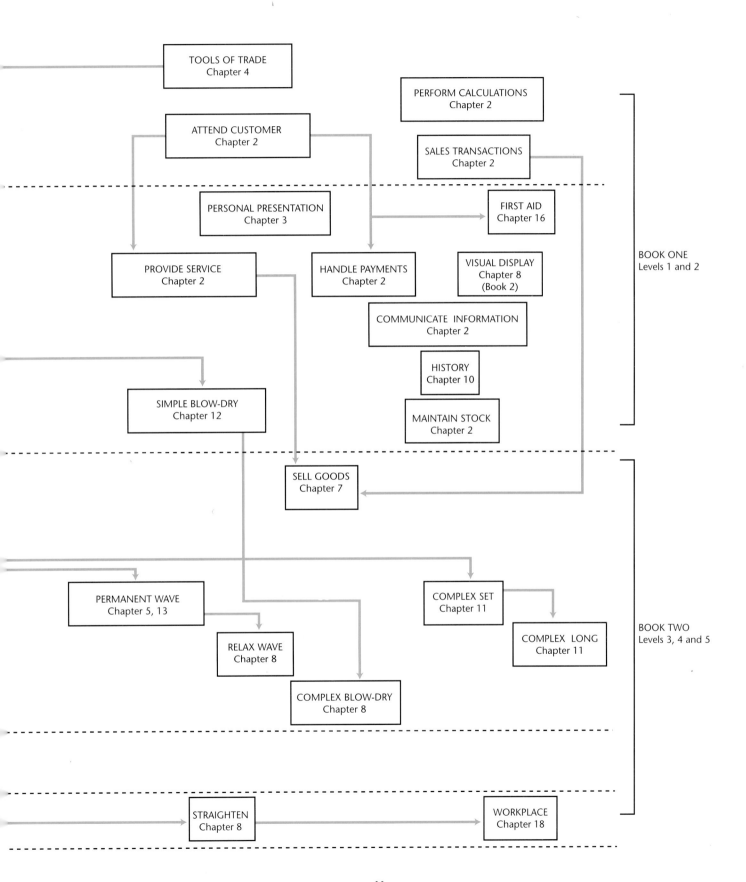

TOOLS OF TRADE
Chapter 4

PERFORM CALCULATIONS
Chapter 2

ATTEND CUSTOMER
Chapter 2

SALES TRANSACTIONS
Chapter 2

PERSONAL PRESENTATION
Chapter 3

FIRST AID
Chapter 16

BOOK ONE
Levels 1 and 2

PROVIDE SERVICE
Chapter 2

HANDLE PAYMENTS
Chapter 2

VISUAL DISPLAY
Chapter 8
(Book 2)

COMMUNICATE INFORMATION
Chapter 2

HISTORY
Chapter 10

SIMPLE BLOW-DRY
Chapter 12

MAINTAIN STOCK
Chapter 2

SELL GOODS
Chapter 7

PERMANENT WAVE
Chapter 5, 13

COMPLEX SET
Chapter 11

BOOK TWO
Levels 3, 4 and 5

COMPLEX LONG
Chapter 11

RELAX WAVE
Chapter 8

COMPLEX BLOW-DRY
Chapter 8

STRAIGHTEN
Chapter 8

WORKPLACE
Chapter 18

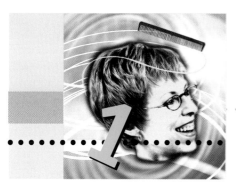

Cutting the hair with scissors and clippers

Once you have shown proficiency in skills such as pincurling, fingerwaving and roller placement, you will be getting a feel for the hair; this only comes with experience. You will begin to know what natural tendencies are and to understand nape growth patterns, the hair's natural fall and growth lines. All this you will have observed when shampooing, and you will have acquired a knowledge of different types of hair texture and of waves and curls. You will also have learned, by watching senior stylists when they are setting and permanent waving. By now, too, your hands and fingers will be more dexterous, your manipulative skills will be more co-ordinated. Only when you have reached this stage should you be ready to handle the scissors and practise cutting the hair. It will take time and practice before you become skilful at cutting.

Your employer should encourage you to attend workshops, seminars, and demonstrations on cutting. These will help develop your cutting skill.

Using the correct tools

Comb and clips

The first thing you need when practising cutting is a good cutting comb. Cutting combs should be made of vulcanite and be saw-cut to help pick up the hair strands. This type of comb is the only one suitable for hair cutting as it is an all-purpose general cutting comb, with the teeth wider at one end than the other. The wide end takes the sections and the narrow end combs while cutting, except in the case of bob haircuts, when you use the wide end to distribute the hair. Don't use a comb with missing teeth. Narrower vulcanite saw-cut combs can be used for different cutting effects such as shingling or fine tapering.

You will also need sectioning clips which are invaluable for clipping large sections of hair so you can cut systematically.

Scissors

Invest in a good pair of scissors (see the section on buying scissors in *Hairdressing: A Professional Approach – Levels 1 and 2*). Hairdressing suppliers have overcome many of the restrictions that used to inhibit the importation of good quality cutting scissors. Look out for names such as Jowell, Yasaka and Nic, all of which are excellent scissors.

The money you invest in scissors is well worth it as, if they are looked after, they will last for many years. The cost of a good pair of scissors may be more than $300, but the scissors will be sharp, well-balanced and precisely engineered so that they feel comfortable in your hand. Buying quality scissors will encourage you to learn how to cut. Always keep the scissors sharp.

Figure 1.1

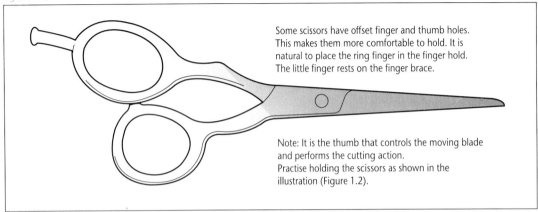

Some scissors have offset finger and thumb holes. This makes them more comfortable to hold. It is natural to place the ring finger in the finger hold. The little finger rests on the finger brace.

Note: It is the thumb that controls the moving blade and performs the cutting action.
Practise holding the scissors as shown in the illustration (Figure 1.2).

The *first step* towards good hair cutting technique is, therefore, to use the correct comb and sharp, precision scissors of high quality.

The *second step* is holding the scissors correctly. The scissors are to be held as shown in the diagram, using the tip of the thumb and the third finger, with the little finger resting on the brace (if the scissors have one). When you are not cutting, but are combing the hair, take your thumb out and fold the fingers securely around the scissors in the palm. Note the position of the comb while you are actually cutting. Practise this technique for holding the scissors – thumb in and cut; thumb out and fold in the palm. Continue this until you do it without effort or having to think.

When you cut a hairstyle, it is made up of a series of lines joined together. These lines should look good from all viewpoints – front, profile and back. You must consider the following:

a   The shape around the perimeter of the haircut.
b   The angle at which it will project from the head.
c   What the silhouette will look like if all the hair stands out from the head.

The cut style will be made up of:

a   line – around the perimeter.
b   structure – the length of the hair within the style.
c   texture – whether the surface will be rough or smooth.
d   direction – how the line of the haircut flows.

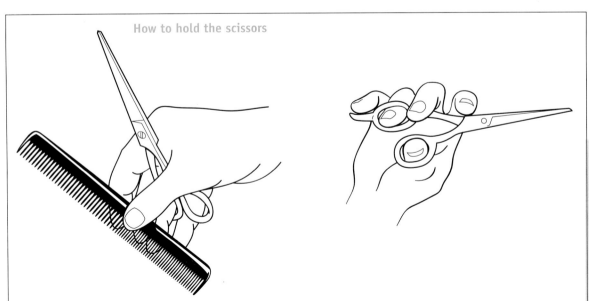

How to hold the scissors

Figure 1.2

When you are not cutting, slip your thumb out of the thumb hole and fold your fingers around the scissors in the palm of the hand.

Client consultation

Step three in becoming a good haircutter is handling the *preliminary client consultation and the hair analysis* well. This involves talking to your model or client. Before you do anything else – even caping and shampooing – seat the client and assess a number of factors. The first part of the consultation involves assessing the psychological and physical characteristics of the client. For example, observe what type of person the client is – age group and body structure (i.e. height and weight). If possible, determine the client's personality. Is the client an outgoing type who could carry off a strong style, or a quieter personality who doesn't want to draw attention to him- or herself? The way clients dress may help you to decide about their personality; are they conservatively dressed or extremely fashion-conscious? Discuss the client's lifestyle and ask questions to help you assess personality.

Take into account face and head shape, particularly cheekbone structure, forehead depth, size of ears (do they stick out?), size of nose and length of neck. Notice also the contours of the skull, especially in the parietal area.

The consultation is almost a cross-examination, you *must* perceive the style that will be suitable for the client.

Choosing the style

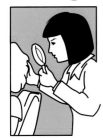

1 Don't cut the hair very short unless the client asks you to do so.
2 Make sure the client understands fully what you intend to do before you start.
3 Don't give your client the haircut *you* want to see; you will only lose his or her confidence. If your client has chosen a style with which you don't agree, be tactful when expressing your recommendations, so that next time he or she visits the salon, he/she may listen and take your advice.
4 Sometimes I ask the client, 'What don't you want done to your hair?' The answer can very often assist you in your consultation.

Hair analysis

This involves *feeling* and *looking* at the hair. Feel the texture as this will determine:
1 cutting technique – scissors, razor, blunt or taper;
2 thinning procedure – where thinning should commence on the hair strand;
3 type of cut – whether the hair will sit according to the style desired.

The hairline growth pattern

Comb the hair and observe its natural fall. See how it grows along the front hairline. Are there any cowlicks, widow's peaks, natural partings or any other natural growth tendencies? See how the hair grows at the sides – forward, down or back? Check the nape growth pattern. How does it appear? Will it conform to the client's desired style? Is it tidy or untidy?

Determining the way the hair falls naturally will influence your cut and the finished style. It is always better to work with any hair growth than against it. If the client requests a style that is against the hair's natural fall, then you must find out if the style is going to be looked after regularly (i.e. using blow-drying, tonging, curling brush, etc.) to maintain it. If the client indicates that this will be the case then you can compromise and achieve the style. If the

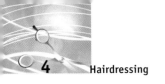
style is not going to be looked after regularly, then it would be better if you advised the client to reconsider the style. Alternatively, you could suggest a permanent wave or a style support to help maintain the finished look.

The type of hair

Observe what type of hair the client has. Is it straight, wavy or curly? If it is curly, is the curl natural or has it been permed and, if so, how long ago? Sometimes when the hair is dry it looks as though it has certain qualities, such as bounce and volume, but when it's wet and cut these are lost. The client may have straight hair but have put in heat rollers that morning or the night before. Problems that might arise can usually be avoided by asking questions. Consultation and hair analysis will help you determine the style suitable for the client. Don't start to cut until you have consulted the client and analysed the hair.

Haircutting tips

The following tips apply regardless of what style is chosen. Be sure you have the finished look in your mind before you start.

1   Buy a good comb and sharp, good-quality scissors.
2   Hold the tools correctly.
3   Spend time consulting, asking questions and analysing the hair BEFORE shampooing.

By following these points you will be well on the way to becoming a good haircutter.

Figure 1.3

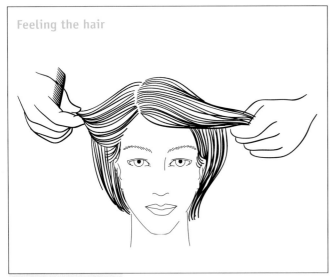

Feeling the hair

Feel the texture and weight of the hair.

Figure 1.4

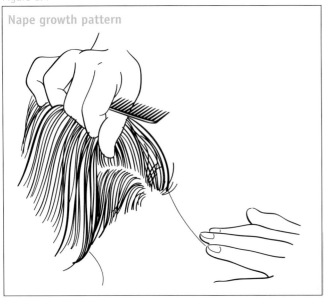

Nape growth pattern

Observe and analyse the nape growth pattern. See how it grows.

Analysing the haircut

Perceiving the style

'Perceiving the style' means trying to imagine what the finished style is going to look like. This is also important in the case of many other hairdressing services apart from cutting. Many expert hairdressers say if you can picture what the finished style will look like, chances are it will come out as you have imagined. But, start a style without a picture in your mind (the 'We'll-see-how-it-turns-out' approach) and the chances are that you will end up looking as if you don't know what you are doing. This does not instil confidence in your client. So an important aspect of good cutting technique is analysing the haircut in your mind.

A haircut is made up of three major *design* elements, namely:

a shape or form;
b surface texture;
c structure.

Before you start cutting try to imagine the following:
a What will the shape look like? Imagine the shape of the haircut, around the perimeter (much like the black silhouette of the girl with the magnifying glass, on page 3).
b Imagine what *abstract shape* the hair has – that is, the hair standing out from the curve of the head at a 90° angle.
c What the client will look like in *reality* when they he/she leaves the salon, i.e. the finished haircut.

Shape or form

This is the line or weight of the haircut. This line will give the haircut its shape (form). The line should be viewed from two perspectives.

a The line around the outside (silhouette) of the shape.
b The line around the 'inside'; that is, around the face.

Haircuts can be 'identified' by their shape or form.

Surface texture

This is the appearance that the surface of the haircut has. There are two types of surface texture, 'unactivated' and 'activated'.

Unactivated surface texture

This gives a smooth surface appearance such as that seen in a bob hairstyle. The ends of the hair are not visible. They all end at one particular line so therefore give the surface a smooth look. A bob haircut (solid form) is a good example of a haircut with the texture totally unactivated.

Activated surface texture

This gives a rough surface appearance such as that seen in a uniform layer hairstyle. The ends of the hair are visible.

A haircut can have a *combination* of the two types of surface texture. A graduated haircut would be an example of this. In Figure 1.13, you can see that the interior of the hair cut is smooth and unactivated, while the exterior is activated. The dividing line between the two surface textures is called the ridge line.

Note: The interior of the head form is divided from the exterior by the crest line. The crest line is the widest part of the head all the way around the head form. It is similar to a line that goes around a tennis ball.

Structure

The structure is the length arrangement of the hair within its shape or form. Structure can be viewed in two ways. It can be viewed by imagining all the hair projected out from the head at a 90° angle from the curve of the head (as shown in the illustrations); this is called natural projection. Or it can be viewed with the lengths falling naturally down; this is called natural fall.

In hair cutting there are FOUR classic structures. They are:

a   the bob (solid form);
b   graduation;
c   increase layer;
d   uniform layer.

The bob (solid form)

When you analyse a bob, you find that all the hair ends end at one particular line. This is a line of weight. A bobbed haircut has the heaviest line of weight in any of the four classic structures. The heavy line of weight will give the haircut stability. In Figure 1.17, the diagram of the bob, note the structure analysis (length arrangement) in natural projection and compare it to the finished look. See how the length is longer in the interior and shorter in the exterior in natural projection. In its natural fall all the lengths end in one line. This will give the haircut a smooth, unactivated finish.

Graduation

A graduated haircut gives the second heaviest line of weight. This is because a lot of hair ends in a weight line – but not all of it. View the structure of graduation in natural projection and observe the length arrangement (see Figure 1.13). It has longer length in the interior and gradually becomes shorter towards the exterior. In natural fall, the lengths 'stack' upon one another. Note that the interior lengths do not reach the exterior lengths; this makes the weight line less stable. This will give the interior a smooth unactivated look while the perimeter will be activated. Can you visualise what you would have to do for all the hair ends to meet in one line (weight line)? (Answer: Project all the hair out until all the ends meet.)

Increase layer

This is the opposite to a bobbed haircut – it's like an upside-down bob. This time the structure in natural projection has the short lengths on the interior and the long lengths on the exterior. In its natural fall, the lengths are short at the top and increase in length towards the back and sides. This will give an activated surface texture. For all the hair ends to meet in one line you would need to comb all the hair to the top of the head. This is the line of weight of an increasing layer. The longer the interior length on the crown, the further the exterior back lengths have to travel to meet the top hair. Therefore, in natural fall the hair will be longer at the back. The opposite will occur if the crown hair is cut short. The hair at the back has less distance to travel to meet the top hair and therefore the increase layer is shorter in natural fall. There can sometimes be confusion in analysing the difference between a graduated haircut and an increasing layered haircut, particularly if it is a long increasing layer. The difference is simple to define: if the hair has been projected and cut higher than the crest line, it is layered.

Uniform layer

A classic uniform layer has no line of weight because when they are viewed in natural projection, all the hair lengths are equal. This type of cut will produce a round shape. Even though the hair may be cut only 1 cm all over (e.g. with clippers) this is still a uniform layer. Nowhere will the hair ends meet in a line (although there are variations of this type of cut in which the ends may meet, e.g. flat top). In natural fall, all the hair ends are visible. This will give the surface texture a totally activated look.

Cutting the hair

The hair can be cut in several different ways: using blunt or club cutting, tapering and thinning.

Blunt or club cutting

In this technique, the ends of the hair are cut straight off. Hold the hair between the first and second fingers and cut the ends straight across with scissors.

This is a popular method of cutting. Hold the knuckles together tightly to grasp the hair evenly so that the cutting line is straight (and you don't cut the knuckles by mistake). And for precision, NEVER cut past the second knuckle. Blunt or club cutting will make the ends of the hair appear thicker and bulkier so is best suited to fine and medium-textured hair.

Shingling

This is also a method of *blunt* cutting the hair and can be described as cutting the hair close to the nape of the neck and leaving it gradually longer toward the crown, without showing a definite line. It is achieved by cutting the hair over the comb. Shingling can be used on male and female hairstyles. The hair should always be at the bottom of the comb when cutting or a step will show. Hold the scissors parallel to the comb and work up from the nape. The same effect can be achieved using clippers. Shingling can be performed on wet or dry hair.

Tapering

The *ends* of the hair are tapered with the scissors which are used with a slithering action. The short hairs of the strand are usually pushed toward the scalp first. Each time the scissors move towards the scalp, the scissors close slightly. This action tapers the end. Tapering with the scissors is usually done on dry hair. Tapering is also possible with a razor. The angle at which you hold the razor will determine the amount of taper; a short taper is a sharply sliced end.

Tapers can also refer to what the individual mesh strand (or section of hair being cut) looks like on the ends. Compare the short taper, with perhaps 1 cm of taper, with the long taper which has about 2 cm of taper or more (see Figure 1.8 on p. 9).

You can see that a long tapered mesh could be difficult to set or permanent wave. Try and keep your tapering to the short variation. There is a place for the longer taper, perhaps in a fringe or in the nape area, but at this stage of learning it is important to get the hair ends as even as possible. You can experiment with tapering at a later stage of training. Since tapering removes bulk from the ends, it is ideal for clients with thick, coarse hair.

Thinning

Thinning means the removal of bulk from the hair. This can be done in a number of ways, using either specially designed thinning scissors or regular scissors.

Using thinning scissors

Designed to remove bulk, thinning scissors have either one or two serrated edges; the single serrated edge removes more bulk. If thinning scissors with one serrated edge are used, ensure that the serrated edge is on the top when you're cutting. If scissors with two serrated edges are used, make sure the 'V' in the teeth is on the bottom.

If you're using the thinning scissors the texture of the hair will determine where the thinning should start on the hair strand. As a general rule, if coarse, strong hair is thinned too close to the scalp, it will stick up, whereas fine-textured hair will sit much closer and flatter to the scalp if thinned. (Although it is fine, such hair may still be bulky and heavy.) Remember, there is more hair per cm^2 in the case of fine hair. Ensure that coarse-textured hair is thinned at least 5 cm from the scalp, medium-textured 3 to 4 cm from the scalp, and fine-textured 1.5 to 2.5 cm from the scalp.

Figure 1.5

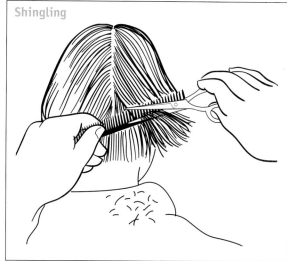

Shingling

In shingling, the hair is cut over the comb. The hair must always be at the bottom of the comb when it is cut or a step will show.

There are also certain areas where it is not advisable to thin the hair: on the ends, along a natural parting, on the top layer of hair, above the ears, on the crest of a wave and along the front hairline. Reducing bulk in these areas will either make the hair shapeless (that is, leave it the same shape but with less hair to work on) or cause the hair to stick up.

Using regular scissors

Removing bulk can also be achieved by using regular scissors. This is referred to as texturising, chipping or slithering. Small strands of hair are removed with the scissors. The blade is closed either when moving towards the scalp or towards the ends, depending on where the bulk is to be reduced. If you remove the small strands closer to the scalp, a cushion will form if the hair is back combed. The shorter strands will be pushed towards the scalp, helping to create volume. The method involves skill, well-supported and balanced scissors, and requires you to move quickly within the strands of hair.

Specially designed thinning scissors are now available to give hair texture for special effects. These have serrated teeth spaced at irregular intervals.

Figure 1.6

Slithering or chipping (tapering)

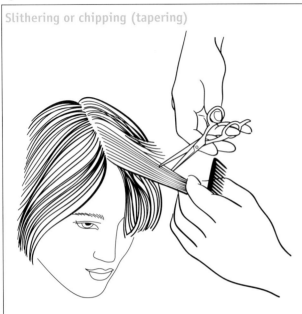

Removing bulk with regular scissors is referred to as slithering or chipping (tapering). In this technique the scissors take on a chipping motion and close slightly when they move towards the ends. This reduces the weight of the hair where necessary.

Figure 1.7

Differences in cut

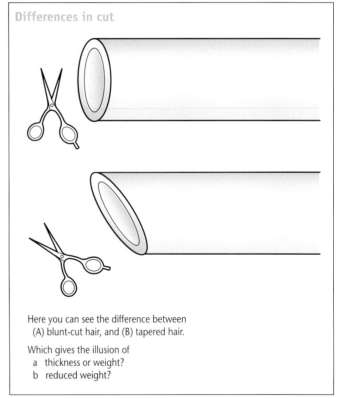

Here you can see the difference between (A) blunt-cut hair, and (B) tapered hair.

Which gives the illusion of
a   thickness or weight?
b   reduced weight?

Whether to cut the hair wet or dry

You should learn to cut hair when it is wet, for the following reasons.
1   Hygiene: no dirty strands of hair will fly up into your face.
2   The hair is easier to control as it will not slip through your fingers.
3   Any natural wave movement is easily recognisable. (Any curl induced by heated rollers will disappear!)
4   The shape of the head is more clearly defined, especially the parietal area.

Figure 1.9

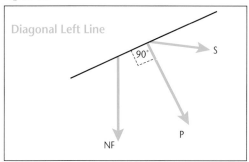

Diagonal Left Line

 # Distributing and sectioning the hair

The direction in which the hair is combed from its base parting is called distribution. There are three ways in which hair can be distributed or combed from its base parting:

a natural fall distribution;
b perpendicular distribution;
c shifted distribution.

Natural fall distribution

This is the fall of the hair if it is left to fall naturally. If you take a horizontal line at the nape, then the hair's natural fall distribution would be perpendicular (at right angles) to that horizontal line (a popular way of achieving a bob).

Perpendicular distribution

This is where the hair is combed at right angles (a 90° angle) to the base parting.

Figure 1.10

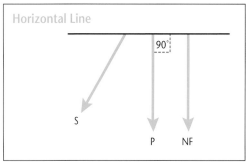

Horizontal Line

Figure 1.8

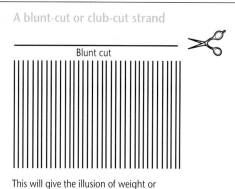

A blunt-cut or club-cut strand

Blunt cut

This will give the illusion of weight or heaviness at the ends of the hair.

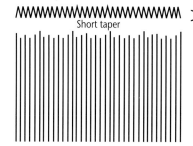

Short taper

Short taper

A short-tapered strand gives the illusion of lightness and reduced weight at the ends of the hair.

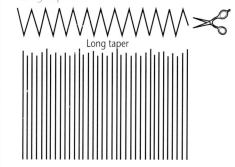

Long taper

Long taper

A long-tapered strand will reduce the weight from the ends even more than a short taper.

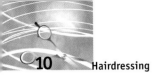

Shifted distribution

This is neither natural fall nor perpendicular (90° angle) distribution but any other angle of distribution.

Figure 1.11

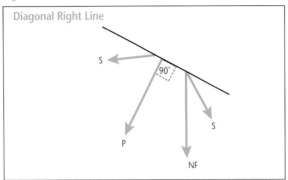

Shifted distribution creates a length increase and is used to blend the hair. These three methods of distribution are used in hair-cutting techniques.

The different types of distribution

LEGEND: NF = Natural Fall
         P = Perpendicular
         S = Shifted

Note: On the horizontal line, both perpendicular and natural fall are the same. Shifted can be at any angle except perpendicular or natural fall.

Cutting angles

You must know the correct angles for cutting, projecting and distributing the hair:

90° – the most common angle;
45° – the second most common angle;
22.5° – the next most common angle (half of a 45° angle);
0° – the hair is not lifted out from the head at all – no projection.

The cutting angle can vary and will influence the final result. Different hair cuts are achieved by cutting hair at different angles. Show skill in cutting styles using these different angles.

Projection angles

Projection refers to the amount by which the hair is held out from the head when cutting to create the line or shape. Projection can vary from 0° (usually natural fall) to 180°. *Low* projection (for longer lengths) is where the hair is not projected out from the head very much, e.g. at 45° while in *high* projection (for shorter lengths), the mesh is lifted away from the scalp, e.g. at 90°.

Since the head is spherical, there are many ways you can hold the hair out from the head to achieve an angle. In the diagram (Figure 1.12) you will see that the curve of the head allows for different angles. If the hair is brought out at right angles, this creates 90° projection (natural projection).

The classic bob is achieved by cutting with no projection. The hair is not brought out from the head at all. This is called 0°, baseline projection or natural fall, and produces a paintbrush look. *All* the meshes and sections are cut when the hair falls naturally. This produces a very heavy line of weight.

There are, of course, variations to all these classic cuts, such as the graduated bob, which is a combination: graduation at a low projection. The underneath hair is almost a shingle at the nape only. There is no projection (degree of lift) at the sides.

Figure 1.13

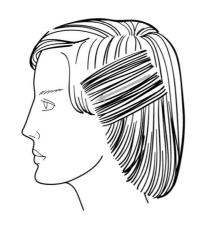

Graduation

To achieve a graduated effect, the hair is combed at a 90° angle from the sectioned line (perpendicular distribution). When the hair falls, it is graduated.

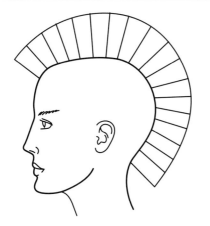

Uniform layer

In a uniform layer, each strand of hair is brought out from the head at 90° and is cut the same length all over the head.

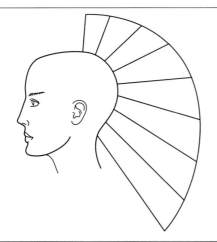

Increasing layer

In an increasing layer, the short layers are on top, with the sides, back and nape sections becoming gradually longer.

Figure 1.12

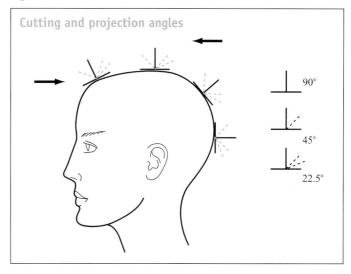

Cutting and projection angles

Projection for graduation

The one thing that you should remember is that, because heads are round, as soon as you project (lift) the hair away from the head, there will be some degree of graduation (or layer). The amount of lift is called 'projection'; the effect is called 'graduation' or layering. The more you lift the hair, the greater the projection. Graduation is the *grade* (projection or lift) that you have used to achieve a *gradual* effect. When the hair is brought out to one point this produces a graduated effect, and a line of weight.

Graduating can also be achieved without actually lifting the hair out from the head form. Combing the hair perpendicular or at right angles (90°) to a diagonal sectioned line will achieve graduation, even though there is no projection. In addition, a greater degree of graduation can be achieved by combing the hair perpendicular *and* projecting it at the same time. IF THE HAIR IS PROJECTED HIGHER THAN THE CREST LINE, THE RESULT IS A LAYER.

Projection for layering (uniform and increasing)

Uniform layer

90° projection: Holding the hair at right angles to the curve of the head gives a 90° angle of projection. If each mesh is brought out at a 90° angle all over the head and then cut, this results in a uniform layered effect. The hair will be the same length all over the head; it would have a perfect round silhouette if it stood out from the head. A 90° angle is commonly used to achieve a uniform layer cutting.

Figure 1.14

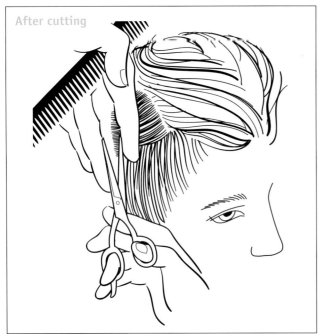

After cutting

Check the cut for any protruding ends when you have finished and again once the style has been dried and completed. Remember: do not cut past your second knuckle.

Increasing layer

This is achieved by projecting the hair to a particular point above the crest line. The first cut section on the crown could be projected, for example, at a 90° angle. Subsequent sections are all brought up to this original design line. Understandably, the length towards the nape has further to travel to the crown section. Therefore, the layers increase, or become longer, towards the back. The result is an increase layer effect. The original design line can have variations to achieve an increase layer – it can even be variable during the cutting procedure.

Tips when cutting hair

Regardless of what style is chosen, these tips are useful.
1 Keep the client's neck free from jewellery, bulky collars, jumpers, towels and anything else which may inhibit the cutting line.
2 Keep the sections fine enough to be able to see the previous cut line.
3 Always retain a section of the previous cut line as your guide.
4 Always work in the direction of hair growth.
5 While cutting, use your eyes to 'visibly' cut the hair. Look at the shape which is evolving. Stand back and observe.
6 Use only the first 6 mm of the scissors (the tip).
7 Never cut past the second knuckle when the hair is held between the fingers.
8 Keep the hair wet – the wetter, the better.
9 Check the cut:
   a stand behind the client and feel the hair length on each side to ensure that the lengths are the same. (You don't even have to look; just feel.)
   b Check the outline. The entire perimeter of the head – the outside of the haircut – is what gives the style its shape.
   c Now check the inside of the haircut for weight and evenness.
   d In the case of a bob, ask the client to stand up, and then observe the precision of the line. On graduated bobs, a mirror placed facing upward on the hairline will show the graduation clearly and reveal any unevenness.
10 Ask your senior to check your work.

Figure 1.15

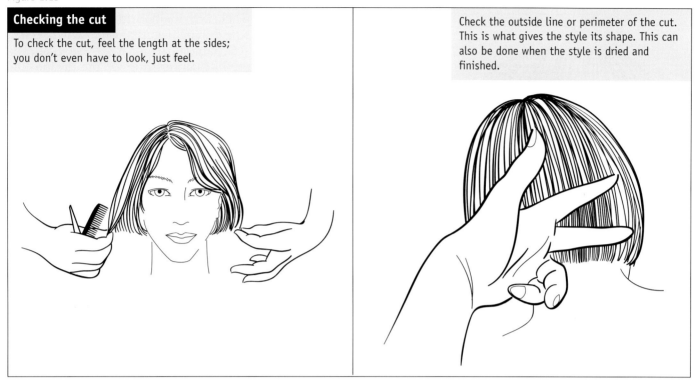

Checking the cut

To check the cut, feel the length at the sides; you don't even have to look, just feel.

Check the outside line or perimeter of the cut. This is what gives the style its shape. This can also be done when the style is dried and finished.

Cutting the hair with scissors and clippers

 # Cutting the bob (solid form)

Determine whether the final design line is to be horizontal or diagonal. If it is to be diagonal, consider:
a the degree of angle of the diagonal;
b whether the diagonal is a forward line or a back line, i.e. does the length increase towards the face or towards the nape?

Preparation

The client's neck must be free from jewellery, clothing, towels and cape to achieve precision in the cut.

Shampoo the hair and subsection the head for easy control. Subsection the hair using the same base partings as for the final design line. This will include sectioning the sides as well as the back. You may need up to 10 section clips to subsection satisfactorily – having only two section clips is clearly not adequate!

Ask the client to keep his/her head in an upright position. This will give you an exact indication of the final length. If the client inclines his/her head forward, this will produce variations in the final length.

Method

Start at the nape and, taking a 0.5 cm base part, distribute the hair in its natural fall using the WIDE END of the comb. Whenever you cut a bobbed haircut, always use the wide end of the comb. The narrow end of the comb could put tension on or stretch the hair; when the hair dries, the weight line will shatter, giving the effect of graduation.

Using the first 6 mm (the tip) of the scissors, cut the design line parallel to the base parting. Keep the shoulders, scissors and fingers parallel to the base parting whether it be horizontal or diagonal. Do not project the hair or shift

Figure 1.16

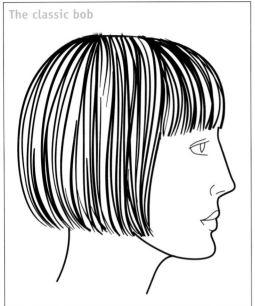

The classic bob

A bob haircut (solid form). A good example of a haircut with the smooth texture totally unactivated.

Figure 1.17

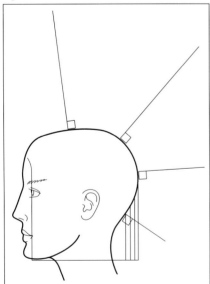

The length arrangement of a bob.

the hair away from its natural fall or you will shatter the weight line. Keep the hands and the scissors close to the head throughout the hair cut; this first cut section will be the design line. All the hair will be cut to this length. Next take another 0.5 cm base parting across the nape. The parting should not be so thick that you cannot see the design line underneath. Always take 'see-through' sections. Look up to establish that the hair is distributed in its natural fall. If the base parting is horizontal, the distribution will be perpendicular, that is, at right angles to the base parting. Using the wide end of the comb, distribute without stretching or putting on tension. Cut the hair between the middle and index finger – do not cut past the second knuckle – *using only the first 6 mm of the scissors*.

It is best not to leave the hair longer than the bone that you can feel on the centre at the base of the client's neck (any longer and the hair will flick up).

Do not alter the base parting as you proceed up the back of the head: the sections must remain constant at all times. Do not hold too large a section in your fingers as the hair may be pulled out of its natural fall.

Continue taking the sections up the back of the head and cutting the hair in its natural fall.

Now move to the side and continue to blend the sides to the back. Take the same base partings, horizontal or diagonal, as you did at the back. Avoid tension or projection over the ear. Use a portion of the previously cut back section as a guide to cutting the sides. Continue cutting the sides. Stand directly in front of where you are cutting, keeping everything parallel – that is, body, shoulders, fingers and scissors – to the base parting.

If a fringe is to be cut, section the frontal triangle – make sure the hair is falling naturally. It may take time to determine its exact position. Cut the hair square to the temporal hair line, just below eyebrow level. Do not cut into the hair line.

When the cut is complete check for any loose ends. These may be found if the hair has not been distributed naturally. Check also that both sides are even. Blow-dry and take the same base section as the haircut and dry the hair under. When the hair is dry, check again for any loose ends.

The bobbed haircut is a classic cut – practise cutting horizontal and diagonal lines to achieve a sound technique.

Tips when cutting the bob

1 Keep the neck free from obstructions.
2 Take 'see-through' sections.
3 Do not cut past the second knuckle.
4 Use NO tension, pressure or stretching.
5 Do not project the hair at all.
6 Distribute the hair in its natural fall.
7 Cut parallel to the base parting.
8 Keep the body, shoulders, fingers and scissors parallel to the base parting.
9 It is best not to leave the hair longer than indicated by the bone at the centre nape.
10 Check for loose ends.

How to achieve graduation

Graduation means that there is a 'gradual' change in hair length from the interior to the exterior of the head form. The hair ends appear to 'stack' upon one another. The interior lengths do not quite reach the exterior lengths in natural fall. Graduation can be achieved by using two techniques:

a projection;
b distribution.

Graduation by projection

Method

When the hair is projected out from the head and then cut, graduation will occur. The more the hair is projected, the shorter the lengths become and the greater the graduation will be. This is why it is important to determine the amount of graduation the client wants. The 'wedge' and 'firefly' are classic examples of graduated hair cuts. The effect of graduation will give an activated rough surface appearance around the perimeter. The hair's texture will also influence the finished result. Fine, blonde, textured hair has the tendency to 'bell out' more. The important thing to remember when graduating is not to project the hair higher than the crest line. This will 'shatter' the line of weight and give a layered look in the interior. Typical angles of projection would be 22.5°, 45° and 90° (low, medium and high projection). Low-projection angles create a heavier line of weight and therefore less graduation, whereas high-projection angles create more graduation by producing a steeper 'stacked' effect (line of inclination). While you are cutting the hair by projection, all the hair ends will be of an equal length; although you may 'feel' the graduation developing between your fingers, it is only seen when the hair falls to its natural position. Either a stationary or a variable projection angle can be used to achieve graduation.

Graduation by distribution

Method

When the hair is distributed perpendicularly (at right angles) to its base part and then cut, graduation will occur. However, this is only the case when the base partings are diagonal. A horizontal base parting distributed perpendicularly in natural fall will have to be combined with projection to achieve graduation. When cutting graduation by perpendicular distribution, the ends of the hair all finish equal in a solid line. This is only seen when the hair falls naturally. The hair can be distributed other than perpendicular to its base parting. This is where you 'shift' the hair away from its base parting and cut the hair non-parallel to the base parting. This effect will create a length increase. This 'shifting' technique is done when you wish to blend the short sides of a haircut to create a length increase behind the ear and down into the nape. Distribution can also be 'combined' with projection to produce even shorter lengths and more graduation.

Shapes of graduation

A graduated haircut can take on many different designs. Parallel graduation is a common hair cutting technique in the salon. This is where the graduation is apparent between two parallel lines. The lines can be horizontal or diagonal – at 22.5° or 45° (especially going back off the face). Graduation can also be non-parallel on diagonal lines. This is when the graduation increases towards the nape, leaving the front area heavier. Or the graduation may decrease towards the nape, leaving the sides more graduated and the nape heavier.

Tips when projecting for graduation

1 Use the wide end of the comb to take the sections and the narrow end of the comb for distributing.

2 If a 'soft' design line is required, project the first cut section – when it falls, the line will be 'soft' (shattered).

3 If a 'hard' design line is required, do not project the first cut section, but cut the hair in its natural fall. This will leave the perimeter line heavier.

4 The higher the projection angle (90°), the shorter the lengths and the greater the graduation.

5 The lower the projection angle (22.5°) the longer the lengths, the heavier the line, and the less the graduation.

6 Keep the body, shoulders, fingers and scissors parallel to the base parting to create parallel graduation.

7 Do not project the hair higher than the crest line.

8 Variable projection angles can be used when cutting graduation. The projection angle does not have to be constant.

9 A stationary projection angle produces classic graduation as seen in a 'wedge' or 'firefly' haircut.

10 'Feel' the graduation develop between your fingers.

Figure 1.18

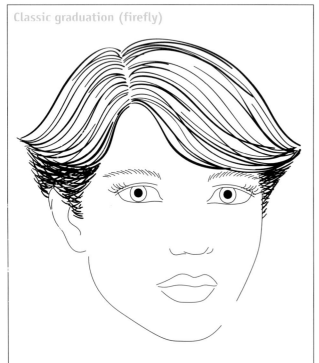

Classic graduation (firefly)

Note the line of inclination, the smooth interior and the activated perimeter.

Figure 1.19

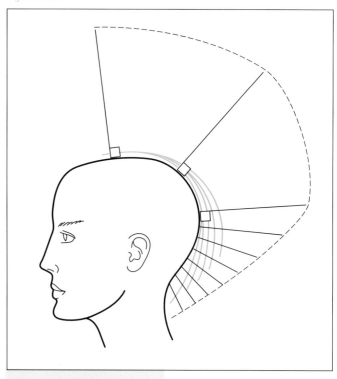

The length arrangement of graduation.

1 Perpendicular distribution (generally) is only used on diagonal lines.
2 Keep the hands and scissors close to the head form.
3 The graduation is only apparent when the hair is left to fall naturally.
4 Take 'see-through' sections.
5 If you shift the hair away from the base parting this will create a length increase and blend short lengths to longer lengths.
6 Keep the fingers, shoulders and scissors parallel to the base parting.
7 Perpendicular distribution can also be combined with projection for shorter lengths.

Layering

There are many variations to layering the hair. Two classic variations are:
a   increase layer;
b   uniform layer.

Increase layer

So far, we have been working up the head from the nape to the crown. The increase layer haircut starts on the crown and you work your way down the head to the nape. The hair lengths increase toward the nape of the neck. There are a number of ways to achieve an increase layer and they all involve projecting or distributing the hair above the crest line.

Method

Subsection for easier control; divide the back and sides.

The design line is usually cut on the crown. A horizontal section is taken and projected at a 90° angle from the head. The final length of each of the increase layers is determined by the length of this design line. All the remaining sections are brought up to this design line so the longer it is, the further the hair has to travel up the back to reach it. There are many variations when cutting the design line as it need not always be projected at a 90° angle; also, the design line need not always be stationary. Variable design lines may be used. This will help blend in lengths that do not reach the original design line on the crown, thus producing shorter layers. Remember, though, that to produce a layer you must project or distribute the hair higher than the crest line. If all the hair lengths are equal when cut on the crown, the hair will fall in a perfect classic increase layer.

Figure 1.20

Increase layer

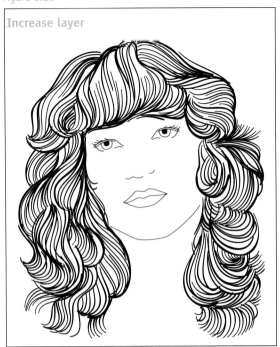

Can you imagine what the
structure of this haircut
would look like? Draw it.

Figure 1.21

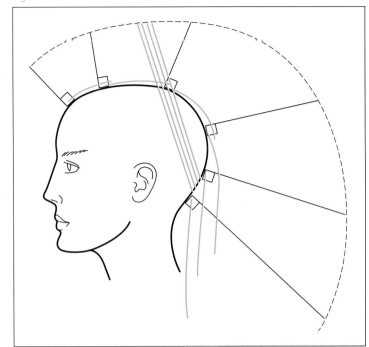

The length arrangement of
an increase layer.

Tips on increase layering

1 The length of the design line will determine the final length of the increase layer at the nape.
2 Always stand in the opposite position to the intended length increase when cutting, i.e. always distribute hair towards you.
3 A stationary or variable design line can be used.
4 The hair must be projected or distributed higher than the crest line.
5 Work from the interior to the exterior, i.e. down the head form.
6 Increase layering can also be achieved by perpendicular distribution where a vertical design line is taken in front of the face.

Uniform layer

In a classic uniform layer, all the lengths are equal. There are no points, corners, or areas of weight (variations to the uniform layer can have points, corners or weight areas, e.g. a flat top). If all the hair were projected out from the head at 90° angles, the silhouette would be round.

Method

Subsection from forehead to nape and from ear to ear over the crown. Take a 0.5 cm or base parting around the perimeter. This will become your design line. Find out whether your client wants a 'hard' design line or a 'soft' design line. This effect will determine whether you cut the design line in natural fall (hard) or project the section at a 90° angle (soft). Vertical sections can be taken and each section is projected out at a 90° angle from the head. Lift the whole section including the design line out from the head. For a precise result do not cut past the second knuckle. As you work your way up the head from the bottom nape, sections will be falling free from your fingers. Ensure your fingers and scissors are always parallel to the base parting. Blend the back to the sides, taking a piece of the previous design line as a guide. Cross-check the layering on each side. Your fingers should follow the contour of the head shape. Cut the top section, holding the sections at a 90° angle. Once the top has been cut, cross-check, checking for any ends protruding in the entire cut.

Tips when uniform layering

1 Determine whether the design line will be a hard or soft line.
2 Take vertical sections and cut parallel to the base part.
3 The fingers and scissors should follow the curvature of the head shape.
4 Do not cut past the second knuckle.
5 Use only the tip (i.e. the first 6 mm) of the scissors.
6 Check for any weight. Sometimes, if the hair is combed in the opposite direction to the natural fall, it will show up weight.
7 Do not confuse saturated wet hair with the appearance of weight.
8 A classic uniform layer should have no points or corners.
9 Cross-check to ensure all the layers blend in.
10 Variations to a uniform layer are possible.

By learning how to cut these four classic lines – the bob, the graduation, the increase layer and the uniform layer – you will develop a sound knowledge of cutting angles, distribution of hair and degrees of projection.

Many variations can be adopted using the same techniques but altering the angles, the distribution or projection at which the hair is held. All haircuts are merely combinations of these lines. Practise cutting these classic lines.

Figure 1.22

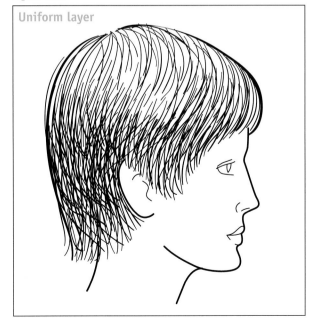

Uniform layer

Figure 1.23

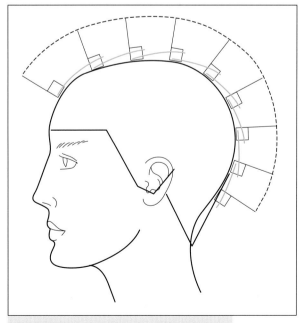

The length arrangement of a uniform layer.

Styling men's hair

A large proportion of salon clientele nowadays are men. Some of your first haircuts may well be on males who are models for your practice evenings. This section will cover cutting men's hair – the traditional 'scissors-over-comb' technique, clipper technique, and cutting in lines – and trimming beards and moustaches.

The majority of hairdressers today are women hairdressers and often their skills do not include sharpening a razor, clipper setting, shaving, or using an open razor against the skin. Indeed, it is difficult today in some countries to buy a cut-throat razor or straight razor, or to buy the strop and hone which are used to sharpen them. Stropping, honing and shaving have become the true art of the barber or men's stylist. There are specialist books covering barbering skills.

The use of an open razor against the skin is not advocated in this book. The skill is used in barber salons to define lines in men's cutting, particularly around the sideburns, and ear-to-nape area. This technique requires barbering skill, and problems can arise if the skin is broken by the razor, in particular the danger of passing on infection or disease. The technique is not associated with women's hairdressing.

 # Scissors-over-comb

Ensure your client is well protected and caped. A small paper towel can be tucked into the nape area as an extra safeguard to prevent hair going down the neck. Some clients (for example, the writer!) are particularly fussy about getting hair down their necks as it can be terribly itchy for the rest of the day. The scissors-over-comb technique is one that causes hair to fly in all directions and you will be surprised where it can end up.

Scissors-over-comb gives a shingle effect. This refers to hair being cut short at the nape and being left gradually longer toward the crown without showing a definite line. Using this technique, you can cut the hair extremely short and for many years it has been the traditional way of cutting men's hair.

A fine, pliable, saw-cut vulcanite barbering comb is used. This flexible comb allows the hair to be cut as close to the scalp as possible. It is also possible to work it around the ear arch, a definite advantage of this fine, flexible comb.

The hair is combed from the nape up toward the crown and the hair that sticks through the comb's teeth are cut off. The scissors rest along the bottom of the comb, and open and close quickly while the comb moves up the head. If the scissors are not held at the bottom of the comb, or if the action is too slow, or if the scissors are not held parallel to the comb, then steps can be cut. The length of the shingle or graduation is controlled by positioning the comb at different angles.

Lying the comb flat against the head will mean that the hair is quite short; angle the comb out, and the length will increase. Hold the comb out and the length will increase even more. The quick open-and-close action of the scissors ensures that the pivot and blade are kept free of hair and do not inhibit or impede the action. The open-and-close action can and should continue, even though you may not be cutting the hair at the time, for example, when you comb the hair down from the crown. This gives a professional sound to the technique. Continue to move around the head, cutting all the hair that protrudes through the teeth of the comb. There should be no demarcation line or shadow between the short and long hair. Each section should get progressively longer from the nape to the crown. Move the comb gradually up the head, moving it out as you get to the crown. When you get proficient at scissors-over-comb, you will only need to go over the area once. (Professional men's hairdressers and barbers can do these haircuts in a matter of minutes.)

Clippers can also be used (clipper over comb) in place of the scissors. Clippers can also be used free-hand around the lower nape area. The lower the clipper number, the shorter it will cut.

Stand back occasionally and observe the effect. Look for any shadowing, which may indicate an imperfection. Although the scissors-over-comb technique should be carried out using a quick action, make sure the scissors do not fall off the comb or cut under the comb by mistake. A hole or step will result if this happens.

Defining the line

The line in a men's haircut is usually 'harder' and squarer than in a women's cut. The line differs from a woman's line, which may be rounder, softer and possibly not so tight, although just as defined.

The line definition can be cut with scissors or clippers (electric or rechargeable). Do not cut into the natural hair line with the scissors or clippers. Cutting into the natural hairline will cause holes or steps. This sometimes happens when cutting from the ear arch to the nape. The result is not pleasing.

Defining the line – scissors

Sideburns

Determine the length the client would like the sideburns. Hold the scissors as in the illustration (Figure 1.26) and steady the blade with the index finger. Always ensure the points of the scissors are facing away from the face. Cut the sideburn at the desired length.

Now comb the sideburn hair back toward the ear. Supporting the scissors with the index finger, cut the excess hair, moving the scissors up and over the ear peak. The index finger supports the scissor all the way to the ear peak and the point of the scissors are used to cut the hair. Use scissors-over-comb to take any weight or excess hair from the sideburn. At the ear peak, hold the ear down so that you can see the hair that needs to be cut. Comb the hair over the ear, including any growth that grows horizontally above the ear. Move the points of the scissors around the ear and cut off the excess hair.

Defining from ear to nape

Avoid cutting too high over the ear as the resulting line is not pleasing. Comb any excess hair over the natural hairline. Remember, do not cut into the natural hairline in this area – take care, this can happen quite easily.

Rest your index finger against the nape as shown in the illustration (Figure 1.29) and very steadily cut the line. You can work either way – from ear peak to nape (working down the shoulders will parallel the line being cut), or from nape to ear (working up). If there is a lot of hair on the neck, keep the scissors moving and cut through the hair to continue the line. This will define the area of shingle. Remove these hairs with clippers, as you should do with all hair outside the natural hair line.

A similar technique is used to define the other side (the left side, if you are right-handed); the sideburns are cut holding the scissors in a backhand position as shown in the illustration (Figure 1.27).

Figure 1.24

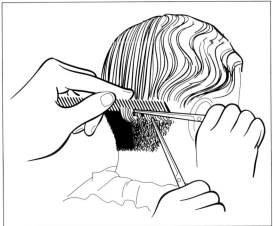

Figure 1.25

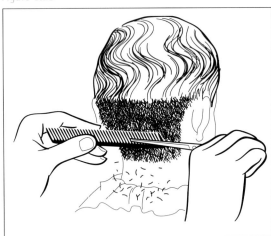

Ensure both sideburns are even. Place your finger immediately below each sideburn and check the length in the mirror.

The line from ear peak to nape can also be cut backhand on the left side (if you are right handed) – the shoulders should be parallel to the line being cut, from ear peak to nape.

Defining the line – clippers

Both electric and re-chargeable clippers can be used to define the lines in a men's haircut. Electric clippers can puncture the skin if too much pressure is applied when defining the line, so in all cases only light pressure should be used.

The clippers are reversed so that the clipper head can be brought down and rested against the skin. Once the sideburn length has been cut, move the clipper down slightly.

Now use the clipper the correct way up to remove the hair from under the sideburn. Move the clippers up and out, to the bottom of the sideburn.

The electric clippers are not a good tool to use to clean the line around the ear arch, especially when you are learning or beginning. There is a danger that you will cut into the natural hairline and leave a hole. The head of the electric clipper may be too large for you to handle around the confined space of the ear arch. The re-chargeable clipper head is smaller and may be more suitable. It is important that you do not get carried away with the clippers around the ears.

Use the clippers to cut the line between the ear peak and nape. Reverse the clippers and use them to edge the line. Support the clipper head with your hand and cut the line precisely. This line is an important part of the cut so make sure you are accurate. Ensure all hairs are combed over the natural hairline. Hairs can grow in different directions and the line can be lost after just a few days of growth.

Remove any neck hairs with the clippers, using them the right way up.

Figure 1.26

Figure 1.27

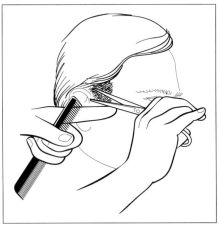

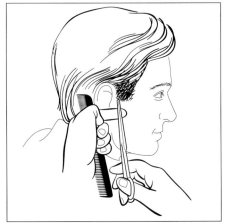

Other clipper uses

Clippers can also be used to 'square off' the centre nape. This is an individual preference and will need to be discussed with the client before the cut. If a straight line is to be cut, reverse the clippers and etch out the straight line at the nape. However, it is important to decide beforehand whether a straight line is a possibility!

There are many neck growth patterns and some may not be suited to the 'square cut' effect. Do not cut into the hairline to achieve the look as the resulting line is not pleasing. You may be tempted to cut a 'V' hairline growth pattern off to achieve a straight line. Resist the temptation and advise the client that the effect is not suitable for his hairline. This nape growth pattern is best tapered into the neck gradually, with no line.

Use the clippers to taper the hair tightly into the nape, as shown in Figures 1.32 and 1.33. Adjust the taper on the clipper head, lay the clippers against the neck and lead the clippers up and out, away from the head. This procedure also needs a steady hand as it is easy to start cutting into the hairline. Remember, lead the clippers out and away from the head as you work up to the hairline.

The heads of moles, pimples, spots, or blemishes can be taken off with the clippers if you are not careful. Work around moles carefully, as they tend to bleed if caught with a clipper head. Spots, blemishes and rough skin can also catch in the clipper head and cause discomfort to the client. It can be unpleasant for the hairdresser to work on skin with acne, but you will just have to tolerate this. If the skin surface is not smooth, then it is best to work around the area with the scissor tip, but you still need to be very carefully not to catch moles or spots; stretching the skin with fingers when using the clippers will stop the clipper head catching. This is another reason why using a razor on the skin is best left to an expert barber.

Powder can be used to dust away the fine hairs that remain on the neck. A slight dusting of talcum powder (some neck brushes come with talcum powder in the brush handle) around the neck and sides will remove hair that sticks to the skin.

Figure 1.28

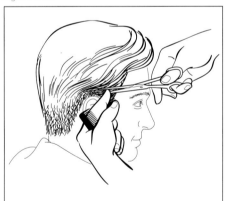

Figure 1.29

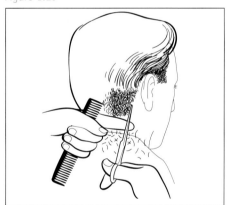

Figure 1.30

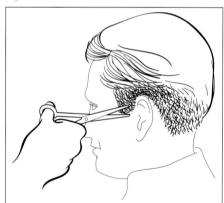

Figure 1.31

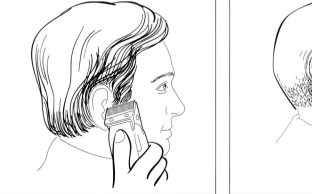

Figure 1.32

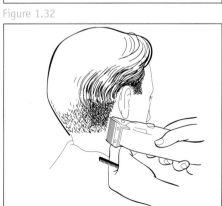

Figure 1.33

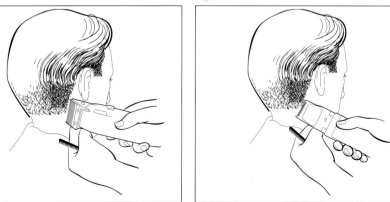

Figure 1.34a

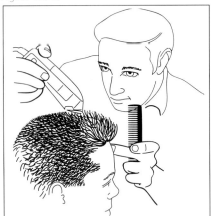

Figure 1.34b

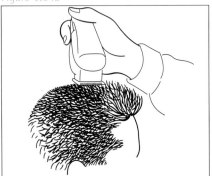

Figure 1.34c

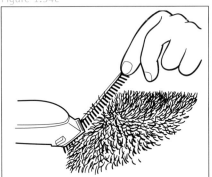

Figure 1.34d

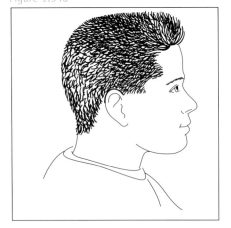

How to cut a flat-top

This men's haircut is an adaptation of the crew cut and was popularised by American 'G.I.s' (the G.I. cut) in the 1940s. It may also have an origin in Europe, particularly Germany. From time to time it comes back into vogue, often because a popular musician or film actor adopts the style. It is still asked for frequently today, and was extremely popular in the early 1990s. In women's hairdressing, the face of the 80s, Grace Jones, wore a flat-top.

All hair types can be cut into a flat-top, although Asian hair is perhaps best suited to the style as the line can look particularly sharp. But even curly African hair can be cut to have a flat-top look. It is the shape of the cut that decides the flat-top, rather than the hair type. Use the electric clippers to achieve this look (although they may get hot) rather than re-chargeable clippers or scissors. Scissors can be used, but it takes a long time to achieve the result.

The shape

There are a number of key factors in cutting a flat-top and the first is to get the shape right. Use a drier to blow the hair upwards before cutting, especially if the client has worn a cap or hat into the salon. It is best to cut the flat-top dry, as wet hair tends to collapse. If you wash the hair, still blow-dry the hair upwards and leave a little moisture in the hair as you work with the clippers.

Flat-tops can be cut to different lengths so you will need to establish the length your client desires. A size-3 clipper head is a good start, with perhaps no attachment for the sides or back (or just the long taper on the clippers).

A second key factor is to keep the crown really short. Bring the clippers up to the crown. Just forward of this crown area is the starting point for the flat-top. Take this down to almost a No. 1 or the long taper on the clippers. The hair does not stand up at the crown.

Bring the clippers straight up the sides, do not round off the corners.

Now determine the length at the front. The shortness of the front marks the length of the flat-top. Work with a small comb and use scissors and clippers to establish the front length. Keeping the hair brushed up, work from the front to the back. Use the clippers 'freehand' to flatten the top. Clipper-over-comb the whole top area.

Work the clippers in the opposite direction, i.e. stand on the side and bring the clippers across from the other side towards you.

Look at the flat-top from all angles; it may look fine on one side but not when you move around to the other side. When looking straight at your client from behind, it can be an advantage to be wearing a white or light-coloured shirt so that the line is shown in silhouette against it in the mirror. Take into account the different angles from which you are looking at the cut. You may be looking down at the line whereas the client will be looking at it on the level.

Naturally, the more flat-tops you do, the better and faster you will be able to do them. Key factors include the following.

- You must get the shape right – this is what determines a flat-top.
- Keep the crown short – the flat-top starts forward of the crown.
- Establish the front length and work back to the crown.
- Take a lot of the moisture out or cut the hair dry.
- Blow the hair upwards to establish the line.
- Work the clippers across the top toward where you stand.
- Use the clippers 'free hand' or clipper-over-comb.
- Look at the line from all angles.

Common moustache types

Pencil line moustache (Latin)

This moustache is shaped between the nose and the lip. It gives the appearance of being drawn with a pencil. It is reminiscent of the moustaches worn by actors in films of the 1930s and 1940s.

Figure 1.35a

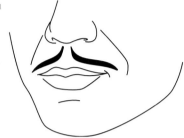

The walrus or soup strainer

A popular moustache type which has a tendency to trap particles of food. Often the upper lip is completely covered.

Figure 1.35d

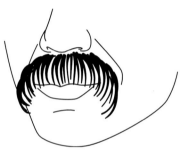

Handlebar moustache

Associated with the air force and barber-shop quartets, this moustache is shaped to resemble the handlebars of a bicycle. It is often waxed and shaped into position. The handlebar moustache needs to be worn with confidence and aplomb.

Figure 1.35b

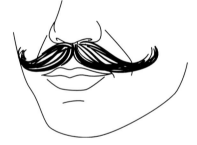

The lip rester

Any type of moustache that reaches the upper lip and does not extend past the corner of the mouth. It covers a variety of different types and is associated with military styles. However, if the lip rester extends to the nose, it becomes a brush.

Figure 1.35e

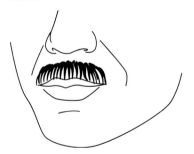

The brush (Hitler or Charlie Chaplain)

The brush covers a wide variety of moustaches. Hitler and Charlie Chaplain both wore brush-type moustaches, which include any type of moustache that covers the entire area of the upper lip but does not extend beyond the corner of the mouth.

Figure 1.35c

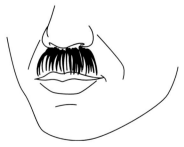

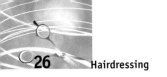

 # Common beard types

Full beard

This type of beard is allowed to grow willy-nilly. I often ask clients with this type of beard, 'Are you growing a beard, or just not shaving?' Is there a difference? There could be!

However, a full beard can be maintained and kept meticulously. Although it may seldom be cut or trimmed, it can still be combed to look neat and tidy.

Figure 1.36

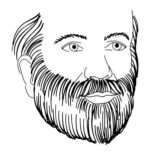

Lincoln beard

This beard requires that the upper lip be shaved. Often, scuba divers who want a beard select this type as it does not interfere with the use of the mouthpiece when diving. The beard was named after the American president, Abraham Lincoln.

Figure 1.37

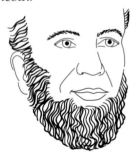

Ring beard

A short beard, with the moustache and beard forming an almost perfect circle around the mouth.

Figure 1.38

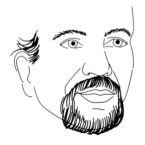

Van Dyck beard

This beard is named after the Dutch painter, Antoon Van Dyck. A Van Dyck beard is a chin beard; any short beard that covers most of the chin can be termed a Van Dyck or variation.

Figure 1.39

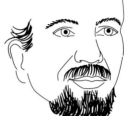

Goatee beard

These beards closely resemble the 'beards' of goats – hence the name. A long Van Dyck can be called a goatee. Goatee beards have no side whiskers.

Figure 1.40

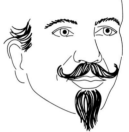

Mutton chops

Side whiskers, rounded at the ends, resembling mutton chops.

Figure 1.41

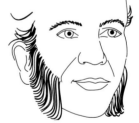

Medium-full beard (partial or short beard)

This type of beard is shaved in some areas for definition. For example, it may be shaved on the cheeks, around the lip and around the neck.

Figure 1.42

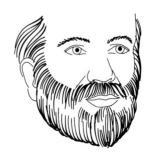

How to trim a beard

Considering the beard type

A good idea is to ask the client to bring a set of small passport photographs and sketch on them the beard and moustache combinations to see what suits. The size and shape of the face need to be considered as does the stature of the wearer. For example, a small, close beard may not suit a large, round-faced wearer; conversely, a full, long, heavy beard may not suit a short, small-faced man. A Van Dyck-type beard or goatee would suit a round face whereas a square beard is more suited to a triangular face. A rounded beard can correct a long chin.

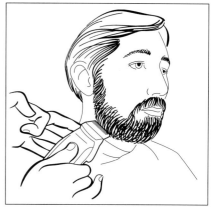
Figure 1.43

Beards should be washed regularly. The beard can be cleaned with shampoo or soap and thoroughly rinsed. Beards need to be combed if they are short or brushed if they are long.

Preparation

Gown the client well as the coarse clippings have a tendency to fly everywhere (the client should be told to keep his eyes and mouth closed). Brush or comb the beard to eliminate tangles and knots, and comb the beard into the general shape that the client wants.

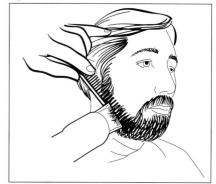
Figure 1.44

Method

Starting at the sides, use scissors or clippers-over-comb from the ear down to the chin. (Sometimes re-chargeable clippers are not powerful enough for coarse, strong, full beards and may get jammed; this type of clipper is not designed to cut full beards but merely to trim sideburns and neck lines, so it may be best to use powerful electric clippers.)

The clippers can be used to cut close to the skin if this is the look the client desires. Reverse the clippers and clean out the line under the chin and around the jawline. Tilt the client's head back and take out the bulk and weight of the beard under the chin with scissors. If the hair is long enough it may be picked up between the fingers and club cut. Ensure that both sides of the beard are even and that an equal amount of bulk is removed from each side. Look in the mirror to ensure the balance is correct. Trim the beard around the chin with scissors or clippers to define the shape. The scissors or clippers can be used freehand to remove protruding hairs. Use the clippers if the client wishes the hair around the neck under the beard to be removed. (As mentioned previously, this book does not cover the use of an open razor against the skin – it is not a technique used in women's hairdressing and there is a danger of passing on infection or disease should the skin be broken. A barber may be trained to clean this area with an open razor, but the danger of infection and disease will still exist.) Use the clippers to remove all hair to around the area of the collar. Ask the client whether a definite line is preferred or a gradual taper (reverse the clipper if a definite line is preferred).

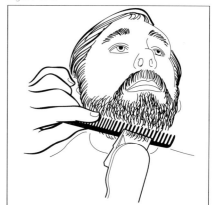
Figure 1.45

Clear the mouth area of all stray hairs. Frequently, the client may wish the 'underlip' area of the chin to be clipped quite short. The client may need to 'stretch' the bottom lip to force the hair out to be cut. This can be cut with scissors or clippers. As a courtesy, from time to time the neck brush should be used to remove all the short clippings from the client's face, especially around the eyes, nose and mouth. Cutting the hair closely with clippers and scissors around lips, nose, neck, and chin needs to be done with care. Take care not to cut the skin. Finally, refrain from asking your client questions while you are trimming his beard (this is a trick my dentist enjoys playing on me while working on my teeth).

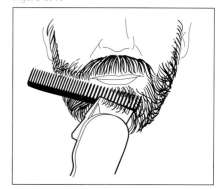
Figure 1.46

How to trim a moustache

Figure 1.47

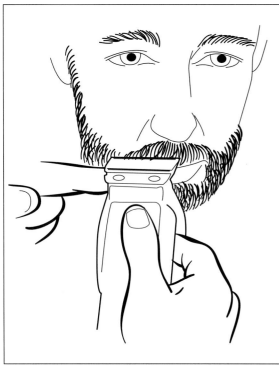

First, make sure the client has closed his mouth. If the moustache is in a style that requires the ends to stand away from the face (such as a handlebar moustache), then direct the growth with the comb to emphasise this. Comb the hair straight down over the upper lip and carefully trim along the outer boundary of the moustache with scissors or clippers (support the scissors with the first finger to avoid cutting the lip). Determine where the moustache is to start standing away from the face and trim to this point.

Now comb the moustache horizontally from the centre towards the ends. Trim off any excess hair hanging over the top lip; define the line of the lip with the clippers. (A Walrus moustache will completely cover the top lip and might only be trimmed by its owner.) Lift the hair with your comb at the corner of the mouth and clean out any protruding hairs with clippers or scissors. Clippers can also be brought down (reverse the clipper head) on the moustache to keep the moustache and hairs flat and straight. Snip off any hairs that extend below the line where the upper lip begins. If the client wants the moustache cut short, then the bulk can be removed by the scissors or clipper-over-comb techniques. Use the tip of the scissors to achieve this. Moustaches that stand away from the face may also be controlled with moustache wax (sometimes beeswax is used for this purpose).

Common terms used in hair cutting

activated texture	a rough surface such as a uniform layer
angle	a corner line measured in degrees
base part	a parting taken against the scalp
blunt cut	lacking a pointed end, cut straight off
bob	a style achieved by cutting each section at 0°
chipping	removing small strands using regular scissors
clippers	a tool used to cut the hair and also to obtain the shingled look at the nape
club cutting	lacking a point, cut straight off, also known as blunt cutting
crest line	the widest point of the head which divides the interior from the exterior areas
cutting comb	a comb narrow at one end and wide at the other, preferably saw-cut or narrow-set comb used to shingle the hair close to the nape
degree of angle	the angle at which the hair is held out from the head and cut or the angle at which the hair is distributed
design element	one of three components (shape, texture and structure) which make up a haircut
design line	the shape of the cut or the outside of the haircut at the perimeter
diagonal	a slanting line, e.g. 45° from corner to corner
elevation	the degrees, from 0° to 180°, at which the hair can be lifted or raised from the scalp

exterior	the area of the haircut below the crest line
geometric	a regular, symmetrical angle or shape, e.g. square, diamond
guide strand	the first section of hair cut to the length desired
graduation	the grade at which all the hair will be cut
guideline	a line which is followed throughout the entire haircut
horizontal	at right angles to the vertical, level with the horizon, flat
interior	the area of the haircut above the crest line
layering	cutting the hair to achieve a layered effect
natural fall	the way the hair grows and falls naturally
natural projection	hair projected at a 90° angle from the curve of the head
neckline	the shape of the hair growth at the nape hairline
parallel graduation	graduation between two parallel lines, whether horizontal or diagonal
perimeter	the outer edge of the haircut
perpendicular	at right angles (90° angle) to a given line
precision cut	an exact, accurate haircut
projection	the degree of lift out from the head
ridge line	a line which separates two surface textures
right angles	90° (perpendicular)
shape	the line, construction or form of a haircut
shifting	neither perpendicular or natural fall but at any other angle of distribution
shingling	using scissors over the comb to cut the hair short at the nape, leaving it gradually longer toward the crown without showing a definite line
silhouette	the profile or outline of the haircut
slithering	the action of the regular scissors when used to remove bulk from the hair
structure	the lengths in a haircut
taper	to become gradually sharper at the end; the opposite of blunt
texture	the surface appearance of a haircut
texturising	removing weight or bulk from the hair
thinning	removing bulk from the hair
unactivated texture	a smooth surface such as that of a bob
variation	a change in the technique, something different about the same version, an alternative
vertical	upright, at right angles to the horizon
volume	bulk, a large amount, height, fullness
weight	heaviness, bulk in a certain area of a haircut, a point

Questions – Cutting women's hair

1 What type of comb is best suited for general cutting purposes?

2 How should the scissors be held for control and balance?

3 Name two ways in which the finished cut should be perceived.

4 Name three design elements that make up a haircut.

5 List three considerations in your analysis of:

a the client;

b the hair.

6 What is meant by 'the hairline growth pattern'?

7 What are the three ways in which hair can be cut?

8 What is shingling?

9 Using illustrations, describe tapering.

10 **a** What physical characteristic will determine where thinning will start on the hair strand?

_____

b Why should coarse hair be thinned further from the scalp than fine hair?

_____

_____

_____

11 Name four areas where it is inadvisable to thin the hair.

_____

_____

_____

_____

12 What is slithering?

_____

13 List three advantages of cutting the hair wet.

_____

_____

_____

14 Using profile sketches, show the following angles:
   a 90° angle;

b 45° angle;

c 22.5° angle.

15 How should you analyse a hair design in your mind before you start a haircut?

_____

16 What are the four classic haircuts?

_____

_____

_____

_____

17 What type of surface appearance does the following have:

a a bob?

_____

b a uniform layer?

_____

18 Which type of haircut gives:

a the heaviest line of weight?

_____

b no weight line?

_____

19 What is the major difference in cutting technique between graduation and a layer?

_____

20 Describe the crest line and the ridge line.

_____

21 What is meant by 'cutting the design line parallel to the base line'? Use sketches to illustrate your answer.

_____

22 What is the difference between natural fall and natural projection?

_____

23 Using sketches, show a structural analysis of a bob and a uniform layer. Describe the surface appearance.

_____

24 What is meant by the following hair-cutting terms:

   a interior;

   _____

   b perpendicular;

   _____

   c base part;

   _____

   d 0° projection;

   _____

   e weight line;

   _____

   f increasing layer;

   _____

   g design element;

   _____

   h shape.

   _____

Questions – Cutting men's hair

1 Describe the scissors-over-comb technique.

_____

_____

_____

2 What other word can describe 'scissors-over-comb'?

_____

3 What two items are used to sharpen a straight razor?

_____

_____

4 What can cause a 'step' in a man's haircut?

_____

_____

_____

5 Why are clippers not ideal for cleaning the hairline around the ear arch?

_____

_____

_____

6 Other than the neck brush, what can be used to remove the fine hairs that stick to the skin after a haircut?

7 Describe the action of the clippers when closely tapering the hair at the nape line.

8 Name and illustrate three moustache types.

9 **a** What is the difference between a full beard and a partial beard?

b What is the difference between a Van Dyck beard and a goatee?

10 Describe how to trim a moustache.

11 What are the dangers of using an open razor against the skin?

12 Describe two key factors in cutting a 'flat-top' hairstyle.

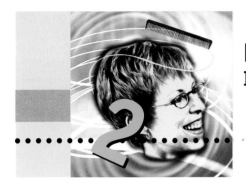

Razor cutting
Introduces: 'Cut the hair with a razor'

In this chapter, you will learn about:

- elevating with the razor;
- the conventional razor-cutting technique.

An important part of general hairdressing, razor cutting is a skill which should be practised for at least eight months before your final practical assessment. It is used to achieve a tapered look, to reduce weight and to texturise the hair, and is ideal for clients with thick, coarse hair. In your practical assessments, you may be required to give your client a complete razor cut; only the occasional end will be allowed to be cut with scissors. Although there are many methods of giving a razor cut, the technique which gives a clean precise finish to the hair is known as 'elevating with the razor'.

 Elevating with the razor

Elevating is a technique used under the hair strands. Hair, hand and razor are brought up and out in one unit to achieve a very clean, precise, tapered line. It is a sound technique. Since some razors come without a razor blade guard, be very careful with the open blade.

Preparation

Ensure that your razor has a new blade. Your client's hair must be shampooed and rinsed and a water sprayer should be on hand to moisten the hair regularly. It is important that you make a correct assessment of the hair in your preliminary consultation. Try to cut the hair in the direction of its natural growth.

Method

Hold the razor as shown in diagram A, Figure 2.2, with the fingers wrapped around the handle and the thumb in the groove. Hold the razor firmly. Once you have decided on the style, section the hair – the cut can be started on any part of the head. Select your guide strand and hold the razor flat under the guide strand, as in diagram A. Stand directly behind the section you are cutting. Now rest the razor on the middle finger. Don't apply undue pressure on the razor but hold the hair firmly

Figure 2.1

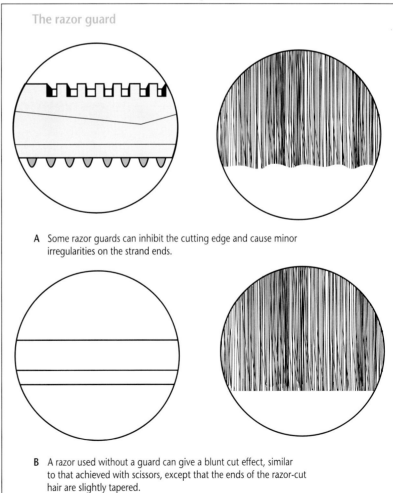

The razor guard

A Some razor guards can inhibit the cutting edge and cause minor irregularities on the strand ends.

B A razor used without a guard can give a blunt cut effect, similar to that achieved with scissors, except that the ends of the razor-cut hair are slightly tapered.

Figure 2.2

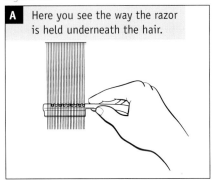

A Here you see the way the razor is held underneath the hair.

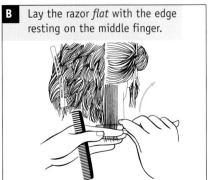

B Lay the razor *flat* with the edge resting on the middle finger.

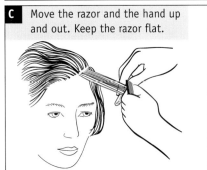

C Move the razor and the hand up and out. Keep the razor flat.

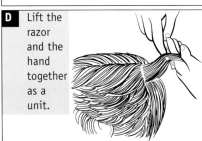

D Lift the razor and the hand together as a unit.

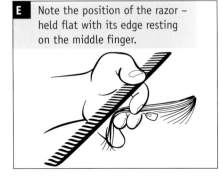

E Note the position of the razor – held flat with its edge resting on the middle finger.

between the first and middle fingers, as in diagram B, Figure 2.2. Note the placement of the comb.

Keep the razor flat and slightly edged in towards the fingers. A razor guard can be used but it tends to inhibit the cutting action. Now lift the razor, hands and hair, as a unit, up and out in a small arc, as in diagram C, Figure 2.2. Don't lift the razor off the fingers but keep it turned in toward the fingers. The hair is cut by the razor when the hands are swung up and out. If the style is to be layered, lift the hair higher than the section being cut. Styles which require only graduating need be lifted only to the level of the section being cut. Make sure the width of the section is no longer than the razor blade. Continue to cut the guide strand.

Check for precision. Note in diagram D how close the hair has been cut to the fingers. Now, take the next subsection and comb down; you should be able to see the previous guide strand. Lift and comb the hair the way it is to fall. Don't stretch the hair when combing. Place the razor and hands under the next section, slide the fingers down and wait for the guide strand to drop away, as in diagram E.

Keeping the razor flat and slightly turned in, lift it in an arc up and out toward your chin. This technique is used to razor cut the rest of the hair. If you are layering the top and crown area, make sure you can get above the sections.

Cross-check for precision. The occasional end may be trimmed with the scissors. If the client complains that his/her hair is being pulled, check:

- razor blade for sharpness;
- that the hair is wet enough;
- that the razor is held flat.

Like most other cutting techniques, this one will require practice. There are other ways to razor cut; ask your senior stylist to help you.

The conventional razor-cutting technique

This action involves the traditional razoring technique in which the razor lies on top of the hair strand or mesh and the razor travels in short strokes toward the ends of the hair. The finished effects of this technique are not as precise as those obtained with the 'elevating' technique, but nevertheless it is commonly used in the salon as a way of cutting the hair using the razor.

Generally, the action creates a short-to-long taper on the ends of the hair and gives an overall soft, 'wispy' effect. Coarse, strong hair is ideally suited to the conventional razor-cutting technique as the removal of bulk from the ends of the hair allows the hair to be more 'pliable'. This softens the effect for the client, which is ideal in some cases.

The degree of tapering and ultimately the removal of bulk is affected by three major elements. Assuming the razor blade is sharp, the first is the angle of the razor when held against the hair mesh combined with the second, the degree of pressure put on the razor. Generally it is accepted that the flatter the razor is held against the mesh with pressure applied, the longer the taper will be (and the easier the mesh will be cut). On the other hand, the more upright the razor is held against the mesh and the gentler the pressure, the less or shorter the taper. The third element is also combined with the first two and that is the length of the razor stroke. Naturally, long, flat, heavy strokes will produce quite a considerable taper. Conversely, shorter, gentler strokes with the razor held more upright will produce a short taper. As you become more proficient you will be able to feel the amount of taper being created. You will sense how much the razor is removing in the way of bulk – and thus learn at what angle the razor should be held, how much pressure should be applied, and how long the razor strokes should be.

Sections can be taken vertically, with the razor also positioned vertically. This style is a common way to cut the hair with a razor (refer to the illustrations in Figure 2.3 for this technique). Remember you can also combine the elevating technique with the conventional technique when you want a harder, more precise line. The conventional razor-cutting technique definitely gives a softer, feathered, tapered effect.

Prior to trying the conventional razor-cutting technique, practice your razor strokes on a vertical hair strip. Alter the angle of the blade against the hair mesh, vary the pressure and the length of stroke of the razor on the ends. For a short taper, try to confine the razor strokes to the last 1 cm to 1.5 cm of the hair ends. Now, maintaining the same angle, lengthen the stroke to 3 cm of the hair ends. Observe the effect of the taper. The longer the taper, the more difficult it will be to place a perm rod or roller around the ends. So, prior to a permanent wave or set a long tapered razor cut may not be ideal. It would be better to give a shorter taper in this instance. A long taper would be ideal for a scrunch-dry, diffuser or blow-dry, or perhaps set on large velcro rollers.

In a practical assessment it is best to show a shorter taper.

Practical exercise

Show skill in elevating with the razor:
1   a graduated/bob haircut;
2   a layered haircut.
Try and achieve these haircuts within 45 minutes.

Cutting with the razor held at a more vertical angle will ensure a taper.

Figure 2.3 (a and b)

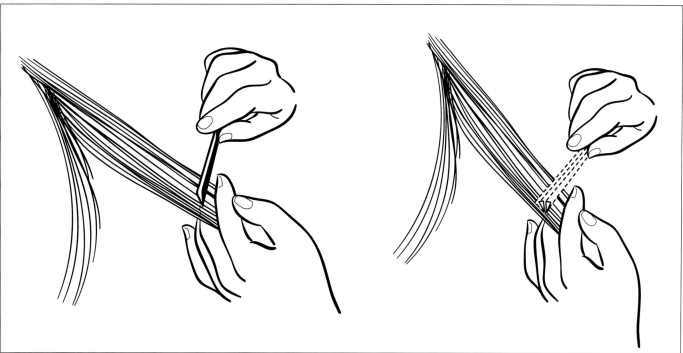

The angle of the razor against the mesh can affect the length of the taper.

Figure 2.4

Razor cutting

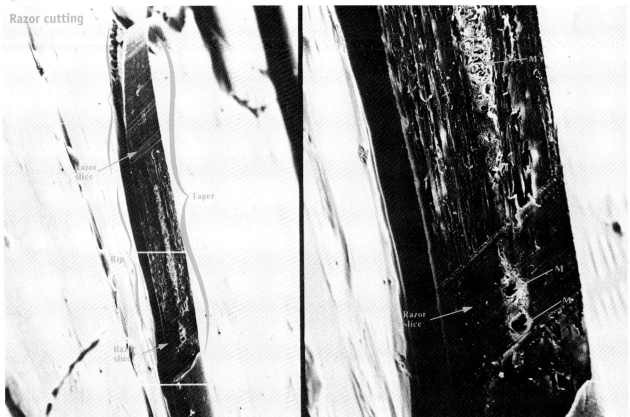

In this interesting photograph, notice the following:

A   the degree of taper indicated;
B   the razor has sliced the fibre in the medullated area and the
    fibre has ripped. The razor has then cut again toward the tip
    of the hair;
C   the medulla – the hollow structure, intermittent along the
    fibre. The razor has sliced along the medulla then through
    the other side (as indicated).

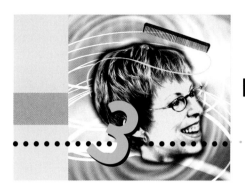

Product knowledge

In this chapter, you will learn about:

- hair care and advice;
- select treatments;
- hair products – the chemistry and effect on the hair;
- hydrogen peroxide;
- hairdressing products and the environment.

 ## Hair care and advice

Lanolins, anionic detergents, hydrolised proteins, cationic conditioners, emulsions, polymer, alcohol resins PVP – are you confused by all these terms? What do they all mean?

Hairdressers are becoming very aware of the need for hair care and most salons offer advice and special services on general hair care and health. Unfortunately, some products used in the hairdressing salon can cause hair damage, especially if they are used constantly, abused or if the instructions are not followed.

If you are giving a client any kind of service, whether it be a blow-dry or a permanent wave, your first priority is to ensure that the hair is in the best possible condition. You won't achieve good results otherwise, no matter how good a hairdresser you are.

The chemicals used in permanent waving, colouring and bleaching, chlorine and salt water can all damage the hair.

Constant application of such chemicals will cause:

- *harshness*: hair is rough to the touch; feels as though something is coating it;
- *dryness*: a damaged cuticle will give the hair a dry feel and appearance;
- *loss of elasticity*: no bounce or stretch in the hair causes it to become limp;
- *brittleness*: the hair is fragile, delicate and easily broken;
- *splitting*: the hair has split and frayed ends;
- *breakage*: the hair looks fractured, frayed and imperfect.

Damage can also be caused by physical factors or by tools and appliances.

1 Excessive blow-drying or overuse of curling tongs or heated rollers can all harm the hair. Over-hot appliances can burn the hair, which can also be damaged through being stretched too much with a brush.
2 Brushing the hair when it is wet can cause loss of elasticity, and tugging the tangles out of wet hair causes breakage.
3 Drying the hair by an open or electric fire causes dryness and a lack of natural lubricant.
4 Pulling elastic or rubber bands from the hair leads to breakage and split ends.
5 Overexposure to sun causes harsh, dry hair, lacking in shine.

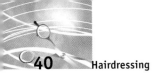

Whatever the problem is, you as a professional hairdresser will have to advise the client on the best product to remedy the situation. Manufacturers are constantly developing products which enable you to improve the quality of your clients' hair. Every month they produce new formulas with new ingredients that claim to do wonders. You must keep up to date with all this new information and be familiar with what is available. You will then be in a better position to give clients advice.

 # Select corrective treatments for the hair and scalp

(Information on treatments is further covered in Chapters 6 and 13 in Book 1.)

Analyse the hair and scalp for corrective treatment

An important part of selecting treatments is the analysis of the hair and scalp (generally, treatments are specifically for the hair rather than the scalp). The analysis is done to confirm what work needs to be completed. The hair analysis should involve physically touching the hair and visual observation to establish the characteristics and hair condition. Check for abrasions on the scalp, scalp sensitivity, and whether there are any disorders.

Selecting the treatment

- Conditioning treatments are ideal for hair which is dry, chemically treated or unmanageable. There are a number of conditioners on the market that are quickly applied to the hair with a brush and are left on the hair either for only a few moments or for longer, with the addition of heat. They are quick acting and coat the hair fibre instantly. Those that are left on for longer penetrate the hair fibre and rebuild its strength. Conditioners are rinsed off and no trace of the product should remain in the hair.
- Porosity fillers are specially formulated treatments designed to reduce the porous nature of the hair. They are simply applied by spray bottle directly to the hair and left in the hair. Porosity fillers are one of the few treatments that are left in the hair after being applied. The conditioning properties 'fill' the cuticle and make it less porous. This effect slows down the development of any processing product applied to the hair, such as permanent wave lotion.
- Hot oil treatments are designed for hair that is excessively dry, over-porous or damaged due to too much processing. Details of types of oil and their application are described in Chapter 13, 'Recognising and advising on simple scalp and hair problems' in Book 1.

 # Hair products – the chemistry and effect on the hair

(More advanced information on the chemistry of products can be found in Chapters 12 and 14 of this book.)

Advice and hair care services offered in the salon should include information on shampoos (also referred to as surfactants – surface active agents). There are two main categories of shampoo, soap and synthetic (soapless). Of these, synthetic shampoos are used far more often than soap shampoos in hairdressing salons.

Both types of shampoo look the same and it can be difficult to distinguish between them. Sometimes the label may tell you what chemicals have been used in the shampoo's preparation; it is becoming more common in many countries to include such information on labels. More than 95% of shampoos available through hairdressing salons or pharmacies are soapless.

Shampoos constitute one of the main products for personal care. A shampoo's primary function, regardless of type or cost, is to cleanse the hair, removing accumulated sebum, scalp debris and any hair preparations (hairspray, mousse, etc). Most detergents will do this; however, the cleansing should be selective and should preserve some of the natural oil in the hair and skin. Problems that could arise if all the oil were removed include: difficulty in combing, lack of lustre, 'fly-away' hair, roughness to the hands. Shampoo which cleanses and conditions should be chosen with care, bearing in mind the balance that should be maintained between cleansing and conditioning, and also the following:

a the ease with which the shampoo can be spread on the hair;

b lathering ability;

c efficiency in dirt removal;

d ease of rinsing – some shampoos rinse away quickly, others continue to lather after endless rinsing;

e ease of combing the wet hair – will the hair be difficult to comb and become tangled after shampooing?

f Lustre – the hair must feel and smell clean and fresh once it has been shampooed;

g speed of drying – some shampoos leave the hair very wet (and slow to dry), others tend to shed water fairly quickly;

h non-irritant – the shampoos should not irritate the eyes or skin or cause any other scalp discomfort.

In other words, simply removing the sebum from the hair shaft is not the whole story!

Figure 3.1

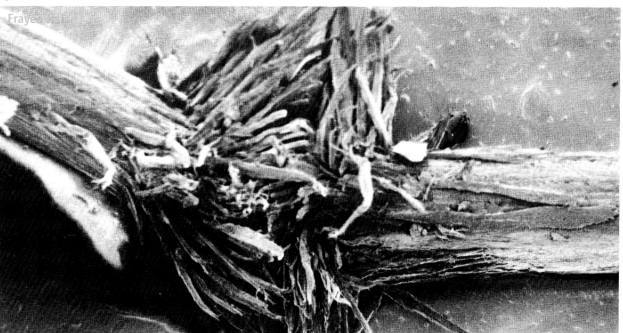

Frayed hair

Do you do this to your clients' hair? This hair has been damaged by incorrect permanent wave winding (rubber tension). The hair has become frayed, exposing the cortical fibres. The cuticle has also been removed as a result of harsh chemical treatment.

Figure 3.2

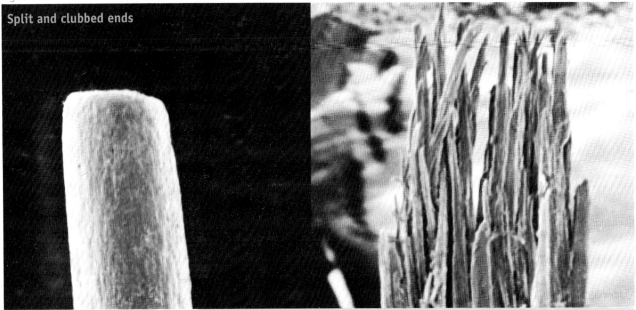

Split and clubbed ends

The classic split end on the right, exposing the frayed cortical fibre. Compare it with the better conditioned clubbed end on the left.

Synthetic detergents (soapless shampoos)

These are made from chemicals such as sodium or triethanolamine lauryl sulphate, mixed with animal fats, lanolin or tallow, or vegetable, coconut or olive oil, which have been boiled with sulphuric acid. These are highly processed formulas, which have a pH of 2 to 7 (although this has no relationship to the shampoos' effectiveness).

Soapless shampoos remove grease from the hair very effectively because they are good wetting agents. Sometimes, however, they degrease the hair too much, and their greatest disadvantage, as far as the hairdresser is concerned, is that they can cause skin irritations such as dermatitis. There is, therefore, little point in changing from one shampoo to another if they are both soapless.

Typical ingredients that go into a shampoo include:

- surfactants (cleaning and foaming agents);
- conditioning agents;
- special additives;
- preservatives;
- thickening agents;
- opacifiers;
- perfume – essential oils such as rose, lavender, jasmine, herbs or lemon;
- colour.

Shampoos can also be classified as either anionic, cationic or non-ionic detergents. These terms refer to the electrical charge of molecules which make a solution a conductor of electricity.

Anionic shampoos are characterised by negative charged ions; cationic are characterised by positive surface-active ions, while non-ionic detergents have uncharged polar molecules.

Soapless shampoos nowadays contain any number of ingredients which claim to revitalise the hair. Fractionated or hydrolised proteins are proteins broken down to be effective as conditioners for the hair. Other ingredients include lemon, cream, egg, almond, honey, fruit and nuts. These shampoos are advertised as being suitable for oily, dry, normal and processed hair. Many such ingredients are merely advertising gimmicks, designed to arouse the consumer's interest in a particular product. These ingredients are of little benefit to the hair; they cannot 'feed' the hair but can make the shampoo thicker or more acidic or make it smell nice.

Soapless shampoos will give a lather in salt-water and can remove artificial colour. Such shampoos are tested to determine whether they sting the eye by the 'rabbit test' (Draize test): a solution of the shampoo is dropped into the eyes of rabbits and the effect is noted. (This kind of testing is not carried out in all countries.) Although some shampoos, such as baby shampoos, have a low eye-stinging characteristic, they are still made from a synthetic detergent but they have a neutral pH. Whether a shampoo stings or not depends on its pH. If it has a pH of 7, it doesn't sting; if it is an acid or alkali, it will sting.

Soap shampoo (soft-soap detergent)

These are really old-fashioned shampoos and have been used very successfully for hundreds of years, long before the new formulated synthetic preparations came on the market. Soap shampoos are made from animal wax (lanolin) or vegetable oils such as olive oil, almond oil and coconut oil, boiled with caustic soda/potash – sodium or potassium hydroxide. This process is called saponification, which means converting to soap.

All soaps are alkaline. The soap liquid is diluted and used successfully as shampoo. Soap shampoos do leave a scum, if used with hard water. Hard water can leave a coating of calcium or magnesium salts on the hair shaft, making the hair dull and unattractive. The traditional soap shampoo is a green soft soap available at pharmacies or health shops. An advantage of soap shampoos is that they rarely cause dermatitis.

Soap shampoos do not lather in salt water. They also contain preservatives to prevent the oil or fat from going rancid. (Hard soaps are toilet soaps manufactured from animal wax or fats (tallow) and caustic soda.)

Anti-dandruff shampoos

There are many anti-dandruff shampoos available, most of which have an antiseptic action and contain zinc pyrithione, selenium, sulphide, tar, sulphur or cetrimide BP. These chemicals are antibacterial germicides and they are used in an attempt to reduce the collection of scales and micro-organisms which have formed on the surface of the scalp. Shampoos for dry, flaky scalps contain similar ingredients. Such shampoos are recommended for clients who have difficulty in accepting that they have dandruff. Try different anti-dandruff shampoos until the client finds one that is suitable.

General conditioners – cream rinses or revitalisers

Conditioners are cationic (positively charged) emulsions which attach to the predominantly anionic (negative) regions of hair keratin. (For this reason, conditioners cannot be completely removed from the hair by rinsing alone; their coating attraction needs to be shampooed off.) A fat, lanolin or oil (almond, avocado, wheat germ) is added to increase the hair's wet combing ability. Conditioners also contain preservatives (to stop the fat or oil from going rancid) and antistatic additives to make hair manageable.

A conditioner must provide gloss, softness and smoothness, must prevent tangling and should help to repair hair damage such as split ends. The anionic detergent in the shampoo must be thoroughly rinsed out before conditioning; if it is not, the positive cationic (conditioner) will combine with the negative anionic (shampoo) and create scum.

Conditioners are almost always acid, with a pH from 2.5 to 5.5. As conditioners work very quickly, they should be left on the hair for less than 30 seconds.

Conditioners are ideal for weakened hair or over-porous hair resulting from chemical treatment such as bleaching, permanent waving, tinting, too frequent shampooing, mechanical abuse (curling tongs, blow-dryers) and over-exposure to the sun. A conditioner will act as a substitute for natural sebum and provide a softer, smoother feel to the hair. In addition, a conditioner will protect against further damage, 'fill' the cuticle and flatten the cuticle scales and make the hair easier to comb.

Special conditioning treatments

Lanolin

A common ingredient of many hairdressing preparations, lanolin is purified wool wax, and it is one of the best emollients (skin softeners) available, since it preserves, softens and smooths the skin and hair. There is little evidence of lanolin causing irritation.

Glycerine

Also used in many hair and skin preparations, glycerine is a by-product of soap manufacture. It improves the spreading property of creams and lotions and is non-irritant.

These special conditioners are formulated in the same way as general conditioners but are presented differently. They may be thicker and have a higher concentration of animal fats and vegetable oils, and they come in punnets, sachets or tubes. When worked into the hair, they are left on for approximately 20 minutes, and treatment usually incorporates heat from lamps or a steamer. The heat helps to open up the hair cuticle so that the conditioning treatment will be absorbed, add some external protein, and realign the cuticle scales. This coating will help to protect the hair against further damage. Because the cuticle will lie flatter, it will reflect the light and give the hair greater sheen and lustre.

Setting lotions, sprays, gels, mousse and foams

Setting agents are essentially resins, either vegetable or alcohol. They coat and leave a film on the hair shaft, preventing moisture from penetrating the hair and thereby creating a longer-lasting style.

There are two types of setting lotion. The first is known as a mucilage, made from gum obtained from trees; gum tragacanth is commonly used. This is dissolved with a splash of alcohol and mixed with distilled water, perfume and a preservative (formalin) to stop it from going mouldy. Mucilage setting lotions tend to be sticky and tacky when dried on the hair, and are not commonly used nowadays in the hairdressing salon. Gum setting lotions used to be characterised by the gum which formed around the end of the applicator nozzle. This had to be chipped away before the setting lotion could be used. Hair lacquers behaved in a similar way.

The second type of setting agent, which is used in most salons, is the spirit plastifier resin. Plastifier contains a plastic resin called PVP (polyvinylpyrrolidone) which is dissolved in industrial alcohol, a small amount of glycerine (a thick viscous liquid), distilled water and perfume. Colour can be added – browns, reds, yellows or blues. These are called coloured setting lotions and the colour is only temporary.

Mousse and gels

Is there a difference between mousse and gel? Yes. Mousse looks and feels like shaving cream but acts as a combination of setting lotion and hairspray. It controls hair, adding volume and lift. Gel is thicker and can be used to mould, sculpt and give a wet look to hair if a lot is used. The hair type will influence your choice of product. If the hair is fine, a super-hold or a super-control is required. Wavy hair needs a regular formula, and thick curly hair should have a built-in hair tamer.

Lacquers and hairsprays

Like setting lotions, lacquers and hairsprays help to keep moisture from getting into hair and collapsing the set or blow-dry style. They also keep the hair in place. Their composition is similar to that of setting lotion.

Lacquers

Lacquers are not used much in hairdressing salons nowadays, although they were common many years ago. They are often thought of as something harsh, which coats the hair and causes flaking. This is true to a certain extent; the majority of today's final dressing fixatives are hairsprays which do not contain the harsh coating gum.

Lacquers are made from shellac, a coloured resin produced on tree bark by insects, which is also an ingredient of polish and varnish. Shellac resembles 'cornflakes' and is mixed with alcohol, spirit, lanolin and water. Lacquers are difficult to remove because shellac is not water soluble, although it does dissolve in alcohol. Lacquers used to be removed with borax – a white soluble salt – or a shampoo which contained this.

Hairsprays

Hairsprays must provide style support without causing harsh, dry build-up. They should be water-soluble (wash out in water) and be easily brushed out without flaking. They should be mildly perfumed and contain moisture-repellent agents to help hold the set or blow-dry style in place.

Hairsprays are made from plastifier PVP (polyvinylpyrrolidone) which forms the protective moisture-repellent film. This PVP is usually dissolved in alcohol with glycerine added to keep it soft and non-flaking. Perfume is also added. No water is added as this will rust the can.

Hairsprays are usually produced in aerosol pressurised cans. The propellant is usually freon or butane. Freon is said to break down the ozone layer of the earth's atmosphere which protects us against ultraviolet rays. Freon and butane turn into gas quickly at room temperature. This gas creates pressure and forces the hairspray out of the can when the nozzle is depressed.

Advice to clients when using hairsprays

1 Read the instructions before use.
2 Shake the can to mix the propellant and the hairspray.
3 Hold the can at arm's length to get a finer spray and better coverage.
4 Brush the hair free from spray before reapplying to avoid build-up.
5 Use a water-soluble spray, that is, one that washes out in water.
6 Do not store hairspray cans near a source of heat, such as heaters (as they could explode).

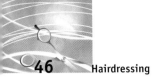

Dressing-out creams and hair shines

Dressing-out creams and hair shine sprays usually contain a mineral oil (silicone). Kerosene oil, paraffin wax mineral oil and liquid paraffin are obtained by distilling petroleum, vegetable oils and a white wax found in sperm whales. These ingredients, plus perfume, are the major constituents of these hair dressings. Such elements also prevent moisture from entering the hair shaft, close the cuticle and help to give the hair a better shine by reflecting the light.

Reducing and rebonding products

Permanent waving lotion

The main ingredient in cold permanent waving lotion is ammonium thioglycollate, a salt which is a reducing agent. The salt is produced by neutralising thioglycollic acid using ammonium hydroxide. The ammonium hydroxide makes the hair swell and acts as a wetting agent which allows easy penetration of the solution into the cortex. The reducing agent, ammonium thioglycollate, breaks the hydrogen and salt linkage. This chemical reaction, which involves the addition of hydrogen to a substance, is known as reduction.

Straightening lotion

Straightening products contain a higher concentration of ammonium thioglycollate than that in permanent waving lotion. As a result, they have higher pH value. Strong or 'afro' hair may require an even stronger straightening lotion and this may contain sodium hydroxide, which is a caustic solution and must not come in contact with the skin. As in the chemical action of permanent waving, the linkages are broken by reduction.

Neutraliser

The neutraliser used in permanent waving is an oxidising agent. The chemical used is hydrogen peroxide or sodium bromate and is formulated as a cream or liquid.

Colouring and lightening products

(see also Chapters 4 and 10)

Temporary rinses

The molecules of the temporary rinse are large and unable to enter the cortex. They only stain the cuticle layer. There are two types:
- cationic rinses which are water-soluble and are diluted with water before use;
- anionic (acidic) or azo-type rinses.

These rinses come as water rinses, coloured shampoos or plastic setting lotions.

Semi-permanent rinses

The molecules of the semi-permanent rinse are small enough to penetrate the cortex. They last longer than temporary rinses.

Semi-colours are referred to as 'nitro' colours and contain red and yellow pigment. They are mixed with benzyl alcohol which assists in dispersing the molecules into the cortex. Emulsions are sometimes added and are formulated as colour shampoos.

Permanent colour

These are known as oxidation dyes or para-dyes. They contain para-phenylenediamine or para-toluenediamine. A wide range of other substances are now added to permanent colours. These light-coloured compounds are small enough to enter the cortex. They are mixed with hydrogen peroxide before use, which creates the final colour, by oxidation.

Lightening agents (bleaches)

These products lighten the hair by oxidation. Bleach consists of an oxidising agent, hydrogen peroxide, and an alkali, ammonium hydroxide or ammonium carbonate. They are mixed and thickened to form a paste or cream. Once mixed, the alkali assists in the release of the oxygen from the hydrogen peroxide and this lightens the melanin and pheomelanin in the cortex.

Hydrogen peroxide (H_2O_2)

Hydrogen peroxide is one of the most commonly used chemicals in the hairdressing salon and comes in either a liquid or a cream form. It was first used on hair by a Parisian hairdresser at the Paris Exhibition in the 1890s and has been used ever since. Its chemical formula is H_2O_2.

Hydrogen peroxide is a compound, that is, it is made up of two different elements – two hydrogen (H–H) and two oxygen (O–O) molecules. Once the O_2 is exhausted, it becomes water on the hair.

Hydrogen peroxide (H_2O_2) is used to obtain the O_2 gas for oxidising purposes such as the following.

- *Tinting*. It is the hydrogen peroxide that lightens the natural melanin colour pigment of the hair and helps in opening and softening the cuticle. It also reacts with the chemicals in the tint to make them permanent.
- *Bleaching/highlighting*. Lighteners which are mixed with stronger hydrogen peroxides will brighten and lighten the hair as many shades as desired.
- *Permanent wave neutralising*. The oxygen gas in the hydrogen peroxide rejoins the broken cross-linkages.
- *Lightening rinses*. These are diluted, weak hydrogen peroxide solutions which affect the melanin pigment, and also make the hair porous.

Pure hydrogen peroxide has a pH of 7. It is unreactive at an acidic pH relative to its reactivity under alkaline conditions. Its pH value does not depend on its strength. However, its reactivity depends on both its pH and, of course, its strength. There are a number of ways in which hydrogen peroxide will give up its O_2 content. The easiest way to liberate the O_2 gas is to mix it with something which contains ammonia (NH_3). The ammonia will help release the O_2 for oxidising purposes. Twenty years ago or more hairdressers used to add extra ammonia to the bleach solutions to get a faster action and to eliminate the red/gold tones. The additional ammonia was harsh on the hair. Nowadays the ammonia content in bleach is controlled in the powder and combines with the O_2 when it is mixed.

When the hairdressing salon purchases hydrogen peroxide, it will be in the form of volume or percentage. It is bought in the following strengths:

Volumes:	10,	20,	30,	40,	or even 60.
Percentages:	3,	6,	9,	12,	or even 18.

Volume strength means the potential O_2 that can be released. For example, 20 volume strength means that for every volume or cc of H_2, 20 cc of O_2 will be released. The higher the volume, the more O_2 it releases and the faster it functions (often with more hair damage).

In some countries there is no regulation about the strength of hydrogen peroxide that can be used in the hairdressing salon. Nevertheless, hydrogen peroxide in excess of 30 volume should be used with the utmost care and every precaution. In certain countries in Europe, 33 volume H_2O_2 is the maximum strength that can be used and in some American states there are laws pertaining to H_2O_2 strengths. Precautions are necessary because strengths above 30 volume H_2O_2 can be dangerous and damaging to skin and hair. (Boosters can be added to H_2O_2 to increase the lightening action, but these are not available in all countries.)

All hairdressing manufacturers supply hydrogen peroxide in a stabilised form; this means that it contains glycerine or phosphates to stop it from losing its O_2 content. It is the glycerine content which gives some hydrogen peroxides their creamy texture. Stabilised hydrogen peroxide still needs to be stored correctly.

Storing hydrogen peroxide

As previously mentioned, the O_2 content could be liberated from hydrogen peroxide in a number of ways. Adding ammonia is one method; the other alternatives concern the storage of hydrogen peroxide.

1 Heat and light will accelerate the liberation of O_2 from hydrogen peroxide. If the hydrogen peroxide is stored near a heat source – a radiator, electric heater or in direct sunlight – then it will lose its strength. Sometimes when you open a bottle of hydrogen peroxide you may hear a hiss or a pop. This does not mean that it is fresh (as with a fizzy drink) but that, in actual fact, it is losing its O_2 strength. The fizz and pop was the liberated O_2. The only reason for using hydrogen peroxide is to obtain its O_2; so store hydrogen peroxide in a cool area and preferably in dark bottles. Ideally, hydrogen peroxide bottles should not have overtight tops, because of pressure build-up.

2 Dust entering the bottle will decompose or break down the O_2 content of hydrogen peroxide. Hydrogen peroxide will also lose its strength if you leave the cap off the bottle, because the oxygen will escape to the air, so replace the cap immediately. It is not good practice to pour leftover hydrogen peroxide back into the bottle as this, too, will decompose the O_2.

Note: Stabilised hydrogen peroxide has the advantage of storing much better because it contains certain stabilisers to prevent O_2 loss. Therefore oxidation processes need longer to liberate the O_2. Remember, it is the O_2 you want from the hydrogen peroxide and manufacturers are putting in chemicals to stop its release (for storage purposes). Hydrogen peroxide which is not stabilised stores poorly but oxidation processes are quicker because there are no chemicals to stop O_2 loss. It takes only 20 minutes for unstabilised hydrogen peroxide to release its oxygen; stabilised products may take up to twice as long.

Always store hydrogen peroxide in the same place in the stockroom and not in bottles that are commonly used for beverages. Keep bottles well labelled. Purchase small quantities frequently to ensure fresh supplies.

Dilution of hydrogen peroxide

There may be times in the salon when you need to dilute hydrogen peroxide. Be accurate in measuring your quantities and, if possible, use pure distilled water. (The strength of hydrogen peroxide is reduced by adding water.) A hydroxometer or peroxometer is invaluable for measuring the volume strengths if the hydrogen peroxide is liquid. Salons which specialise in colouring use hydroxometers quite frequently to check hydrogen peroxide strength when tinting or lightening. Salons are encouraged to procure hydroxometers as they are also extremely useful for determining the strength of hydrogen peroxide which may have been stored for some time. Any hydrogen peroxide that is diluted is best not stored or at least kept for a limited time only.

How to dilute hydrogen peroxide

There is a simple method for working out hydrogen peroxide dilution. Ask yourself, for instance: how do I dilute 30 volume hydrogen peroxide to get 20 volume hydrogen peroxide?

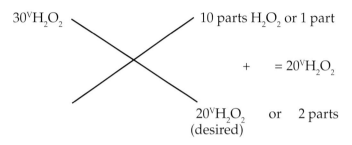

$30^V H_2O_2$ ⟍ ⟋ 10 parts H_2O_2 or 1 part

+ $= 20^V H_2O_2$

$20^V H_2O_2$ or 2 parts
(desired)

Q: What have I got?
A: 30 volume H_2O_2.

Q: What do I want?
A: 20 volume H_2O_2.

Q: What is the difference between 30 and 20?
A: 10.

So the answer is 10 parts or cc of distilled water and 20 cc of the 30 volume hydrogen peroxide (1 part distilled H_2O and 2 parts H_2O_2) = 30 cc of 20 volume hydrogen peroxide.

Another example: How do I dilute 60 volume hydrogen peroxide to get 20 volume hydrogen peroxide?

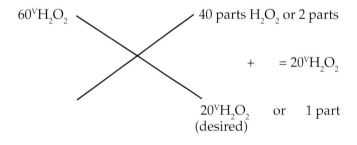

$60^V H_2O_2$ ⟍ ⟋ 40 parts H_2O_2 or 2 parts

+ $= 20^V H_2O_2$

$20^V H_2O_2$ or 1 part
(desired)

Q: What have I got?
A: 60 volume H_2O_2.

Q: What do I want?
A: 20 volume H_2O_2.

Q: What is the difference between 60 and 20?
A: 40.

So the answer is 40 parts or cc of distilled H_2O and 20 parts or cc of the 60 volume (or 2 parts distilled H_2O and 1 part H_2O_2) = 60 cc of 20 volume hydrogen peroxide.

- The hydrogen peroxide available is volume 60 H_2O_2.
  To get 40 volume – 1 part distilled H_2O and 2 parts H_2O_2.
  To get 30 volume – equal parts distilled H_2O and H_2O_2.
  To get 20 volume – 2 parts distilled H_2O and 1 H_2O_2.

- The hydrogen peroxide available is 40 volume H_2O_2.
  To get 30 volume – 1 part distilled H_2O and 3 parts H_2O_2.
  To get 20 volume – equal parts distilled H_2O and H_2O_2.
  To get 10 volume – 3 parts distilled H_2O and 1 part H_2O_2.

- The hydrogen peroxide available is 30 volume H_2O_2.
  To get 20 volume – 1 part distilled H_2O and 2 parts H_2O_2.
  To get 10 volume – 2 parts distilled H_2O and 1 part H_2O_2.

- The hydrogen peroxide available is 20 volume H_2O_2.
  To get 10 volume – equal parts distilled H_2O and H_2O_2.
  To get 5 volume – 3 parts distilled H_2O and 1 part H_2O_2.

Figure 3.3

Measuring the strength of hydrogen peroxide

10
20
30 — 30ᵛH₂O₂
40
50
60

Pour a quantity (100cc) of hydrogen peroxide into a test tube and simply place the peroxometer into the liquid. Once the peroxometer settles, read the measurement at the top of the hydrogen peroxide. This will give you an accurate reading of the volume strength of your hydrogen peroxide.

Experiment

1 Take four samples of hair which are the same colour. Mix 30 volume hydrogen peroxide with bleach and leave on the hair for 30 minutes:
   a apply to the hair;
   b apply to the hair with added ammonia;
   c apply to the hair with added acid, e.g. vinegar or lemon juice;
   d apply to the hair with additional heat.

   Check the effectiveness of the lightening action in each case.

2 Dilute hydrogen peroxide and measure its strength with a hydroxometer.

 ## Hairdressing products and the environment

Acid rain, the depletion of the ozone layer, pollution, toxic gases, the greenhouse effect, changing climates, smog: these are the messages that mother nature is sending us. Today, many hairdressers and clients are 'green', i.e. environmentally conscious, and products have been amended accordingly. As long as clients and hairdressers are willing to persevere, manufacturers will continue to research and develop efficient alternatives to products that can be harmful to the environment. The majority of manufacturers have re-thought their policies with regard to the environment but will only continue to respond to a market force. Many companies have developed totally 'green' ranges in response to demand for either more natural or environmentally friendly products. Phasing out CFCs has been a gradual process, which has involved searching out alternatives (some authorities claim that the alternative propellants contribute to the greenhouse effect). Such research and production have a cost in financial terms and if hairdressers and clients are unwilling to pay extra to protect the environment, then manufacturers will not provide the products.

What you and your clients can do

If you want to be 'green', you need to do more than just get rid of CFCs.

1 Ensure both products and packaging are biodegradable, i.e. able to be broken down by bacteria or other living organisms. (This includes posters, bottles, packages, and ingredients.) It should be possible to dispose of products without causing the emission of toxic gases.

2 Encourage clients (and manufacturers) to use re-fillable bottles for shampoos, conditioners and hairsprays.

3 Avoid products that have unnecessary packaging material. Products should at least have packaging that is recyclable.

4 Recycle your rubbish – plastics, paper, glass, and cans should be separated and dropped off at recycling bins.

5 Have a non-smoking policy in the salon (for both staff and clients).

6 Re-use empty bottles.

7 Display ozone-friendly products.

8 Cease using or control the use of plastic bags.

9 Buy recycled paper.

10 Buy stock that states that the final product and its ingredients have not been tested on animals.

11 Display show cards or promotional material on recycled card or paper.

12 Use recycled client record cards.

13 Use air-propelled pumps for hair fixatives.

14 Avoid the use of petroleum-based products as they may have an effect on the recycling of water.

Conforming to these 'green notions' will help create a healthy environment. Consider these options – they can be combined with your commercial business decisions. Being environmentally aware is crucial for the planet's survival and possibly the survival of one hairdresser over another!

Questions

1   Give three examples of hair damage caused by

    a   chemicals;

_____

_____

_____

    b   physical causes.

_____

_____

_____

2   Name the two categories into which shampoos are divided.

_____

_____

3   What hairdressing products contain the following chemicals:

    a   triethanolamine lauryl sulphate?

_____

    b   zinc pyrithione?

_____

    c   cationic emulsions?

_____

    d   polyvinyl pyrrolidone?

_____

    e   shellac?

_____

4   What can be a major disadvantage, particularly for the junior apprentice, of the use of a soapless shampoo?

_____

_____

_____

5   Name a vegetable oil and animal fat used in the formulation of shampoos.

_____

6   Are soaps acidic or alkaline?

_____

7 a What is the disadvantage of using a soap in hard water?

_____

_____

b What do soaps contain to prevent the oil or fat from becoming rancid?

_____

8 Explain the effect that conditioners have on the hair fibre.

_____

_____

_____

9 What is:

_____

a lanolin?

_____

b glycerine?

_____

10 Match the words in Column B with the words in Column A.

COLUMN A	COLUMN B
i purified wool fat	**a** soapless shampoo
ii conditioners	**b** anti-dandruff shampoo
iii animal fat	**c** lanolin
iv synthetic detergent	**d** hydrogen peroxide
v antibacterial	**e** cationic
	f mousse
	g tallow

11 Use words from the list to complete the following sentences:

alcohol, butane, plastifier, freon, PVP, mucilage, tormalin

a A setting lotion which is formulated with gum is called a _____.

b These are mixed with perfume and _____ to prevent them from going mouldy.

c _____ contains a plastic resin called _____.

d This type of setting lotion contains perfume, glycerine, distilled water and _____.

e Hairsprays are produced in aerosol cans with the propellant usually being _____ or _____.

12 a What is a dressing-out cream used for?

_____

b What does it usually contain?

_____

13 Match the words in Column B with the words in Column A.

COLUMN A	COLUMN B
i hydrogen peroxide	**a** element
ii oxygen	**b** H_2O
iii hydrogen	**c** NH_3
iv water	**d** compound
v ammonia	**e** H
	f atom

14 What is the equivalent of each of the following in percentages of hydrogen peroxide?

    a   10 volume;

_____

    b   20 volume;

_____

    c   30 volume;

_____

    d   40 volume;

_____

    e   60 volume.

_____

15 a   To what does 'stabilised' hydrogen peroxide refer?

_____

    b   What is the stabilising agent used in stabilised hydrogen peroxide?

_____

16 How should hydrogen peroxide be stored?

_____

17 What chemical is used to liberate the oxygen content from hydrogen peroxide when it is mixed with products?

_____

18 What instrument is used to measure the strength of hydrogen peroxide?

_____

19 Name three hairdressing services which require the use of hydrogen peroxide.

_____

20 If you were required to mix 60 cc of 20 volume hydrogen peroxide with 1 tube of tint and all that was available was 60 volume H_2O_2, what proportions of H_2O_2 and distilled water would you have to mix to obtain 60 cc of 20 volume hydrogen peroxide?

_____

21 Name three aspects of taking a 'green' approach in the salon.

_____

_____

_____

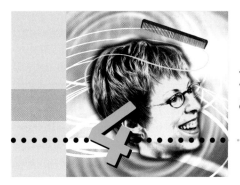

Personal selling
Introducing: 'Selling skills – sell goods and/or services'

In this chapter, you will learn about:

- skills and qualities of a good salesperson;
- suggesting extra service;
- suggesting take-home haircare products;
- legislation affecting the selling of goods and services.

Selling skills

As you are employed in the service sector there is an expectation that you will be able to identify and describe the qualities that create a good salesperson. This chapter describes some of those qualities.

Personal selling means suggesting extra services and take-home haircare products which your clients can purchase. If you want to be the hair fashion leader in your area and keep pace with new trends, you must give your clients new service.

In the first year we talked about personal selling. We mentioned that suggesting treatments which might be of benefit to the client's hair should be the job of the shampooist, as he or she is in the best position to advise on treatment there and then. The treatment can be given immediately after the shampoo and the junior apprentice can propose or suggest it. When it comes to personal selling of extra services such as colour or henna or highlighting, the suggestion should come from the hairdresser who does the client's hair, whether it is being blow-dried, set or cut. Take-home haircare products such as shampoos and conditioners should be suggested by the hairdresser who finishes the service.

Suggesting extra service

One ideal extra service that you can suggest is colour, which is a fast-developing influence on the 'total look' hairstyles of today. Magazines are full of new ideas. Clients are often keen to try exciting new hair colours, so try to encourage your existing clientele to have their hair professionally coloured. It is interesting to consider that most clients who have their hair coloured have not actually made an appointment for this service. The idea of colour usually develops while the client is in the salon. (Conversely, the majority of permanent-wave clients actually intend to have a permanent wave before they reach the salon.)

Develop yourself as a fashion colourist and you will derive tremendous pleasure from the creative results produced on your clients' hair. Read all the new technical information that manufacturers put out on hair colour products. Gain confidence in the use of such products and become familiar with the

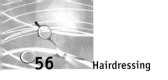

results that can be obtained. Modern technology has made hair colouring much simpler; manufacturers' technicians are always available to give advice and most manufacturers conduct colour courses. Videotapes can also be used to help

If you see colour variation ideas in magazines, cut them out and place them in a folder. Show your clients how their hair could look and explain the benefits of colouring. Explain how easy it is to do, how long it takes to achieve and the cost involved. Be prepared to answer confidently and enthusiastically any questions or objections your clients may have. If they hesitate, suggest subtle changes.

To begin with, aim at getting 20% (two out of every ten) of your clients interested in having their hair coloured. It is best to start with your regular clients, with whom you are more likely to feel comfortable. Choose clients who are well known and who are likely to tell their friends and show off their new colour. Giving shows and demonstrations can also help. Your own hair should be a showcase for clients interested in colour.

Suggesting take-home haircare (THHC) products

Know your products. Read all the pamphlets and instructions that come with haircare products, go to demonstrations and talk to sales representatives. Understand how the products are formulated, what they contain, how they are used and what benefits they have. Know their cost.

The best person to suggest take-home haircare products to clients is the hairdresser who is finishing the hair service – and the best time to do this is when you have completed your hairdressing work, and your clients are looking and feeling good. This also gives you the opportunity to recommend the take-home haircare products that are suited to their hair, and that, in your professional opinion, will help them to keep their hair in this same good condition.

Tell your client how shining, healthy and full body and bounce his/her hair looks, and how ideally suited this particular product is to his/her hair. Maintain eye contact with the client when describing the product, and make sure that you explain the benefits of using it very carefully. Be prepared to answer objections, especially as to why the product, to your mind, is better than any other.

When talking to your client, explain a product's benefits, elaborate on its effects and give the price. Offer to place the product in bag, and make it easy for the client to buy the product by taking a cheque or credit card in payment.

It is best to suggest take-home haircare products while the client is still in the chair, before he/she gets up and goes to the reception desk. Products you can suggest include shampoos, conditioners, setting agents and fixatives, or even brushes.

As a professional hairdresser you can offer good advice on these products and can demonstrate their use. You know your client and their hair types; you know the products and you are aware of the results they can achieve. Be well informed, and you'll outshine other retailers who offer these products. Clients shouldn't have to guess what they should buy.

Sales will come automatically. Failing to show clients how to take care of their new hairstyles and keep them looking good means that your job is only half done. Clients will be influenced by your professional opinion and take your advice on what you think is best for their hair, so that they are buying only what is needed.

Most hairdressing manufacturers offer courses on personal selling of products – you should attend these.

Legislation affecting the selling of goods and service provision

The Consumer Guarantees Act 1994

The Consumer Guarantees Act came into effect on 1 April 1994. In terms of this Act, services must meet four criteria.

1 Work must be carried out with reasonable care and skill.
2 The work must be fit for any particular purpose the client has told you about.
3 If a time for completing the work has not been agreed, the work must be carried out within a reasonable time.
4 If the price for the work has not been agreed, the price demanded must be reasonable for the work done.

For more information, see the Ministry of Consumer Affairs *Business Note*, No. 5.

Other legislative requirements which may effect the selling of goods and/or the provision of services include: the Privacy Act 1993; Health and Safety in Employment Act 1993; Human Rights Act 1993; Sale of Goods Act 1908; Fair Trading Act 1986; Hire Purchase Act 1971 and the Lay By Sales Act 1971.

The recognition of compliance with, function and scope of legislative requirements imposed on business is too complex a subject to cover in a book such as this. For further information on legislation affecting small businesses, refer to: *Principles of Law for New Zealand Business* by Jeremy Hubbard, Cordelia Thomas and Sally Varnham, published by Addison Wesley Longman, 1999.

Questions

1   When is the right time to suggest take-home haircare products to clients?

_____

_____

2   What extra salon service is usually suggested while the client is in the salon?

_____

_____

3   What information should you give to the client when suggesting an extra service or a take-home product?

_____

_____

4   'It's too expensive' is a common objection to purchasing THHC products; list three more objections that you must be prepared to answer.

_____

_____

_____

5   Give two examples of how you can close a sale.

_____

_____

6   Name a criterion for service covered by the Consumer Guarantees Act.

_____

_____

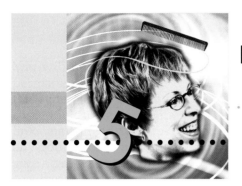

Permanent waving

In this chapter, you will learn about:

- theory of permanent waving;
- general procedure for permanent waving;
- directional permanent waving;
- permanent waving problems.

 ## Introduction

Now that you are in your second year of hairdressing, you will be expected to wind permanent waves in the salon. This service is part of building up your clientele. Unlike your first year when you just assisted the senior, now you may well be responsible for many of the skills associated with the procedure. This chapter will help you understand these responsibilities.

Remember, of course, that if you are in doubt you should ask your senior. You must also get your senior to check your work regularly. This will help you perfect your permanent wave technique. Manufacturers frequently organise permanent wave seminars and you should attend such seminars in order to improve your skill.

 ## The theory of permanent waving

You'll recall that ammonium thioglycollate or thios breaks the cross-linkage that holds the keratin chain in its position. The neutraliser (O_2) is responsible for the reformation of this broken cross-linkage which fixes the curl to the same size as the perm rod.

The chemical action

As soon as the permanent waving solution is applied to the hair, it softens and opens the cuticle to allow the thios to penetrate and enter the cortex. The thios start to break down the cross-linkage on the polypeptide chain. This changes the chemical state of the hair protein.

In its natural state – before the application of the permanent waving solution – the cross-linkage is made up of two sulphur atoms creating a di-sulphide (–S–S–) bond known as cystine. When the permanent waving lotion is applied, it starts to break the di-sulphide (–S–S–) cystine bonds and changes them into two cysteines (–S S–) – a broken sulphur bond. (Cystine and cysteine are two examples of the 19 amino acids that make up the keratin protein.)

This chemical action is known as reduction. Reduction means reducing the di-sulphide (–S S–) bonds. This action occurs because thios contain hydrogen atoms which attach to the di-sulphide (–S–S–) bonds, reducing and breaking the linkages, altering the state from cystine to cysteine (–SH HS–). Once the di-sulphide bonds begin to break and relax, the hair can be moulded into shape – that of the perm rod. When enough of the di-sulphide bonds have relaxed and broken, the thios is rinsed away and the hair neutralised by the process of oxidation. The neutralisers contain oxygen (O_2) which eliminates the H_2 (from the thios). It breaks and eliminates the H_2 and S bond attraction and joins up to the S bonds to fix the broken bond and form cystine again. The oxygen produced by the oxidising agent removes hydrogen from the cysteine molecules to form water, (H_2O).

There are advantages and disadvantages in permanent waving using base solutions (ammonium thioglycollate).

1   Base solutions rely on ammonia to open the cuticle and this can be detrimental to the hair. Many manufacturers have now developed acidic waves, for which heat is required to open the cuticle and so allow the wave to work. This is done either through an exothermic (self-heating) wave or by using preheated clamps. The acidic waves are still made up of thios but they contain no excess ammonia. Acidic waves are far kinder to the hair and leave it in better condition after permanent waving. The danger of overprocessing is not as great because of the milder action and because the cooling effect stops the action from going any further. These products are, however, usually a little more expensive than base solutions.

2   Perm solutions remove artificial (and natural) colour from the hair, and can cause hair and skin damage (and especially eye damage, if splashed) by stripping the hair of its natural oil and the skin of its acid mantle protection.

If the scalp is broken (cuts or abrasions) perm solutions will cause discomfort to the client and can inflame the scalp and even cause dermatitis. The hairdresser's hands are also at risk from the strong ammonia – so wear gloves.

Client consultation (a very important component in the permanent waving procedure)

It is important that you give the client the correct preliminary analysis and consultation. This may take time, especially if clients are unsure of the effect they want; however, TIME SPENT COMMUNICATING WITH THE CLIENT CAN SAVE EMBARRASSMENT LATER. Try to convey to the client the finished look that you have in mind. Sometimes clients will bring in a picture of what they want; this is a good idea as it can help both you and the client to decide whether the result can be achieved. It is not wise even to start the permanent

Figure 5.1

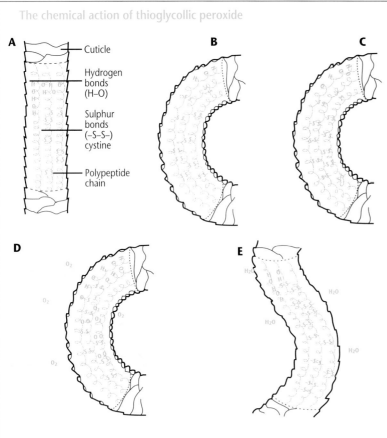

The chemical action of thioglycollic peroxide

A   Cuticle
    Hydrogen bonds (H–O)
    Sulphur bonds (–S–S–) cystine
    Polypeptide chain

A   The hair in its natural state of cystine with disulphide links crossing the main polypeptide chain.
B   The hair wound on a perm rod. The disulphide links are still in a cystine state (–S–S–).
C   When thioglycollic acid is applied, the hydrogen atoms that it contains reduce the disulphide cystine linkage to two cysteine links (–SS–)
D   Oxygen from the neutraliser eliminates the hydrogen atoms and rejoins the sulphur links. The end result is water, H_2O.
    (This is one of the reasons why hair is so wet after permanent waving.)
E   Once the disulphide links have rejoined, they return to their original tate, cystine. The curl is now permanent.

waving procedure until both you and the client are quite sure what the finished style will be like.

Preliminary analysis – important considerations for good results

Permanent waving is a mechanical skill. What is important is the condition that the hair is left in afterwards. To ensure the best possible condition, determine and consider the following as part of your preliminary analysis:

- the strength of the solution;
- the rod size;
- winding technique;
- processing;
- neutralising.

Analysing any of these incorrectly could result in a permanent wave failure.

The strength of the solution

The strength of a solution depends on the percentages of ammonia and thios it contains, and its pH value. Mild solutions contain less ammonia and thios and have a lower pH value.

Manufacturers design permanent waving lotions for different hair types and your salon should have lotions in various strengths. The bottle or package will tell you the type of hair for which the lotion is suited. The lotion strength you use will be determined by the following factors.

1 Hair texture – fine, coarse, medium. The packet wording will read:
   - 'Solution for fine hair – easy to wave.'
   - 'Solution for coarse hair – hard to wave.'
   - 'Solution for normal to medium texture.'
2 Porosity/resistance – the rate at which the hair will adsorb the solution. The label will read:
   - 'Solution for porous – sensitised, easy to wave.'
   - 'Solution for resistant, strong – hard to wave.'
3 Whether the hair has previously been processed – the wording will read:
   - 'Solution for hair which is tinted or mildly bleached/lightened.'
   - 'Solution for hair which is 'sensitised' (sun bleached).'

   Some permanent wave solutions are designed for all types of hair – fine/resistant – tinted/lightened (only with 20 H_2O_2).
4 The type of permanent wave the client wants – manufacturers produce a semipermanent wave in which the solution, combined with the correct perming rods, will give a lift of volume and support the style for only a limited number of washes. This type of wave is often called a *style* support or body wave.
5 Length – a stronger solution is generally used for very long hair although this won't be indicated on the packet or bottle.

Self-timing perms

Generally the application, processing and results of self-timing perms are the same as for other perms. Self-timing perms are designed to be left on the hair for a fixed time – which is usually determined by hair type – whether the hair is tinted, normal or resistant. Timing can vary from 10 minutes for tinted, easy-to-wave hair to 20 minutes for resistant, hard-to-wave, difficult hair. Some manufacturers even specify not to take a test curl.

How they work

The common ingredient in self-timing perms is dithioglycollate. This ingredient allows the thioglycollate to slow down its processing action until it 'stops'.

The timing must allow for complete penetration into the hair fibre and enough time for the curl formation. A similar effect is achieved with exothermic perms when a temperature change slows the rate of perming action so that it effectively stops.

To gain the best results from self-timing permanent waves, you need to be able to analyse the client's hair condition and type accurately. The instructions should also be followed precisely as self-timing products put a time scale around the bond-breaking and re-arrangement processes and this time is controlled by the perm ingredients and hair type.

It is best to use self-timing perms:

- when non-conventional winds are used using different styles of rods;
- when it is difficult to check the result of a perm rod.

Self-timing perms should probably not be used:

- if the hair type falls outside manufacturers' specifications;
- if hair is in poor condition (e.g. very fine or very porous) and a pre-perm guard is used.

This is a typical winding pattern for second-year apprentices, using approximately 60–75 perm rods. Perfect this type of winding pattern before proceeding to the directional technique.

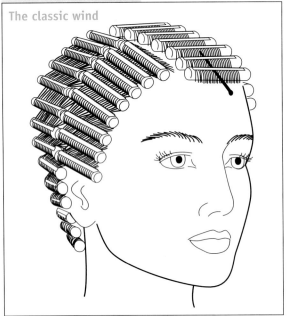

The classic wind

Figure 5.2

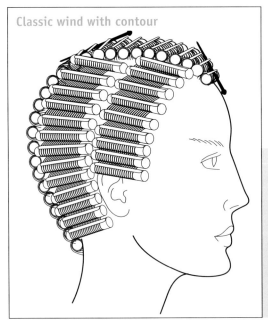

Classic wind with contour

This is a classic winding technique but here you can see the perm rods following the contour to the side of the head. As a variation, the top has been wound forward. Practise this winding pattern.

Figure 5.3

Alkaline versus acid waves

Generally, the pH of alkaline waves ranges from 7.1 to 9.5, whereas the pH of acid waves is 5.5 to 6.9. Alkaline perms process more efficiently than acid waves, as the higher pH softens and swells the hair fibre, making it possible for the 'thios' to penetrate and break the disulphide bonds more quickly and easily.

With acid perms, however, no swelling of the hair takes place, so the finished texture of hair feels more natural.

Try selecting an alkaline perm when the hair is difficult to perm, resistant and coarse or when the client has a history of perm wave failures. These waves are also ideal for long hair or sophisticated winding techniques.

An acid perm is suggested for poorer quality hair, delicate or highly coloured/bleached hair.

The condition of the hair is a key factor in selecting an alkaline or acid permanent wave.

The rod size to use

The size of the perm rod will determine the size of the curl, so the following factors must be taken into account when choosing a rod to use.

1 Type of curl desired.
2 Length of the hair.
3 Texture of the hair – slightly smaller rods are usually used for fine-textured hair. When combined with the correct solution, fine hair generally takes a permanent wave but tends to drop a little more quickly, whereas coarse hair takes longer to process but holds better. (There are exceptions, however.)
4 Some acid waves may specify the use of a smaller rod size than normal.

The winding technique

Determine how the permanent wave is to be wound, as there are many ways of winding and the one you choose will influence the finished design. The classic wind is for the finished curl; the directional wind is for the finished design. Types of direction wind include:

- spiral winding;
- stack winding;
- root perming;
- piggy-back perming.

Processing

Various factors will influence the processing time, that is, the length of time it will take for the curl to develop. These include:

- texture of the hair;
- density of the hair;
- temperature of the salon;
- length of the hair;
- whether the hair is tinted/bleached/lightened;
- type of permanent wave (acid or alkali);
- strength of the solution;
- whether a processing cap is used;
- climate – time of year;
- whether heat is applied;
- whether a porosity filler is used;
- whether the wave has been water-wound or wound with solution;

- winding technique;
- manufacturer's instructions;
- medication taken by client;
- pregnancy (particularly in the later stages).

Neutralising

Ensure that this is completed meticulously according to the manufacturer's instructions. The preceding consultation, analysis, winding and processing could all be of no avail if the neutralising process is unsatisfactory.

Hair and scalp analysis

The scalp must be in good condition. Check it for cuts, sores, abrasions and disorders. If the permanent wave solution is allowed to come into contact with such areas, inflammation could occur, causing discomfort for the client. For this reason, it is not advisable to brush the scalp harshly before permanent waving as the scalp could become scratched and tender. Light brushing of the hair is, however, acceptable.

Check the hair condition. If it is not in good condition, good results cannot be expected. In such a case, it is professional to advise the client to postpone the permanent wave and to suggest a series of conditioning treatments to improve the hair's condition. Any permanent wave from previous treatments should be cut away.

Protecting the client

Permanent waving involves thorough dampening and saturation of the hair with shampoo, water, solutions and neutralisers. Clients must be adequately protected to ensure that they don't get any of the chemicals on their clothing. Protective capes and plenty of towels should be on hand. It is good idea to place a towel on top of the cape to catch the occasional drip. Giving a towel to the client is a professional touch. The salon is responsible for protecting clients, so avoid staining their clothing.

It is also wise to protect the client's skin with a barrier cream, especially if the skin is sensitive. Apply the cream to the areas you feel need protection – usually the forehead and ear area. Don't get any on the hair as this will stop or slow the action of the permanent wave lotion. If the client is wearing any pieces of jewellery such as bulky necklaces or large earrings, it is best to remove them.

Sectioning the hair

The hair should be sectioned before winding as this will ensure a systematic and methodical approach.

The method shown in Figures 5.4 and 5.5 is an extremely good one. Secure the hair with large sectioning clips. The sections should not be any wider than the length of the perm rods. Note the angle of the side sections, which are taken slightly back to behind the ear. Make sure the partings are straight.

Read manufacturer's instructions

All permanent waves are slightly different in their general procedure and technique.

When you are first learning to permanent wave, it is best to start to wind using water. Later, when you get quicker, you can wind with the solution. Practise perm wave winding on your manikin block.

The advantages of water winding include:

1 it's ideal for slow winders;
2 manufacturers recommend water winding;
3 it controls processing in hair with uneven porosity;
4 it's good for tinted or lightened hair as this hair is porous;
5 hair that is to be coloured and permed on the same day benefits from water winding;
6 the water-winding technique suits particularly complicated winds.

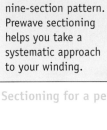

This is the classic nine-section pattern. Prewave sectioning helps you take a systematic approach to your winding.

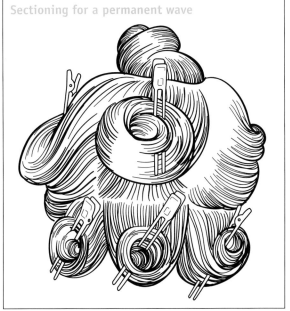

Sectioning for a permanent wave

Figure 5.4

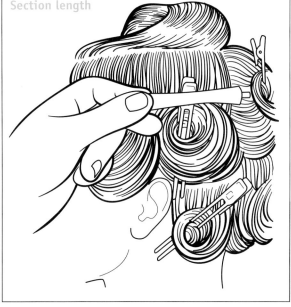

Section length

Make sure no section exceeds the length of the perm rod being wound.

Figure 5.5

How to achieve a successful permanent wave

- Good client communication – find out what the client wants.
- Correct hair and scalp analysis.
- Read the instructions.

By keeping these three major points in mind, you will be well on the way to producing successful permanent wave results.

General procedure – permanent wave winding

Shampoo the hair using a non-nutritive shampoo (including a 2-in-1) and towel dry. If you are predampening with the solution, use a sponge or brush and moisten the strand 0.5 cm from the roots of the hair.

1 Start to wind each rod, starting at the nape first, since this area is usually more resistant and takes longer to process because it is not generally exposed to the elements.
2 Select a mesh which is not deeper nor longer than the rod size: the mesh size is determined by the rod size.
3 Comb the hair to a 90° angle from the scalp.

4 Ensure that the ends are neatly combed and that they are not buckled.

5 Place an end paper neatly around the ends of the hair. The ends will converge slightly, but they should not buckle. Keep the section parallel to the scalp.

6 Proceed to wind with an even tension and without pulling the hair (keep the elbows level).

Figure 5.6

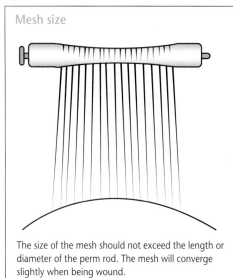

Mesh size

The size of the mesh should not exceed the length or diameter of the perm rod. The mesh will converge slightly when being wound.

7 Slide the perm rod up to the end of the hair and tuck the ends around neatly, using the lull length of your finger. The tail comb can also help tuck the ends around.

8 Don't buckle or 'fish hook' the ends. Rocking to and fro will distribute the hair uniformly along the rods to avoid buckling.

9 Don't stretch the hair as this can cause damage and pull burns. Pull burns occur when the hair is pulled and permanent wave lotion is allowed down the mouth of the follicle, burning the skin. Fasten the band of the perm rod, ensuring

a that it is not twisted;

b that it does not lie across the base of the mesh and cut into the hair.

These are common mistakes resulting inevitably in hair damage.

10 Continue to wind each section individually, winding the sides and the top sections last.

11 Once you have finished winding, check to see that all the perm rods are in the correct position. Check that the perm rods bands are positioned correctly.

12 Dampen with solution. This is an important stage of the permanent waving procedure which must be carried out with care and accuracy. Permanent wave lotions are usually applied from the applicator bottle, but a small sponge or brush and bowl can be used. Cut the top of the lotion bottle finely with old scissors. Try not to cut too big a hole or the solution may pour out uncontrollably.

Figure 5.7

Processing a permanent wave

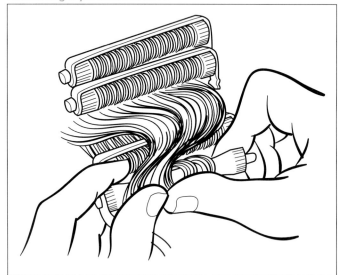

In processing, the curl is ready when the depth of the 'S' movement is the same size as the diameter of the perm rod. Is this permanent wave ready to be neutralised?

If you place cotton wool around the client's forehead for protection, it must be removed after the dampening-down procedure, otherwise it will absorb any excess solution and this will start to burn the client's forehead. You may need to replace it two or three times – keep an eye on this.

Starting at the nape, dampen all the perm rods with solution, making sure that the solution is fully adsorbed by the hair. Don't saturate to the extent that the solution starts to run onto the client's scalp. Make sure no rods are missed. Lift the perm rods slightly to allow adequate adsorption of solution. The hair will look shiny when it is adequately dampened. If any excess lotion does drip onto the scalp, remove it immediately with a tissue. Dampen evenly or the permanent waving result could have an uneven curl.

13 Once dampening has been completed, set the timer.

14 Place a processing cap over the perm rods. The cap should fit snugly over all the rods and should not disturb them. The processing cap has a number of advantages.

a It retains the heat from the scalp and accelerates the processing.

b It maintains an even temperature, free from draughts.

c It helps to contain the permanent wave solution odour.

15 The processing time is influenced by a number of factors (see pp. 63–64). If you have given the client a non-automatic permanent wave, then you will need to check processing at two- to five-minute intervals. When checking, do the following:

a remove the processing cap;

b go to the perm rod that was first wound or dampened;

c undo the band and unwind the perm rod $1^1/_2$ times;

d gently move the hair toward the scalp;

e look for 'S' movement at the same depth as the circumference of the perm rod.

f do the same for the sides and top.

Bear in mind that sometimes the weight of the permanent wave solution can help the hair to give a false 'S' movement. The circumference of the rod determines the size of the curl.

For automatic permanent wave techniques, follow the instructions; sometimes it is not even necessary to check a test curl. Automatic waves depend on the correct preliminary analysis, selection of solution and winding technique. If these have been done properly, the result should be good.

When the desired amount of curl has been achieved, neutralise. Once the permanent wave has been completed, make a record of the method and procedure that you used.

17 This client record card serves several useful purposes.

a It can be used as a guide for any future permanent waves.

b It records accurately all information on the client's permanent wave history.

c It makes clients feel that the salon is taking a long-term interest in their well-being.

d It eliminates any guesswork if the client requests a similar finished style at a later date.

These record cards should be filed alphabetically.

Figure 5.8
Dampening down

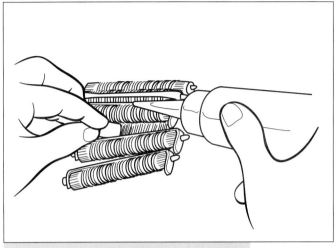

When dampening down, lift each perm rod and dampen the hair evenly with the solution. Don't over-saturate as the solution will run onto the scalp. Catch the occasional drip with cotton wool. The hair will take on a shine when it is adequately dampened.

Client Permanent Wave Record

Name:

Address:

Lotion used:
Processing time:

Rod sizes: Top   Front   Sides   Nape

Condition of hair
General comments

Date   Stylist   Cost

The procedure of permanent wave winding

Figure 5.9

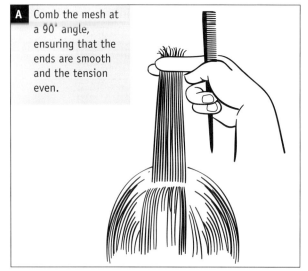

A Comb the mesh at a 90° angle, ensuring that the ends are smooth and the tension even.

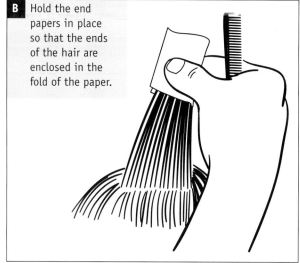

B Hold the end papers in place so that the ends of the hair are enclosed in the fold of the paper.

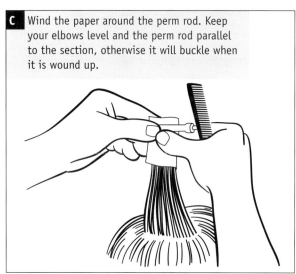

C Wind the paper around the perm rod. Keep your elbows level and the perm rod parallel to the section, otherwise it will buckle when it is wound up.

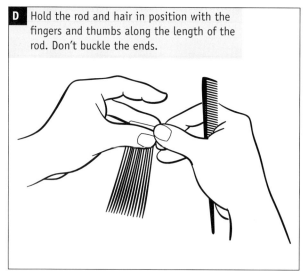

D Hold the rod and hair in position with the fingers and thumbs along the length of the rod. Don't buckle the ends.

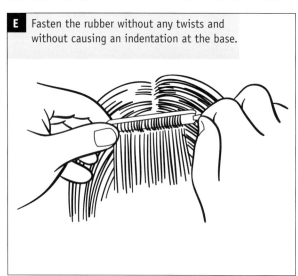

E Fasten the rubber without any twists and without causing an indentation at the base.

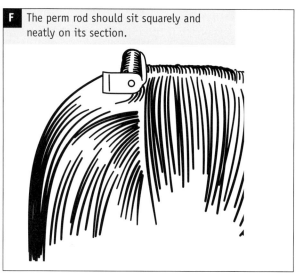

F The perm rod should sit squarely and neatly on its section.

Figure 5.10

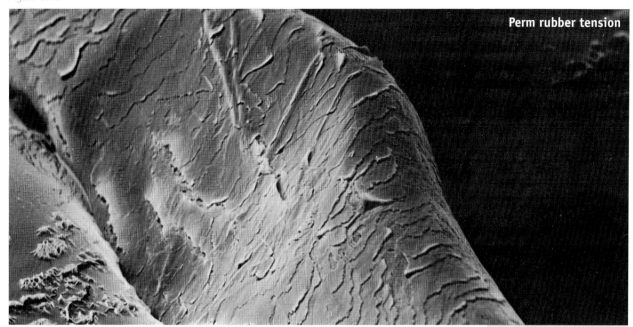

Perm rubber tension

Tension on the perm rubber nearly caused this fibre to break.

Figure 5.11

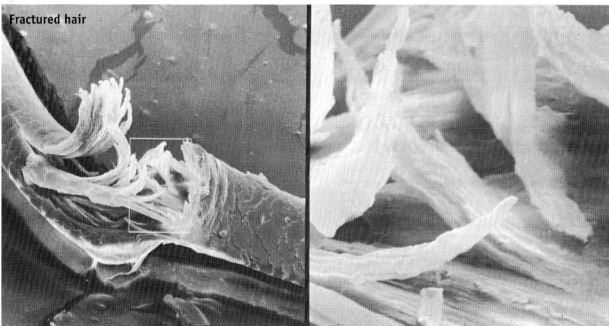

Fractured hair

Incorrect tension on the perm rod fractured this hair.

Figure 5.12

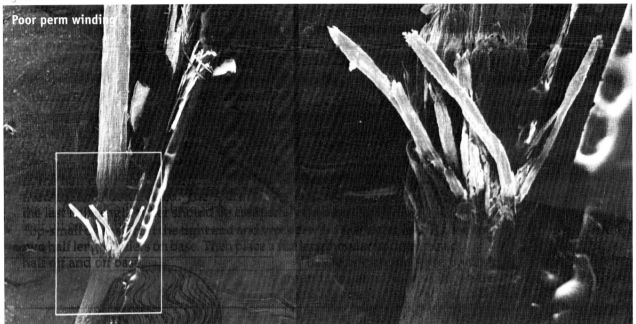

Poor perm winding

Twisted and buckled ends are the
result of poor perm winding. Take
special care when wrapping the ends.

Figure 5.13

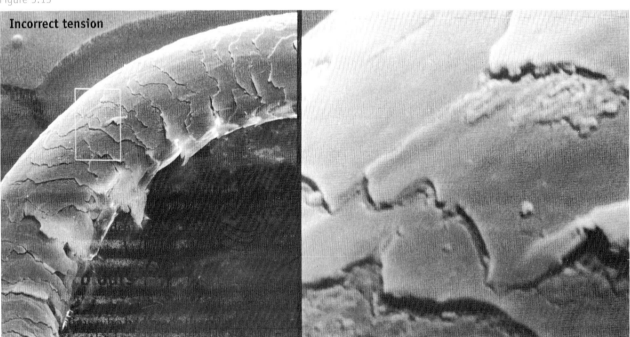

Incorrect tension

Tension during permanent wave winding can
open the cuticle cells. Note in this enlarged
photograph the remains of the cellular
cement which once held a cuticle cell.

Directional permanent wave winding techniques

When permanent waving we can adopt two ways to wind hair: the classic wind and the directional wind.

The conventional classic wind

This is a simple winding pattern (see pp. 65–66) where the top is either wound forward or back. Approximately 60 to 80 perm rods are used and these sit on their base. This technique is used to achieve styles with body and curl which are either set in rollers, blow-dried with a medium-heat dryer or left to dry naturally (like a wash-and-wear). Once you have shown skill in winding the classic wave, you will want to try different techniques of winding to get different results.

The directional wave

There are many ways to directional wind a permanent wave. Directional winding follows the natural line of the hair fall or contours of the head. The hair is usually guided in the same direction as the permanent wave rods have been wound. Directionally wound permanent waves include style supports such as contour winding, foundation waves and stack winds.

Style supports

Style supports support the client's hairstyle between visits to the salon. They usually last 8 to 10 weeks and are ideal for clients whose hair is fine, limp and generally lacks body and bounce. The perm wave lotion is very mild, and usually comes with the system's own perm wave rods, which are larger than average. Sometimes the support wave is an acid or heat wave.

In a variation of the classic wind, the rods move across the front to incorporate a client's side or middle parting. Winding can be done on medium to long layered hair. The rod used are reasonably large or can even alternate in size. To finish the style, set in rollers or blow-dry using a round or vent brush.

Contour winding

Here the rods are placed to follow the contours of the client's head. The top can be wound forward, back or to the sides. The sides of the head show the rods moving around in the direction of the scalp contour. This wind is effective and the client can be assured of a longer-lasting finished dressing. The hair can be set or blow-dried and should fall into a natural shape.

Foundation wave

The foundation wave is best suited to short, precision cuts. On fine, limp hair, this wave produces body without a great deal of curl. Clients with hair like this are usually concerned at having their hair permed and tell how their hair frizzed last time (usually many years ago). You can almost call a foundation wave a semipermanent wave. Manufacturers usually have a product suitable for such clients' needs – perhaps an exothermic-wave heat wave with clamps or special rods which are designed to give bounce and body.

Results achieved with such products are good. The hair feels thicker, is full of volume which can be controlled and is easily blow-dried by the hairdresser or the client. Remember, results won't last long – maybe 6 to 8 weeks. This is ideal for the client (and the hairdresser).

Figure 5.14

The classic wind

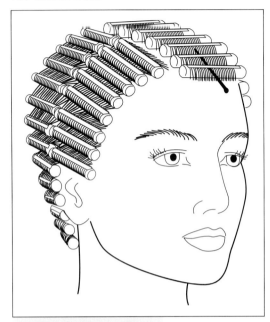

This is the classic wind, using approximately 60–75 perm rods.

Figure 5.15

A directional wave winding pattern

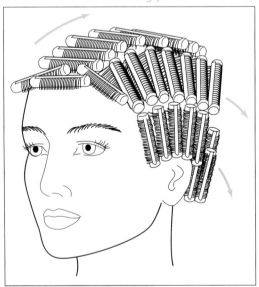

The pattern follows the line of the finished style.

Figure 5.16

Style support

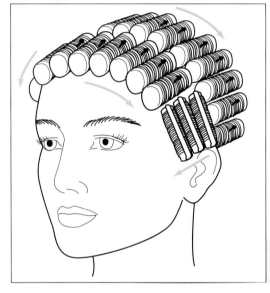

This style incorporates a side parting.

Figure 5.17

Classic wind with contour

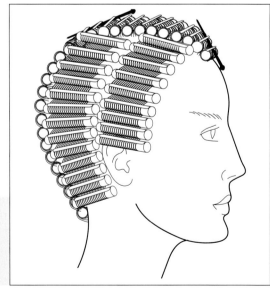

Here the perm rods follow the contour of the side of the head. As a variation, the hair on top has been wound forward.

Figure 5.18
Alternating rod sizes

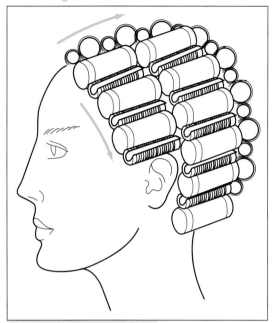

In this foundation wave pattern you can see how various rod sizes have been used in an alternating pattern.

Figure 5.19
Stack winding

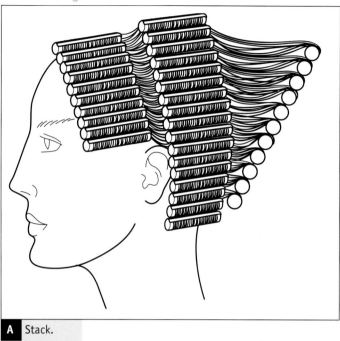

A Stack.

Figure 5.20
Stack winding

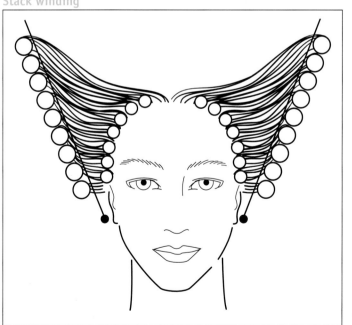

B Stack variation.

Figure 5.21
Stack winding

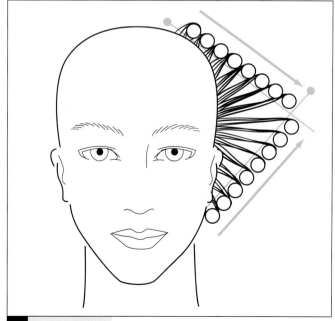

C Stack variation.

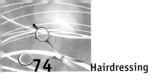

Stack winding

The hair is wound from underneath and each rod is gradually stacked out. The stacked rods can be supported with plastic knitting needles or long plastic sticks. This helps to guide the degree of stacking as each rod is wound, and maintains a methodical approach. Wind each rod through the two sticks and when the rod reaches the sticks, secure the perm rod rubber.

The three diagrams (Figures 5.19 to 5.21) show stack winding variations. Winding is usually begun at the nape area and water winding gives best results. The finished effect is quite strong and styles can be left to dry naturally, be scrunched dried (squeezed dry with the hands and a blow-dryer) or dried with a soft styling attachment. Setting the hair also gives a pleasing, looser line with plenty of movement and flow in the hair.

Practise winding all these directional perm waves in the salon or on the manikin first to see the results.

More winding techniques are discussed on pp. 202–205.

Permanent waving after-care

The back-up service for permanent waving includes giving the client advice on after-care to maintain the health and condition of the hair. You should suggest the correct type of shampoo and conditioner. There are shampoos formulated for permanent waved hair, which are recommended by manufacturers. They generally contain lanolins and coating additives.

Blow-drying after a permanent wave

The correct comb (wide-toothed) and brush (vent brush) should be used after a permanent wave has been applied.

Make sure that the dryer is not too hot and do not use it at a too high a speed. It is best to switch to warm rather than hot, and slow rather than fast. This is particularly important in the case of fine hair, since, if it is dried too quickly and at too high a temperature, the hair tends to 'explode' and becomes fly-away and unmanageable. Take small sections and wind the hair around or through a wide vent brush. Don't pull or stretch the hair unduly or blow-dry it too far from its natural fall. If a 'fonz', soft style or diffuser attachment is used, move the hair gently and apply a gentle heat. It may take a little longer than usual to blow-dry the hair, because it has been thoroughly dampened and saturated with chemicals. Nevertheless, the client's hair should be quite dry before he/she leaves the salon.

Roller setting

Comb the hair carefully and thoroughly; porosity filler conditioners can help. When putting in the rollers, avoid stretching the hair. Remember that spiked plastic rollers leave marks on fine hair. The dryer should be set at a medium heat.

It is essential that the hair should be thoroughly dry before it is brushed and dressed. Even at this point, the results of the permanent wave can be ruined if the hair is dressed while still damp. Gently brush and dress the hair into the desired style; avoid vigorous brushing. A light spray can be used.

Advise the client that strong sunlight and salt water can adversely affect the condition of permanently waved hair. After swimming in the sea or in a chlorine pool, the hair should be rinsed with fresh water. The hair should be trimmed every 5 to 8 weeks as reduced length and weight can enhance the look of a grown-out permanent wave.

Precautions when permanent waving tinted/bleached or highlighted hair

You will need to take a number of precautions if the client requesting a permanent wave has hair that has been tinted or lightened. This is because this type of hair takes a permanent wave much more quickly and is more susceptible to damage because of its already processed state. The di-sulphide links may already be broken. You must analyse the hair carefully; if there is any doubt as to whether the hair will withstand another chemical treatment, give a pre-wave test curl.

Precautions should include the following.

1 Using a permanent wave lotion especially formulated for tinted/bleached hair. This will usually have a low pH value. An acid type of permanent wave lotion may even be recommended.
2 Use a porosity filler. Manufacturers produce fillers which will coat the cuticle and slow down the permanent wave chemical action, making processing more controllable.
3 Wind the rods with water and dampen when winding has been completed. This will produce an even processing time.
4 Wind with extreme care so that there is no stretching, buckling or fish hooks.
5 Check the processing frequently, every two to three minutes.

At no time should you attempt to permanent wave hair which is overporous or in poor condition. If the client has been using metallic dyes in the hair, don't permanently wave. Some metallic dyes like Grecian 2000 or Silvercheck usually come with an 'antidote' which is used during the permanent wave to counteract any reaction, otherwise there can be problems.

Preliminary pre-wave test curls

If you are undecided at any stage during your preliminary analysis regarding the advisability of permanent waving, give the client a pre-wave test curl. This will help you to assess:

- how the hair will react during the processing time;
- the length of processing time;
- resistance;
- whether it is possible to achieve the desired curl.

The test curl is usually given at the back, beneath the crown. If the results are not as expected, then they will be less noticeable in this area.

Permanent wave tips

1 Do spend time communicating with your client.
2 Analyse the hair first. Determine the solution and, if in doubt, give the client a pre-wave test curl.
3 Check for cuts and abrasions on the scalp.
4 Don't brush the scalp.
5 Don't use a nutritive coating shampoo.
6 Read the manufacturer's instructions.
7 Protect the client's clothing – and your own.
8 Cut the hair with precision to the correct length.
9 A barrier cream can protect the client's skin.
10 Use plastic or glass bowls and anodised clips.
11 Prewave sections for a systematic approach.
12 Water wind if you are slow at winding.
13 Watch your winding:
    a no fish hooks;
    b even tension – no stretching;
    c don't buckle the hair.
14 The diameter of the perm rod determines the circumference of the curl.
15 Mesh size should be no longer nor deeper than the rod size.
16 Secure the perm rod band correctly – don't let it indent the root section.
17 Don't miss any perm rods when thoroughly dampening with solution.
18 Don't let the solution come into contact with the skin. Blot with tissues and cotton wool if it does drip on the scalp.
19 If cotton wool absorbs solution, change it immediately and during processing if necessary. If the solution does get on the forehead, neutralise with the neutraliser.
20 Check the neck towel for dampness. The client will be uncomfortable if it is damp.
21 Retain heat, avoid draughts and maintain an even temperature by using a processing cap.
22 Keep an accurate check of timing – don't guess.
23 Always check the first perm rod that you put in at the nape.
24 The depth of the 'S' should be the same size as the perm rod.
25 Fill in the client's record card.
26 Heat speeds up processing; cold retards it.
27 Advise the client on how to maintain the permanent wave and keep the hair in good condition

Permanent wave problems

Introduction

There may be times when the permanent wave result is not satisfactory. This can happen for a number of reasons, all of which the hairdresser is usually able to avoid or overcome. Very rarely is there anyone else to blame! Most problems in permanent waving can be overcome by reading and carefully following the manufacturer's instructions. Hairdressing manufacturers have spent time, money and effort on deciding the best approach to take when permanent waving. If you don't follow their advice, you can't expect good results.

Always analyse first

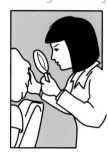

- Know what the client wants; good communication is very important.
- Determine the hair characteristics – texture, porosity, elasticity, density.
- Decide on the solution to use, the size of the rod, the winding technique, the processing and the neutralising. And read the manufacturer's instructions!

A pre-wave test curl should be done if there is any doubt about the result. The test is taken at the back, underneath the crown area, so that if the result is not desirable, it will be less noticeable.

Figure 5.22

Common permanent wave problems

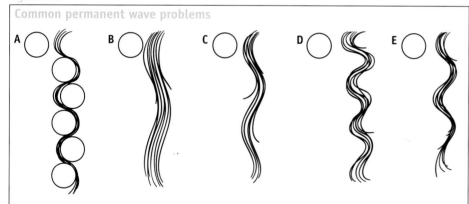

A The perfect permanent wave result, showing the curl formation the same size as the rod's circumference.

B A limp wave result.

C Uneven curl development.

D An overprocessed/overcurled result.

E Buckled and broken/split ends.

Figure 5.23

The perm rod

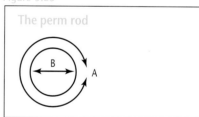

This side view of a perm rod shows its circumference (A) and diameter (B).

Common problems and causes

Limp wave – curl not holding

This can be caused by:

1 sections that are too big, too wide and too thick;
2 solution that is too weak;
3 an insufficient neutralising process procedure;
4 rod size too large;
5 failure to follow manufacturer's instructions;
6 hair that is too wet and dilutes the solution;
7 the permanent wave lotion possibly being old stock;
8 incorrect after-care, such as overstretching the hair during drying;
9 skimping on the application of the perm wave lotion;
10 hair not being correctly analysed prior to permanent wave;
11 the hair needing a longer processing time.

Solution: This problem can be overcome by repeating the permanent waving but, since the hair will be more porous, care will be needed. A milder strength solution, combined with regular test curling, will ensure that the hair is left in the best possible condition.

Uneven wave development

This can be caused by:

1 poor dampening of perm wave solution (uneven application);
2 poor application and coverage of neutraliser;
3 perm rod being wound with uneven tension;
4 bulking or too much hair wound around the rod during winding;
5 perm rod not sitting on its section;
6 slow winding with solution.

Permanent wave too curly

This can be caused by:

1 using perm rods that are too small;
2 sections too fine – too many rods;
3 incorrect strength of perm wave – too strong for hair type;
4 perm wave solution being left on too long;
5 failure to follow manufacturer's instructions;
6 tension during winding being too tight;
7 length of hair too long for the rod size selected;
8 bad communication with client;
9 heat applied during the processing time;
10 perming on hair that is already processed, e.g. bleached, tinted or permed hair.

Solution: The curl can be relaxed by either:

1 setting the hair on larger rollers;
2 leaving the hair to 'relax' naturally after two to three shampoos;
3 relaxing the overcurliness by treating the hair with mild permanent wave lotion as a curl relaxer.

Don't attempt curl reduction if the hair is not in good condition or if there is a possibility of hair damage. You cannot attempt curl reduction if the perm is overprocessed.

No wave development, even after the maximum time indicated by the manufacturer's instructions.

This can be caused by:

1 using incorrect solution – solution too weak for the hair type;
2 poorly dampened hair (insufficient solution applied);
3 hair adsorbing so much solution that it looks dry;
4 failure to follow manufacturer's instructions.

Solution: If this situation does occur, it may be necessary to redampen a second time – i.e. after the solution has been left on for its processing time. You must remember that the hair will be in a porous state as a result of the first application, so the processing time needs to be watched carefully as the curl can develop quite quickly. Redampening a second time is recommended only if any of the above conditions exist.

Broken, fizzy or buckled ends

These can be caused by:

1 porous or damaged ends, which have not been protected;
2 poor winding – fish hooks;
3 too much tension during winding;
4 solution too strong on fine hair;
5 failure to use a porosity filler.

Breakage

This can be caused by:

1 the hair being in a damaged condition prior to application of the permanent wave;
2 not taking necessary precautions (such as porosity fillers) to prevent damage to extremely bleached hair;
3 twisting perm rod rubbers or stretching them too tight, especially on fine hair;
4 solution too strong for the hair type;
5 pulling or stretching the hair during winding;
6 leaving solution on the hair too long;
7 applying excessive heat during the processing.

If the hair looks curly when wet and straight when dry, it is considered overprocessed. Don't attempt to relax it with solution.

As permanent waving is a mechanical skill, what is important is the condition in which the hair is left after the permanent wave. Analyse, ask questions and determine the finished look. Spend time on your preliminary consultation. You will need to determine the hair's characteristics – texture, porosity, elasticity and density – and also the strength of the solution. The strength of solutions are indicated on the label as well as the hair type for which they are suitable:

• tinted or bleached hair;
• fine, easy-to-wave hair;
• normal hair;
• resistant, hard-to-wave hair.

Some manufacturers have developed one permanent wave solution for all types of hair, whether it be tinted, fine or coarse. Read the instructions carefully, and remember that the circumference of the rod determines the size of the curl.

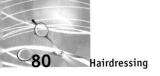

Neutralising procedure

You will spend five to ten minutes consulting with your client, about half-an-hour cutting the hair, twenty to forty minutes winding anywhere between 60 and 120 perm rods and five to twenty minutes processing. That's nearly two hours working on your client to get the correct look, so don't go and ruin all this good work by a sloppy five- or ten-minute neutralising process.

Ensure that neutralising is done thoroughly. All apprentices should appreciate that neutralising is an integral part of permanent wave procedure and that, if it is not carried out correctly or is skimped, the results will not be good. Incorrect neutralising has spoiled many a sound permanent wave procedure. Make sure this doesn't happen to you.

Points to remember

Don't assume that because you have done a permanent wave once you know all about it. You don't. You must check instructions. Keep a folder, so that junior apprentices can readily refer to instructions. There are so many permanent wave products being manufactured nowadays that most hairdressing salons have more than one brand or product in the stockroom. Some salons have quite a selection, so it is even more important that instructions should be available.

Remember, heat from dryers, wall heaters, lamps and spotlights will speed up the development of your permanent wave, whereas cold draughts from windows or open doors, air conditioning units or fans will retard the processing action. These factors can influence the final result of your permanent wave. It is not advisable to use a heat acceleration cold-wave procedure.

Generally, the faster the processing action, the more damaging it is to the hair; it can cause dryness and even breakage. You can lose control of processing time by using accelerators. The processing time for most permanent waves is less than 30 minutes.

Finally, if a permanent wave does require a complicated winding technique – that is, up to an hour or so of winding – wind with water to help maintain an even development.

Questions – General permanent waving

1   Describe the chemical action of permanent wave solution on the hair shaft. Use diagrams to illustrate your answers.

2   Describe what the following terms refer to:
   a   cystine;

   _____

   b   reduction;

   _____

   c   cysteine;

   _____

   d   thio;

   _____

   e   –S–S–.

   _____

3   List three factors that will influence your choice of either an acidic or an alkaline permanent wave solution.

   _____

   _____

   _____

4   Name the three major considerations in your preliminary analysis which are important in obtaining good results.

   _____

   _____

   _____

5   a   Name four factors that will determine your choice of perm wave solution.

   _____

   _____

   _____

   _____

b Elaborate on how two of the above will influence your choice.

_____

_____

6 Name two factors that will determine the size of the perm rod you choose.

_____

_____

7 What is the difference between the 'classic' and the 'directional' wind?

_____

_____

_____

8 List ten factors that will influence the length of processing time.

_____

_____

_____

_____

_____

_____

_____

_____

_____

_____

9 Why is it inadvisable to brush the scalp before applying the permanent wave solution?

_____

_____

10 Name three ways in which permanent wave burns can be prevented.

_____

_____

_____

11 From the list of words complete sentences (a) to (e).

methodical, tension, circumference, stretched, nape, pull burns, dampen.

a The size of the curl is determined by the _____ of the perm rod.

b Presectioning the hair before winding will ensure a _____ approach.

c Wind each rod with even _____.

d If the hair is _____ during winding when the hair is dampened it may cause _____ .

e Start to _____ the perm rods at the _____ area first.

12 Match the words in Column A with the words in Column B.

COLUMN A	**COLUMN B**
i retains heat	**a** weight
ii good results	**b** record card
iii future guide	**c** evenly
iv maintains even temperature	**d** correct preliminary analysis
v 'S' movement	**e** circumference
	f texture
	g processing cap

13 What special care needs to be taken when:

a blow-drying newly permed hair?

_____

b setting after a permanent wave?

_____

14 List the advice you would offer to clients to ensure that their permed hair is kept in the best possible condition.

_____

15 Name four precautions which you should take when permanently waving hair which has been previously coloured.

_____

_____

_____

_____

16 a What is the name of the test that can be given if you are in doubt about the results of a permanent wave?

_____

b How would you give the test?

_____

_____

Questions – Permanent wave problems

17 a   How can most permanent wave problems be avoided? Give three examples.

_____

_____

_____

b   If there is doubt as to whether the final result of a permanent wave will prove satisfactory, what can be done?

_____

_____

18 a   Give five reasons why a permanent wave may not hold.

_____

_____

_____

_____

_____

b   How can this problem be rectified?

_____

_____

_____

c   Illustrate the result of a limp wave that will not hold its curl.

19 a There may be times during the processing of a permanent wave when you need to dampen the rods a second time. List four possible reasons for this.

_____

_____

_____

_____

b Explain a precaution that you will need to take during this procedure.

_____

_____

20 What could be the reason for hair breakage during permanent waving? Name five factors.

_____

_____

_____

_____

21 What are the advantages of water winding?

_____

_____

_____

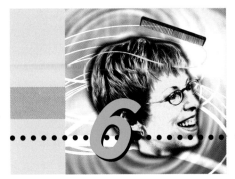

Permanent colouring
Introduces: 'Select and apply permanent and midway hair colour'

In this chapter, you will learn about:

- vegetable colours;
- mineral colours;
- allergy testing;
- hair colour;
- preparation for colouring;
- selecting colours;
- procedure for colouring;
- the chemical action of permanent tint;
- midway colours.

Introduction

Permanent colouring is a skill with which you will need to be completely familiar if you are to succeed as a hairdresser. This chapter is designed to help you obtain a better understanding of colouring. You are also encouraged to attend the colour seminars offered by manufacturers (these are usually of two to three days' duration). Ask your senior to help you develop your colouring skills.

Permanent colours for salon use are divided into three main categories: vegetable, vegetable/mineral and mineral. Manufacturers have still not developed the ideal permanent colour. The ideal permanent colouring should:
1 be harmless to the hair structure (have a low pH value);
2 not cause skin irritation;
3 be easy and quick to apply;
4 not prevent permanent waving;
5 have a good colour range.

Most of the permanent colours available can fulfil at least three of these requirements. Manufacturers are still developing new colour formulas and it will not be long before the ideal dye is developed.

Vegetable colours

Henna is a vegetable colour used in most salons. Henna has been used for many centuries. Muslims who had made the pilgrimage to Mecca would henna their beards to show they had made the journey. Ancient Egyptians used henna to colour their hair; Cleopatra used to sit in the sun with her hair covered in the muddy mixture. It is still used in the East today to dye the body, and to paint the soles of the feet, palms and face for ceremonial rituals such as marriage. Henna has been used in England since the eighteenth century and in New Zealand since the early twentieth century.

Henna comes mainly from Eastern and Middle Eastern countries such as China, Egypt, Iran and Tunisia. It is manufactured from a privet bush or shrub called *Lawsonia* (*alba* or *inemis*) and is harvested much like a tobacco leaf. The top leaves of the henna plant produce red colours, the centre leaves produce a black colourant and the bottom leaves produce neutral henna, which is used as a conditioning agent only. The stem is also crushed and its red colourant used to intensify colours. The leaves are plucked at certain times of the year, left to dry in the sun and then the veins are taken out and crushed into a powder. This crushed powder is henna. In addition to the predominant Arabic hennas, there are also Chinese, Japanese, green, spiced and white hennas.

White henna is really just a bleach pack; no henna, as such, is present, just H_2O_2 and NH_3 (hydrogen peroxide and ammonia). In the 1930s to 1950s, using white henna was known as bleaching.

Traditional Egyptian red henna

This is the natural vegetable colour which, if it is mixed by itself, will colour the hair red or auburn.

Mixing

There are a number of ways in which henna can be mixed. The traditional way in the salon was to mix it to a creamy paste consistency with hot water (as hot as the client could bear). This tended to give a better colouring action, provided that all the powder was well stirred. Nowadays other ingredients are added to the henna mixture. These include: hot black coffee or red wine, egg yolk, lemon juice, yoghurt and chamomile.

Some hairdressers add coins – sometimes up to 30 old two-cent pieces. This is to bring out more red in the final result, but is not recommended as the coins are made of metal and their presence alters the vegetable colour to a vegetable/mineral colour. The metallic film which will be left on the hair will make permanent waving a problem.

When henna was used widely as a colouring method in salons in the 1940s and 1950s, it was mixed in a double boiler. A junior would be responsible for mixing the day's henna in the pot, lighting the gas and placing the pot in another pot of hot water. This was kept going throughout the day and used on the clients as required. Since the main clientele seeking this type of service were prostitutes, other customers were reluctant to ask for henna treatment.

Today henna is mixed up as needed. A 250 g pot is usually sufficient for the average head of hair.

Application

Henna is not the easiest of colours to apply and tends to be messy, so protect the client well. Shampoo the hair and towel dry. The henna will cling better to damp hair so have a water spray filled with hot water on hand. Starting at the nape, apply the henna quite liberally to the hair, from roots to ends. Mulch into the hair with the fingers. Use gloves as henna stains the skin. Work your way up the back and deal with the front last. Mulch and pile on top of the head.

Ensure that all the hair is covered. Plastic wrapping will make certain that it is all contained. The longer the henna is left, the deeper the result, but remember that it will stain the client's skin. Henna can be left on the hair for as long as 6 to 8 hours but it is not advisable to let it dry on the hair as the colour action stops when the henna dries. Dry henna also crumbles and drops onto the client's face and clothes. This length of time is, of course, impractical in the salon, so 40 minutes under a moist steamer is a good alternative. After this time, remove the plastic covering and let the head cool down to close the cuticle. After five minutes give the hair a good shampoo to remove the caked henna. After the treatment, the client's hair will have a pleasant shine and warm glow as henna has excellent conditioning qualities.

Henna first became popular again after a report in the mid 1970s that usual tints caused health problems. Henna is a good alternative to tinting and is recommended especially if a client is sensitive to chemical tints. Henna has both advantages and disadvantages:

1 it is harmless to the hair structure and can improve hair quality;
2 it does not cause skin irritation but does stain;
3 it is not easy to apply and tends to be messy and the smell can be objectionable;
4 permanent waving is not recommended until at least 10 weeks after a henna treatment as henna coats and penetrates the cortex and impairs permanent waving results;
5 the colour range that can be obtained using henna is limited.

General henna tips

1 Applying henna to grey or bleached hair is not recommended.
2 Mix the henna to a paste which drips off the brush or else it will crumble when drying.
3 Results depend on:
   a the level of the natural shade – light or dark (the lighter the natural colour, the more apparent the final result and the shorter the time the henna needs to be left on the hair);
   b the length of time the henna is left on;
   c the texture of the hair;
   d the temperature of the pack.
4 The greener the henna powder, the better the conditioning qualities and, generally, the less intense the auburn or red result.
5 If the henna dries, the colouring process stops.

 # Vegetable/mineral colours

Henna can be mixed with metallic substances, which contain metals mined from the earth (such as silver nitrate). Metallic substances are added to change the shade of henna and give an ash variation to finished results. Copper substances also used to be added (like the two-cent coins mentioned earlier) to achieve variations of red shades. These types of henna were manufactured as compound hennas and, although they are not used often today, they were popular during the 1930s, 1940s and 1950s.

 # Mineral colours

Minerals are natural inorganic substances mined from the earth, and are neither animal nor vegetable. Hair colours can be produced and manufactured from these substances. There are two types of mineral colouring: metallic salt dye and the analine derivative.

Metallic salt dye

The first type, a mineral salt, was also known as a 'progressive-type dye' or 'colour restorer'. Such metallic salt dyes are available today from pharmacies. They are applied daily, by combing them onto the hair 'progressively'. Each day, the hair colour goes darker and eventually, after 7 to 14 days, the client's hair is 'restored' to its pre-grey colour. These dyes form a metallic film on the hair shaft, and in the early days, if the client stopped using them, they tended to fade to peculiar colours, depending on what metal substance was used in their preparation. Tinges of green, violet and gold were often apparent in the hair of clients who stopped using metallic salt dyes. The dyes did, however, allow a wider range of colour choice when lightening the hair was not possible.

The biggest drawback to these dyes in the salon today is that one cannot do permanent waving, tinting or lightening over them. The manufacturers of such hair colours instruct users to inform their hairdresser that they are using a metallic salt dye, and, in some cases, they supply a formula to use when having a permanent wave. If you suspect a client of using a metallic salt dye, don't give a permanent wave. A test can be carried out to establish the possible coating of metallic substances on the hair. This is called a decomposition test (1–20 test).

Decomposition test (incompatibility test)

Mix 25 cc (1 oz) of 20 volume H_2O_2 and 20 drops of ammonia (1–20) into a plastic bowl. Cut a strand of hair and place it in the solution. Watch for any reaction. If there is any bubbling, fizzing or heat emitted, then the hair has a metallic covering. Any reaction should be apparent after 30 minutes. There are chemical strippers which will remove these coverings if necessary.

Analine derivative or oxidation dyes (para dyes)

This second type of mineral colour is derived from coal tar, a black, oily liquid obtained in the coal-gas manufacturing process. The majority of colour work in hairdressing salons nowadays is done using analine derivatives. Product names include Koleston, Majarel and Igora Royal. The chemicals used in such tints are either:

a para phenylene diamine – liquid tints (abbreviated to para); or

b para tolulene diamine – cream tints.

The darker the colour, the more para there is in the tint. In addition to the para agents, the tint will also contain wetting agents, conditioners, ammonia and colouring pigments. These are mixed with oxidants such as hydrogen peroxide to oxidise the pigment in the tint. These dyes are sometimes referred to as oxidation dyes.

The analine derivatives have most of the qualities of an ideal colour except for their major disadvantage – that some clients are allergic to the analine para. Because of this, you should carry out a test every time a para tint is used.

Patch/allergy/skin predisposition/hypersensitivity test

People can have allergic reactions to a wide range of things, including animals, such as cats and horses; fruits, such as strawberries and oranges; and metals. Reactions can vary from occasional sneezing to breaking out in hives or the development of dermatitis. These last two conditions occur because the skin is sensitive and reacts. Unfortunately the same sensitivity can occur with hair tints and clients can develop severe dermatitis of the scalp. Allergies are not predictable; that is, you can't know whether or not a client will react. Clients can build up a reaction, as can happen with the development of hives after eating too much fruit; there is a threshold beyond which the allergy breaks out. You must, therefore, take care – just because a client didn't break out in dermatitis last time a dye was used, is no guarantee that he/she won't have an allergic reaction in the future.

If you suspect an allergic reaction, it is best to give a test. This acts as a safeguard for you and your client, and for hairdressers in general. It is claimed that four out of a thousand clients could be allergic, and a salon's reputation could suffer dramatically if a client developed dermatitis as the result of a tint. It is your responsibility to protect the client from dangerous chemicals and to take all necessary precautions. Take a test every time you use a para tint –

whether as a full head colour, a retouch or a toner. The warning is printed on all packets and bottles. Manufacturers are aware of the possible danger and they protect themselves from liability as should you. Nowadays, even some semipermanent colourants have a percentage of para in their contents.

How to give the test

1 The client needs to undergo the test at least 24 hours before the proposed application.

2 Wash an area the size of a 50-cent piece behind the ear or in the inner fold of the elbow. Use a bland soap in case the client is allergic to ordinary soap. Bland soap is a very mild and non-perfumed preparation.

3 Mix a test solution of the colour to be used – equal parts of tint to hydrogen peroxide. A capful of each should be sufficient.

4 Apply to the cleansed area and leave to dry. The area can be covered with collodion (a type of alcohol mixture). Don't cover with a sticking plaster as this in itself could cause inflammation.

5 Leave undisturbed for 24 hours and then examine the test area for any inflammation or abnormality of any nature. If there is none, proceed with the tint. If there is any reaction, don't use that permanent tint range; the client is predisposed to be allergic to it.

There is a slight possibility that the client may not be allergic to another brand of tint containing another para. Some clients are allergic to para phenylene diamine but not to para tolulene diamine, and vice versa.

Because of the danger of extreme sensitivity, don't use hair tints to colour eyebrows or lashes. There are colours manufactured especially for this purpose. These were discussed in Book 1.

Hair colour

What determines our natural hair colour?

Natural hair colour is determined by two major factors: hereditary traits and climatic conditions. In addition our hair colour is influenced by:

a the type of pigment in the hair;

b the amount of pigment in the hair;

c how this pigment is distributed in the hair.

The two types of pigment are eumelanin – blackish brown, and phaeomelanin – reddish yellow.

Hereditary traits

Our hair colour is passed on to us through our genes from our parents and grandparents. Generally, we have similar characteristics to our parents; e.g. if both parents have brown hair, we will have brown hair. There are exceptions, but these can generally be traced back through the family history, to an earlier generation.

Racial and climatic factors

Racial and climate factors influence hair colour. We come to expect Scandinavians to have blonde hair; Italians, Indians, Chinese and Africans to have dark hair, and the Dutch to have fair hair. The Greeks were originally blonde or fair, but many centuries ago Greece was invaded by dark-haired Turks, so that many of today's Greek community have dark hair. Maori and Pacific Islanders have dark hair. These various races have been around for many hundreds of years and as a result have developed a certain genetic strain, because of genetic isolation.

New Zealand European hair colour has not taken on any particular strain because we are a new society like the United States, with much genetic diversity and it is unlikely that we will ever be characterised by a certain hair colour. Similarly, there is no characteristic hair colour in the United Kingdom because of invasion through the centuries.

What causes grey hair?

The term *grey* should really be *white* since the hair only looks grey when mixed with darker hair. *Grey hair* has, however, become the accepted term. Perhaps, in the salon, a softer and more appropriate term to use when talking to the client is silver.

Silver hair begins to show when the cells in the matrix cease to produce the melanin pigment and are replaced by air sacs or spaces. There is no known reason for this although there is evidence to suggest that hereditary characteristics play a part. Greying is also believed to be caused by the natural aging process which usually occurs from the fourth decade onwards. Although it develops slowly throughout the hair, greying generally starts at the temples and sides. This may be because the hair is more exposed in these areas, getting weathered and falling out more often. This type of greying is traditionally seen as a sign of wisdom and can be very attractive.

Premature greying is said to be brought about by a number of environmental factors such as worry, shock, stress and dietary habits (especially lack of Vitamin B), but there is no proof that a lack of such symptoms stops or retards greying. Hereditary characteristics again play an important role in premature greyness and should always be considered as a primary cause.

Blanching is a term used to describe the sudden silvering of the hair. There are medically attested cases of this occurring, for example, during World War II. There were cases of people going grey within about 48 hours. Shock is thought to be the main cause, but there is no scientific explanation to account for this unusual phenomenon.

Preparation for colouring

Selecting the colour

A number of rules and factors must be considered in selecting the correct shade of colour as the choice can mean the difference between a successful colour and one which fails.

Defining colour

The colours on the colour chart are defined or described by the following two characteristics.

1 Depth, level or base shade

All hair colours are at a certain level, depth or shade. Most modern manufacturers' colour charts have a selection of colours ranging from black to lightest blonde. Your client's hair must be somewhere between these levels. They are usually numbered:

(1) black – the darkest level (0% light reflection, 100% pigment)

(2) darkest brown;

(3) dark brown;

(4) medium brown;

(5) light brown;

(6) lightest brown;

(7) darkest blonde;

(8) dark blonde;

(9) medium blonde;

(10) light blonde;

(11) lightest blonde;

(12) white (100% light reflection, 0% pigment).

These are universal levels of colour and your client's hair will be one of these. Some manufacturers may use the word 'extra' in determining their colour levels, e.g. 'extra light brown'. As an example, dark blonde is one level (shade or depth) *lighter* than darkest blonde, and two levels, shades or depth *lighter* than lightest brown. Dark blonde is one level, shade or depth *darker* than medium blonde. You must always determine the natural level (shade or depth) of your client's hair.

2 Reflect, highlight or character

This means that the level of the colour has a reflect or highlight and manufacturers indicate these down or across their colour charts. The reflects or highlights which are usually numbered include:

(1) gold;
(2) ash;
(3) cendre;
(4) matt;
(5) chestnut;
(6) auburn;
(7) mahogany;
(8) copper;
(9) warm.

You must determine what highlight is reflected in your client's hair. If, for example, your client's hair colours on the level or depth of level (8) – dark blonde – and it has a gold reflect or highlight (1), the colour will be called 'dark golden blonde' (8/1). The dark blonde is the level or depth and the golden is the reflect or highlight. 'Medium golden blonde' would be one shade or level lighter and darkest golden blonde would be one shade or level darker.

Some manufacturers introduce a double reflect, e.g. 8/1.6 – a level (8) dark blonde with a primary (1) gold and a secondary auburn (6).

Reflects or highlights are based on the colours of the colour wheel. Generally, gold is based on orange; auburn, chestnut and copper are based on red; matt or ash are based on blue or green; mahogany and burgundy are based on violet; and colours which determine the level or depth are based on yellow.

You need to know that ashen reflects make the final colour appear darker, while the golden reflects make the colour appear lighter. It is important to remember this if you are eliminating any unwanted gold reflects as the colour will appear darker to the client who usually wants to have brassy reflects removed without going darker.

Texture also plays an important part in colour selection, as it affects the way the colour looks. Coarse, strong hair will not look such a vibrant colour as fine, sleek, glossy hair. The same principles apply when comparing the appearance of a colour in fabrics such as silk and wool; although they may be the same colour, they look different because of the textures. Some manufacturers' instructions allow for textural variations in their colour selections. If the hair is fine, select a colour one level lighter than you would for coarse hair.

Selecting colours

Regardless of the product you are going to use, it is important to analyse the client's hair correctly. When doing this, your judgement may be affected by the lighting in the salon. The best type of lighting for colour work is the natural light that comes in through the salon's windows. In most salons, supplementary artificial light is necessary, either as incandescent light bulbs or as long tube fluorescent or strip lights. The best artificial light is a warm white strip light overhead and white incandescent spotlights shining on the sides of the head. This will light the whole of the head and will give the closest approximation to natural lighting.

Determining the client's natural hair colour

1 Lift the hair up from the scalp and look through it. This will show what reflects or highlights, if any, there are in the hair. It will also help to determine the level or depth of the hair colour. Failure to follow this procedure can result in selecting a colour which is too dark, as hair sitting flat against the head appears darker.

2 Ensure that the hair is thoroughly dry as wet hair appears darker in depth or level. Also, if the hair is greasy, it makes the colour depth or reflect darker. If necessary, wash and dry the hair thoroughly to get an exact colour match.

3 If you half close your eyes one of the colours on the colour chart will 'merge' with the natural colour of the client's hair.

Hair colour and complexion

Certain skin tonings suit certain types of hair colours. It is important, when you assess the client's hair, to pay attention to his/her complexion.

- *Olive* complexions, which have a sallow, yellowish cast (most Europeans, Pacific Islanders and Maori have olive skin), suit dark or ash colours. If the hair is too light, clients can look a little insipid.

- *Florid* complexions, those that are ruddy or have a pinkish cast, suit hair colours that are not too warm, red or gold in their reflects.

- *Fair and cream complexions* suit a wide range of hair colours with most of the reflects, although it is advisable not to make the hair too dark as this can emphasise a paler complexion.

  Elderly clients often want to go back to their pre-grey colour, but it is better to suggest a lighter, more becoming colour as skin tones do become paler with age.

Rules for selecting colour

It is impossible in a text like this to discuss all the possible combinations of colour. A percentage of silver (grey) can influence the final colour choice.

Most manufacturers give instructions on what factors they consider to be important when choosing the colours in their product range. It is important to remember that the colour you apply goes darker on the hair. To allow for this, select colours one or possibly two shades lighter than the required result. (Products differ so read the instructions.) If a medium golden brown colour is applied to medium golden brown hair which has a mixture of 35% grey, the result could well be a dark golden brown. Follow manufacturers' instructions as some consider texture important in deciding final colour selection. All the colours on the colour chart are coloured on 100% white hair and are only a guide as to what colour can be expected. Some manufacturers have colour charts especially created for colouring silver hair.

Procedure for permanent colouring

Preliminary strand test

If there is any doubt in your mind as to the:

- colour to select;
- strength of H_2O_2;
- end result;
- colour formula;
- overall condition of the hair;
- length of time to leave the mixture on,

then give a preliminary strand test.

1   Select an area underneath the back of the crown, cut and secure the ends. Colour the cut strand. (Alternatively the mixture can be directly applied on the strand.)

2   Watch the strand for any reaction, discolouration or damage.

3   Record details on the client's record card.

You may have to perform more than one test if the results are inconclusive or unsatisfactory.

Hair and scalp analysis

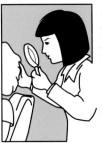

Analyse the scalp for cuts and abrasions which could cause discomfort and, if necessary, discourage the client from having colour treatment. Check the hair's

1   texture – this could influence your colour selection (according to the manufacturer's instructions) and the strength of hydrogen peroxide used;

2   condition – don't suggest a permanent tint if the hair is excessively dry, brittle and fragile or feels harsh to touch; give a course of preconditioning treatment if necessary;

3   porosity – this could determine where your application of colour will begin. Since silver hair is less porous and therefore more resistant and colour treatment on it needs extra time, apply colour to grey areas first.

Client protection

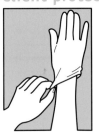

Ensure your client is well protected. Tinting can stain clothing and if this happens, the salon is responsible for replacing the stained garment. Tuck the towel well around the nape and then place the full cape over this. Protect your own clothes by wearing an operator's gown and remember to wear gloves to avoid staining your hands and nails. Remember, any tint spilt on the floor will stain the floor covering, so wipe up any spills at once.

Sectioning

So that your approach is systematic and methodical, section the hair from forehead to nape and from ear to ear over the crown. Use large sectioning clips to secure the sections. In all applications, whether full head or retouch, take 0.5 cm partings. This is important for the success of the colour. Where you begin the application depends on:

1   whether your colouring is to cover silver (in this case start at the front where the silver is more apparent and resistant);

2   whether you are lightening the hair (in this case start where it is darker, at the nape).

Because silver hair is coarser, the colour will take longer to develop and to penetrate the cuticle. You begin at the back when lightening because the hair is generally darker here where it is not exposed to sunlight which fades colour (even natural colour). If the client is lightening his/her hair and also has a percentage of silver, be guided as to which is the most important – to lighten the hair or to cover most of the silver. If there is only a small percentage of silver to colour and the client wants plenty of lightening, start where the hair is darker – at the back.

Mixing the colour

Mixing the permanent colour correctly is important for good results. Generally, a full tube of colour is needed for a full head application. It is mixed with 60 to 90 cc of hydrogen peroxide (H_2O_2). A tint retouch is mixed with half a tube of colour and 30 to 45 cc of hydrogen peroxide.

A cream tint and a cream H_2O_2 can be mixed in together all at once, but a cream tint and a liquid must be mixed little by little. Likewise, a liquid tint and liquid H_2O_2 can be mixed together all at once, but you must mix gradually if a cream developer is used. Use a plastic spoon to mix the products. This ensures a thorough mix and leaves you with a clean tint brush to start your application. Alternatively, you can use a shaker, which should ensure a good mix, especially if more than one colour is used.

When mixing the H_2O_2, measure out the quantity accurately. Place the measurer on a flat surface and pour the H_2O_2 to the required cc or ml level. Measure off on a flat surface. Don't lift the cylinder as you could tilt it and this would give an incorrect measurement. Look at the measurement on the surface at eye level. Ensure you replace the top of the H_2O_2 container and on any remaining tint in the tube or bottle, which should be clearly labelled as 'used'. Mix the products just before they are to be applied. The H_2O_2 will give off its oxygen for a limited time only – 30 to 45 minutes.

In the tube or bottle are the contents which will colour and assist in the development of the product. These include ammonia, para, wetting agent, conditioners and colour pigments. The ammonia content is there for two purposes:

1 it assists in opening up the cuticle so that the new para molecules can get into the cortex;
2 it helps to liberate the O_2 gas from the H_2O_2, thus assisting the development.

Colour formulas will eventually become ammonia-free. The wetting agent helps the colour preparation to adhere to the hair by breaking down surface tension.

Determining the strength of hydrogen peroxide

Determining what strength of hydrogen peroxide to use is influenced by the following four factors.

1 Degree of colour lift

The higher the volume strength of the hydrogen peroxide, the greater the degree of colour lift and the lighter the result. Higher-strength hydrogen peroxide also brings out more warmth in the hair and makes reflects more obvious.

2 Manufacturer's instructions

These may indicate which are the best strengths of hydrogen peroxide to use, and this may depend on the product's formula, i.e. whether it is a toner which is being applied to prelightened hair or a tint lightener designed to lighten the natural hair colour three to four levels. Follow the instructions.

3 Colour selection

Ash or darker colours are best used with low-strength hydrogen peroxide as they will not lighten the natural colour but will make the ash or dark colour more intense.

4 Hair texture

This may influence hydrogen peroxide strength. Fine-textured hair will usually lift satisfactorily with a low volume strength whereas coarse hair may require a stronger hydrogen peroxide.

Figure 6.1
Sectioning hair

Section the hair into four parts and start at the crown with a 0.5 cm parting. This will become the first mesh-strand to which you apply the colour. Keep the partings small.

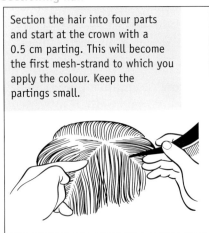

Figure 6.2
Tint tube key

Use a tint tube key to measure accurately the amount of tint required – whether a quarter, a half or three-quarters of a tube. The key will ensure that no tint is wasted by being left inside the tube.

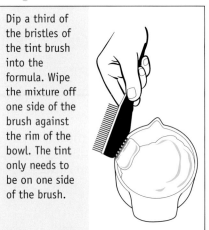

Figure 6.3
Mixing and measuring colour

Mix and measure all formulas accurately. Using a tint tube key and measuring hydrogen peroxide with a cylinder will help. Mix the formula with a plastic spoon for a creamy consistency. *Read the manufacturer's instructions.*

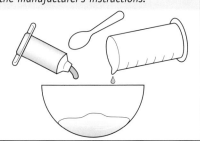

Figure 6.4
Checking measurements

Always check the cc measurement at eye level with the cylinder on a flat surface.

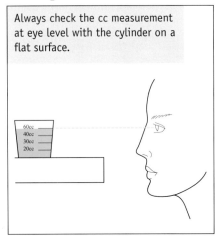

Figure 6.5
Using the tint brush

Dip a third of the bristles of the tint brush into the formula. Wipe the mixture off one side of the brush against the rim of the bowl. The tint only needs to be on one side of the brush.

Figure 6.6
Holding the mesh

Lay the mesh over the palm of the hand.

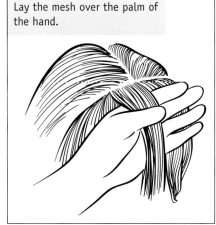

Figure 6.7
Applying the tint

Start to apply the tint mixture 1.5 cm from the roots to the mid-lengths and ends. Apply the mixture generously and work well into the strands with thumb and fingers.

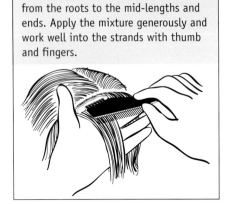

Figure 6.8
Developing the colour

Once the mixture has been applied, leave it to develop. Don't pack the mixture down but lift and open the strands for maximum oxidation. Failure to do this can give a patchy colour result. Make sure that there is no excessive staining of the forehead or ears.

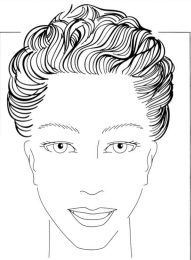

Figure 6.9

Mixing and measuring colour

Mix and measure accurately. A tint tube key and measuring hydrogen peroxide with a cylinder will help. Mix the formula with a plastic spoon for a creamy consistency. *Read the manufacturer's instructions.*

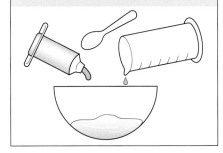

Application to a virgin head of hair

A virgin head of hair is one that has not been coloured before. Ensure that the hair is clean and dry. Don't brush the scalp immediately before a tint as this can cause scratching of the scalp and discomfort when the tint is applied.

1   Start at the back of the head, from the crown. Dip two-thirds of the bristle of the brush into the tint and wipe off one side against the rim – the tint should only be on one side of the brush. Apply the colour to within 1.5 cm of the roots through to the ends on both sides of the strand.
2   Mulch the colour in with the thumb and finger and lay the hair back out of the way.
3   Take the next section (0.5 cm) and do the same 1.5 cm from the roots. Apply throughout to the ends.
4   Once the mid-lengths and ends have been covered over the entire head, check to make sure that no strands have been missed.
5   Leave for approximately 10 to 20 minutes.
6   Now mix up some fresh colour and apply it to the roots which have been left until last. The root area will take more quickly because of the heat generated by the scalp.
7   Check to make sure no area has been left out and leave the tint to develop according to the manufacturer's recommendations.

Steamers do cut down the developing period but by the time the client has been under the steamer for 15 minutes and is then allowed to cool down for a further 5 to 10 minutes, not a great deal of time is actually saved. There is also the disadvantage of diluted tint on the scalp caused by drips from the steamer hood.

It is best to make the client comfortable and to develop for the full 25 or 30 minutes. Aerate the sections – don't pack close to the head.

8   At the end of this time, water can be sprayed on the head to form a mulch and the hair left for a further five minutes.
9   You can check the colour development by drying a small strand with a towel. Reapply tint if it is not fully developed.
10 Rinse and, if necessary or desirable, shampoo. Ensure that all tint is removed from the scalp and hairline.

Retouch application

1   Apply colour *to the regrowth only*, on both sides of each strand. *Don't overlap.*
2   Wipe the brush on the bowl rim so that there is tint only on one side of the brush.
3   Do not stab the bristles into the scalp, as this will cause discomfort and possible inflammation.
4   Lay the tint on – don't keep going over the regrowth area with the brush, as this actually removes the tint mixture.
5   Check the hairline for coverage, and remove any stains from the client's skin. It is important that no areas should be missed either along the front, around the ears or in the parting area.
6   Leave for 30 minutes. Don't pack the strands against the scalp. Also avoid running the tail of the comb along the scalp when lifting sections as this removes the tint from these areas and causes uneven colour development. If the colour needs to be brought through to the mid-lengths and ends, spray warm water onto these areas and apply the remainder of the tint colour, mulching with gloved fingers – don't comb the mixture into the hair. Leave for only five minutes.

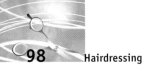

Figure 6.10
Using the tint brush

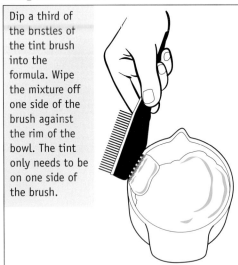

Dip a third of the bristles of the tint brush into the formula. Wipe the mixture off one side of the brush against the rim of the bowl. The tint only needs to be on one side of the brush.

Figure 6.11
Retouch application

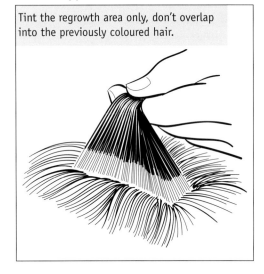

Tint the regrowth area only, don't overlap into the previously coloured hair.

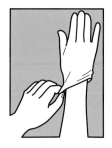

7 Rinse, shampoo if desired and ensure that all colour is lifted from the skin. Don't rub the skin or forehead vigorously with cotton wool or a towel to remove stains. Use a strand of tinted hair to remove colour from the skin.

Adopt a similar method if you are using an applicator bottle with a nozzle. As you squeeze the bottle with one hand, work the mixture in with the thumb and finger of the other hand. You must have adequate control of the applicator. Both techniques are suitable for either full head or retouch applications.

Tinting silver hair

It can sometimes prove difficult to obtain an adequate coverage of silver hair, because of its stronger, coarser, more resistant nature. If a client does need a better coverage, check that:

1 the percentage of silver has not increased so much over the years that the original formula is no longer adequate;
2 the application begins at the silver areas;
3 the stock, product and H_2O_2 are fresh and that the mixture has not been mixed inadequately or too long before the client comes in;
4 the hair is thoroughly clean before the application;
5 the application is thorough and that areas are not being missed by taking over-large sections;
6 enough product is being applied and that the operator is not applying the mixture too sparingly;
7 barrier cream is not coating the hairline every time a retouch takes place and thereby inhibiting the development;
8 adequate developing time is allowed – the full 30 minutes from the end of the application;
9 the sections are not packed down too tightly, causing inadequate oxidation;
10 water from a steamer (if used) is not dripping and so diluting the colour mixture.

If all these requirements have been met and there is still a problem, you can adopt one of two approaches.

1 The silver hair can be presoftened by a double application. First mix up the formula without mixing the H_2O_2 and apply it to the stubborn, resistant silver hair first; NH_3 (ammonia) will help open up the cuticle scale. Now mix up a fresh mixture with the H_2O_2 and apply this in the conventional manner. Because of the first application it may be difficult to see which hair has and which hasn't received its second application, so take care that each section is methodically covered. This technique should help to overcome the resistant silver.

2 Alternatively, a resistant formula can be applied. Mix up a colour which is a shade darker than the desired colour with only half the amount of 30 volume H_2O_2 (if 20 volume H_2O_2 is normally used). This will give a higher concentration of colour molecules for penetration.

The chemical action of permanent tint on the hair shaft (oxidation)

When the colour is applied, the ammonia softens and opens up the cuticle. The para molecules and hydrogen peroxide penetrate the cuticle and enter the cortex. During the developing time, the para phenylene or tolulene diamine colour molecules combine with the oxygen molecules liberated by the H_2O_2. The ammonia helps the hydrogen peroxide to give off its O_2 gas. The O_2 and para colour molecules combine and increase in size. After approximately 30 minutes, they are three times their original size and cannot get out of the cortex the same way as they entered, i.e. via the cuticle. They are therefore trapped and are permanent. They either have to be cut out, bleached out, grown out or reduced in size by colour stripping. In addition, the hydrogen peroxide also lightens the natural pigmentation of the hair. This lightening action, combined with the newly introduced trapped colour molecules, gives the hair a new colour. The application of an antioxidant conditioner closes the cuticle, which has been opened by the ammonia, and returns the hair to its acidic nature.

Permanent colour after-care

As part of the colouring service, the client expects information on maintaining and looking after the newly coloured hair. Advise your client to do the following.

1 Have regular colour retouches, perhaps every four to six weeks, depending on the percentage of silver which needs to be covered and the degree of lightening in comparison to the level of natural colour.

2 Use the correct non-strip shampoo and conditioner. Manufacturers recommend shampoos for hair which has been coloured.

3 Treat the hair carefully, by not pulling or stretching to eliminate tangles, not brushing when wet or blow-drying too harshly. Advise on the use of correct brushes and combs to style the hair, and suggest a porosity filler to help in easing tangles and knots.

4 Protect the hair from the sun and salt water in summer. The hair should be rinsed thoroughly in fresh water after swimming in the sea or in chlorine-treated swimming pools.

5 Have any dry harsh or split ends cut away every six weeks or less.

Maintaining client's records

Of all the records of client services you keep, the colour record is the most frequently referred to. Keeping a record of clients' colour information makes them feel that they are important to the salon. Some salons even send out reminder notices to their clients in the same way as a dentist does, to remind them to visit the salon for their next hair colour treatment. Record cards should be filled in while the client's colour is developing so that exact details of colour formula and application can be recalled.

Figure 6.12 (a–c)
Applying the tint

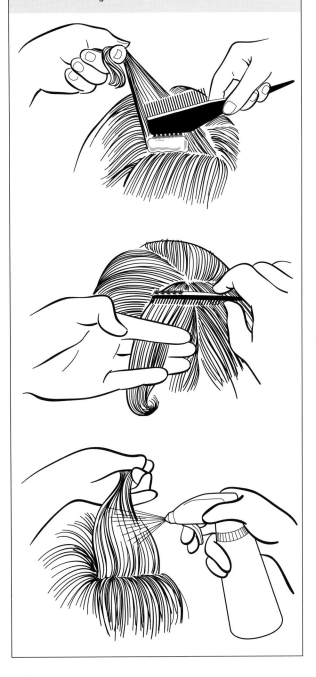

Apply the tint to both sides of the strand. Lay the tint on with as few strokes of the brush as possible.
Don't stab the bristles into the scalp, but lay the tint on, taking care not to overlap the previously coloured hair.
Don't comb the mixture through the hair but mulch any remaining tint (if necessary) with warm water and your gloved fingers. Combing, especially with a tint brush, could cause damage.

Figure 6.13 (a–d)
The chemical action of a permanent tint

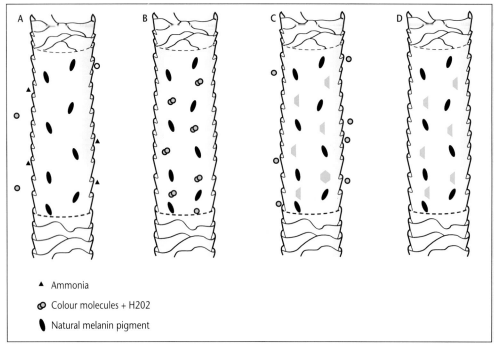

A The small molecules of colour combined with the hydrogen peroxide are applied to the hair. The ammonia in the tint opens up the cuticle.

B Because the cuticle is open, the para colour molecules can now penetrate the cortex, where they begin to swell.

C After approximately 30 minutes the para colour molecules are three times their original size and are trapped in the cortex. They cannot be washed out.

D The hydrogen peroxide also lightens the natural pigment so that the newly introduced and enlarged para colour molecules give the hair its new colour. The cuticle is closed and the colour becomes permanent.

▲ Ammonia

◐ Colour molecules + H202

❚ Natural melanin pigment

Most hairdressing manufacturers have colour record cards available for their specific colour product.

NAME: ADDRESS: PHONE:	SERVICE 1 DATE:	SERVICE 2 DATE:	SERVICE 3 DATE:	SERVICE 4 DATE:
NATURAL DEPTH	Med. brown			
% SILVER	35%			
HAIR LENGTH	Long			
POROUS	Yes			
REFLECT	Gold			
STRENGTH HP	20 v			
QUANTITY	1/2 tube			
APPLICATION	Front-roots			
FORMULA	Light gold brown			
PRICE	$25.95			
OPERATOR	David			

Midway colours

Manufacturers have now developed oxi-semipermanent colourants which contain no ammonia or amounts so small that they do not displace natural melanin during the colouring process. It is this factor that differentiates them from permanent colours that are 'diluted' with a low-volume hydrogen peroxide. Adaptations of a permanent colour, such as making a colour bath, are not true oxi-semipermanent colours.

The decision to choose an oxi-semi colourant will depend on the job or function you want to perform. Oxi-semi colourants are formulated to:

* match current level, or
* deepen current level, or
* brighten or make tonal change.

The benefits of oxi-semi colourants include:

* providing a longer-lasting semipermanent colour without using ammonia;
* finding colour matches or enhancing natural colour – making it warmer or cooler without lightening the hair;
* refreshing colour-treated hair between retouches;
* blending grey hair;
* being gentler on hair with varying degrees of porosity.

Oxi-semipermanent colours are applied in the same way as the traditional semipermanent colours, but usually require a shorter processing time than oxidation tints. These products will also carry a warning about the possibility of skin irritation. The results may give a similar look as the oxidation tints but any reflect intensity may not last as long and grey hair may get coverage but only have a 'translucent' look and show through sooner. However, such products are kinder to the hair than oxidation tints as they contain properties that help maintain the condition of the client's hair.

This colour classification has its advantages in the salon. Clients who are seeking colour to camouflage their grey while growing it out or clients who demand just a little more than a traditional semicolourant will enjoy the benefits of the oxi-semi colours. Clients whose reflects wash out too quickly with the semicolourants should also be advised of the benefits of the oxi-semipermanents.

Most of the major manufacturers market these 'in-between semipermanents'. Ask your local technical representative for an 'in-salon' presentation.

Questions

1   Name three qualities that permanent colour should have.

_____

_____

_____

2   Into which three categories are permanent colours divided?

_____

_____

_____

3   a   What is the name of the plant from which henna is derived?

_____

   b   How is henna harvested?

_____

_____

   c   What countries produce henna?

_____

4   a   Name three ingredients with which henna can be mixed.

_____

_____

_____

   b   From what part of the plant does henna wax come?

_____

5   List three advantages that henna has over a permanent tint.

_____

_____

_____

6   How is henna applied?

_____

_____

7 Give two examples of cases in which the use of henna is not recommended.

_____

_____

8 What is a compound henna?

_____

_____

9 **a** Give another name for colour restorers.

_____

b For what purpose are they used?

_____

_____

c What effect do they have on the hair which creates a major disadvantage for future hairdressing services?

_____

_____

10 Name and describe the test which will determine whether any colour restorers are present on the hair.

_____

_____

_____

11 What are analine derivatives?

_____

12 What is the abbreviated term para short for?

_____

13 What is the major drawback of analine derivative tints?

_____

14 Give another three names for a skin test.

_____

_____

_____

15 How is a skin test given?

_____

_____

_____

Complete the following sentences:

16 The hair's natural colour is made up of black and brown pigment, called _____, and red and _____ pigment, called _____.

17 The colour of our hair is determined in part by _____ and _____ factors.

18 _____ is the term for sudden _____ of the hair.

19 Lack of vitamin B is said to cause _____.

20 Hair colours are defined by their _____ and _____.

21 Match the words in Column A with the words in Column B.

COLUMN A		COLUMN B	
i	are all reflect colours	a	fluorescent, incandescent
ii	the best lighting for colouring	b	texture
iii	fine, sleek glossy hair	c	dark blonde, medium blonde, and light blonde
iv	are all levels of colour	d	ash reflects
v	affects the way the colour looks	e	secondary colours
vi	makes the colour appear darker	f	gives a vibrant colour
vii	artificial lighting	g	gold reflects
viii	appears to make the colour lighter	h	natural lighting
		i	chestnut, auburn and mahogany
		j	primary colours

22 What range of colours suits the following complexions:

a olive complexion?

_____

b florid complexion?

_____

c cream complexion?

_____

23 a What physical property of the hair is important in selecting the final colour?

_____

b What physical property can determine where the application of colour will commence?

_____

_____

24 a How many cc of hydrogen peroxide are mixed with a full tube of colour?

_____

b How is this measured accurately?

_____

_____

25 Describe the mixing of a cream tint with a liquid hydrogen peroxide.

_____

26 Name three ingredients in a tube or bottle of permanent tint.

_____

_____

_____

27 The ammonia content in tint is there for two purposes. Name them.

_____

_____

28 a List and elaborate on three factors which will influence the strength of hydrogen peroxide to be mixed.

   b What is the name of the test you use if you are unsure about the strength of H_2O_2 to use?

29 Complete sentences (a) to (e) below, using the following list of words

discomfort, roots, ends, towel, hair, mid-lengths, drying, root, dilute, scalp, heat.

   a The application of tint to a virgin head of hair is started from the _____ and _____ then applied to the _____.

   b The _____ area will take more quickly because of the _____ from the scalp.

   c Don't brush the _____ immediately before the tint as this could cause _____ to the client when the tint is applied.

   d If the steamer drips onto the tint it may _____ the colour.

   e Checking the colour development can be done by _____ a small strand with a _____.

30 a If a client is having his/her hair coloured to cover the silver, where should the tint application begin?

   b Give reasons for your answer.

_____

_____

_____

31 A client complains that the silver hair is becoming more apparent sooner than expected. Give five possible reasons why this may be happening.

_____

_____

_____

_____

_____

32 Elaborate on three ways to ensure the best possible coverage of silver hair.

_____

_____

_____

33 Using diagrams, explain the chemical action of permanent tint on the hair shaft.

_____

_____

_____

34 What advice would you offer clients to help them maintain the health and condition of their coloured hair?

_____

_____

_____

35 Design a client record card and itemise all the important details that it should include.

36 Name the dye category that lies between semi-permanent and permanent tint.

_____

_____

_____

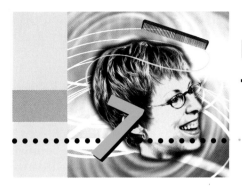

Lightening the hair
– bleach and tone the hair

In this chapter, you will learn about:

- using a lightener;
- bleach and tone the hair;
- correct unwanted colour tones in the hair;
- highlight/lowlight the hair using advanced techniques;
- remove unwanted additives from the hair – colour stripping.

Introduction

Bleaching means removing the natural pigment from the hair to obtain a lighter shade. Bleaching is usually an addition to tinting. Sometimes, when bleaching is mentioned, people automatically have visions of yellow or brassy hair. This is because, many years ago, bleaching was considered a harsh, chemical action which made your hair yellow or gold. In many countries bleaching used to be known as white henna. These white hennas were really just ammonia, hydrogen peroxide and a white powder such as magnesium carbonate or sodium carbonate. They often left the hair gold, orange and brassy. Today, women want more natural blonde colours; a better term these days is hair lightening, which does not sound as harsh to the client. It is also a more appealing term, as lightening can have so many variations in its results.

Lighteners come in a variety of mixtures. At one end of the range there are the mild oil, gel or cream lighteners, which are fun to use and, when mixed with 20 or 30 volume of hydrogen peroxide, have a lightening action range of two to four shades. At the other end of the scale are the stronger powder or crystal lighteners, usually mixed with 20, 30 or 40 volume hydrogen peroxide, which can lighten the hair to the lightest of all blondes – platinum blonde (pale yellow).

Using a lightener

Situations in which to use a lightener

Nowadays, lighteners are used for so many lightening variations that manufacturers have colour technicians who demonstrate new ways of achieving a wide range of interesting and enhancing lightening effects.

1 Lightening can be a new colour treatment in itself. It is used to lighten and brighten the hair either as a full-head application or as a streaking or frosting procedure, lightening from one to seven shades (stages of lightening), from, for example, dark brown to a pale yellow. If an after-colour is used, it is usually a temporary rinse.

2   Lightening may be necessary as a preliminary treatment for a tint which is considerably lighter than the client's own hair or when a client with tinted hair wishes to go lighter. This is not extreme lightening such as that which is required before the application of a blonde toner, but lightening two or three LEVELS, e.g. from a medium brown to a dark blonde. Oil lighteners can be mixed with tint to achieve this.

3   Lighteners can be used as a presoftening treatment before a colour, especially where grey hair proves resistant, but now there are so many ways of overcoming resistant white hair that bleaching is not such a popular softening method. These presoftening treatments are known as mordants (an older term).

4   Lightener may be used as an artificial colour remover, especially after a build-up of colour. (See the section on the removal of artificial colour, pp. 126 –128.)

5   Toning of the hair requires the most lightening. This is where a client requests a delicate pastel colour such as champagne beige, silver beige or platinum blonde. The colours are known as toners (or pastels) and the technique is known as toning. In this case, the lightening is a prelightening procedure.

Figure 7.1

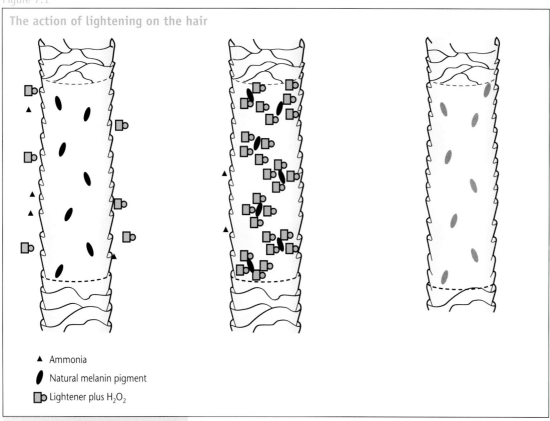

The action of lightening on the hair

▲ Ammonia

❚ Natural melanin pigment

⬚ Lightener plus H_2O_2

The ammonia opens the cuticle and the lightener and hydrogen peroxide lighten the natural colour pigment melanin.

Lightening as a decolouring technique

The texture and degree of lightening required will influence the decision about which lightener and what strength of hydrogen peroxide to use, and the length of time the lightener should be left on.

What lightener to use

Oil, gel or cream lighteners

These are the mildest form of lighteners. The 20 or 30 volume hydrogen peroxide with which they are mixed gives a slow-acting lightening action on medium-textured hair. The finer the texture, the quicker the lightening action. The higher volume strength of the hydrogen peroxide, the quicker the lightening action. Generally you will have a little more time to apply these lighteners than the powder lighteners. They are ideal for lightening before a tint, mixed with tint to get better colour lift or as a colouring cream in themselves when no further colouring is done.

Powder or crystal bleaches

These stronger lighteners are mixed with 20, 30 or 40 volume hydrogen peroxide and have a quicker lightening action. The stronger the lightener and hydrogen peroxide used, the quicker the lightening action and the more hair damage can be caused. The longer the chemical action takes to achieve the required result, the better the hair condition will be. Powdered bleaches are used for high degrees of lightening and usually go through the red/gold stage. Powdered bleaches are suitable for streaking, frosting, tipping and toning. If you lighten a natural head of dark hair you can expect the hair to go through the following stages of lightening:

1 brown
2 red
3 red/gold
4 gold
5 yellow, and
6 (possibly) palest yellow, after extensive lightening.

If you are in doubt as to what lightening agent and strength of hydrogen peroxide to use, cut a strand and test it (preliminary strand test). Remember, however, the quicker the action, the more damage can be done; the slower the action, the better the condition. Read manufacturers' instructions.

Application of lightener for a full head

Preshampooing is not necessary unless the hair is oily, coated with sebum or anything else, such as excessive hairspray, dirt or dust which may stop or slow down the penetration of the lightener.

Preparation

1 Give the client a scalp analysis. Any cuts or small scratches will cause the client discomfort when the mixture is applied. Don't brush the scalp before application, for the same reason.
2 The client's clothes should be well protected with a cape and a towel around the neck.
3 Protect your hands – put on gloves.
4 Part the hair into four sections as shown in Figure 7.2.

Mixing the powder lightener

You will need:

- a plastic bowl;
- a measuring cylinder;
- a plastic spoon;
- an applicator brush;
- hydrogen peroxide;
- lightener.

Read the manufacturer's instructions. Four to six scoops of powder lightener to 60 cc of hydrogen peroxide are the usual proportions. Mix the hydrogen peroxide steadily, making sure that any lumps are removed and that the powder is thoroughly blended, especially at the bottom of the bowl. It is best to mix with a plastic spoon and not the tint brush, because:

1 you will get a better mixing consistency and mixing action;

2 you start application with a clean brush.

The lightener should be mixed into a smooth creamy paste. Mix and measure accurately.

Procedure

1 Start the application where the hair is darkest, usually at the back nape. (This is the area which has had least exposure to the sunlight.) Take 0.5 cm partings and, starting 2 cm away from the scalp, apply the lightener to the middle lengths and ends. If the ends prove overporous during the preliminary strand test, leave them till last. Apply the mixture generously with the brush to both sides of the mesh and work into the section with the fingers. The lightener is applied to the middle lengths first because the heat from the scalp speeds up the lightening action and so the roots take quicker.

2 Place the sections against each other but don't pack them against the scalp. Be meticulous and don't miss any hair.

3 Continue with each section, moving towards the front until the four quarters are covered. Check your work. Don't comb the mixture through the hair length.

4 When the hair starts to lighten (10 to 20 minutes), start to apply lightener to the roots. Starting at the darkest area, lay the mixture on quickly and methodically with the brush. Don't stab the brush into the roots, as this can cause discomfort and, possibly, inflammation. It is not advisable to keep dabbing over the same areas; you will start to take the mixture off the roots with the brush. Continue, finishing with the front top section. (This hair is usually slightly lighter because of exposure to sunlight and therefore more porous.) Keep partings small and check to see if you have missed any spots. If the ends were omitted at the start, because they are overporous, apply the mixture to them now. Pile the hair on top of the head but don't pack it down. The processing time will depend on:

a the strength of the hydrogen peroxide and the proportions of the mixture;

b the degree of lightening desired;

c the texture of the hair.

5 Leave for 10 minutes and do a strand test by wiping a small strand at the nape with cotton wool or tissue. If the hair is not light enough, reapply the mixture to this area. Test every 10 minutes. Avoid sliding the tail of the tint brush along the scalp as this will lift the mixture off and cause patchiness in the root area. Don't attempt to comb the mixture through and don't let it dry on the hair as this can cause hair damage. If dry, the mixture also stops working and a patchy result will be obtained. For this reason, using any form of accelerator, except perhaps a steamer, is not recommended. Steamers do, however, tend to leave the colour too warm.

6 When the hair has reached the required degree of lightening it is important that the mixture be removed correctly. Rinse all the powder mixture thoroughly from the hair; even though the mixture washes readily from the hair, it must still be shampooed out. Rinse and lather again to ensure that the hair is free from the lightener. A temporary rinse can be applied to silver the lightened hair. A conditioner or antioxidant can be applied after the final rinse to assist combing. Pat dry carefully and comb gently from the ends with a wide-tooth comb.

If you are slow in applying the lightener, a double mixing may be necessary as the lightener can become exhausted after 40 minutes or so. Mix only half the lightener first and then apply. Then mix the balance and apply again. This will give a uniform lightening action over the entire head.

Retouch application

Advise your client to have frequent retouches – every three to four weeks if the colour is dark, or four to six weeks if the colour is lighter. The mixing procedure and method of application are the same as for a full head except that less mixture is used, perhaps two or three scoops to 30 cc of hydrogen peroxide.

1　The mixture is applied to the root section only, starting at the darkest area, usually the back. It is important that you don't overlap the lightener onto the already lightened hair as this will cause a line of demarcation and make the hair more porous along this line. Any after-rinse which is applied will be more readily adsorbed into this line of demarcation. Keep the partings small. Check that you haven't missed any areas, especially along the front facial hairline and parting.

2　Ten minutes after the application has been completed, check for degree of lightening by gently wiping back the mixture with cotton wool or tissue. Scraping with a tail comb can cause damage. Reapply the mixture if the colour is not light enough or the result will be patchy.

3　It is not advisable to take the mixture through the rest of the hair; this causes dryness and creates a harsh feel if it is done at every retouch. If, however, after four or five retouches the colour starts to look muddy, mulch the left-over lightener (don't use a fresh mixture) through the rest of the hair and leave for the last 10 minutes of processing. Rinse and shampoo, ensuring that all the mixture is worked free from the roots and shampooed away. Condition and comb from the ends with a wide-toothed comb, preferably made of vulcanite as narrow plastic combs can stretch the hair.

Figure 7.3

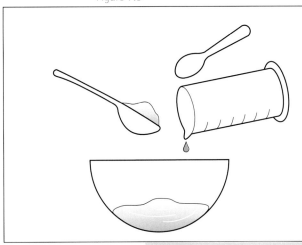

Thorough mixing

Mix the formula with a plastic spoon for a creamy consistency. Ensure that all the powder is mixed thoroughly with the hydrogen peroxide.

Figure 7.2

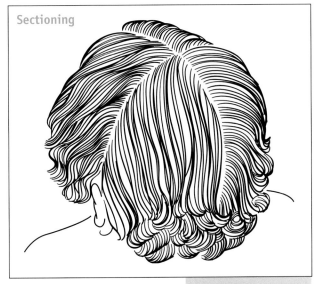

Sectioning

Section the hair into four parts.

General tips for lightening

1 Always ensure that products are fresh.

2 If in doubt, give the client a preliminary strand test.

3 Never use anything made of metal unless it has been anodised. The chemicals will react with the metal.

4 Protect your hands – always wear gloves when applying the mixture.

5 Always ensure that the hair and scalp are in good enough condition to withstand the chemical treatment.

6 If you apply a barrier cream to the client's forehead to protect his/her skin, make sure you don't get any cream on the hairline, as it will prevent the lightener from taking.

7 Keep all partings narrow – 0.5 cm.

8 Don't pack the hair down during the processing as this will inhibit the oxidation action.

9 Don't comb the lightener through.

10 Make sure the rinsing water is tepid and not too hot.

11 After applying conditioner, comb carefully from the ends and don't stretch the hair.

12 Always give the client advice on how to maintain the health and the condition of the hair.

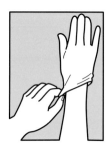

Prelightening for blonde toners (pastel tones)

There may be times when hair needs more extensive lightening and it is then coloured with a tint (toner). This may be done for a competition to show the line of the style or to meet fashion demands. It is a highly skilled technique, involving a lot of the hairdresser's and client's time. To ensure that the results will be satisfactory, you must consider:

* the correct amount of lightening for the toner selected;
* the selection of the correct toner;
* applying the toner correctly.

Obtaining toning results means prelightening the hair to either the gold, yellow or pale yellow stage and then applying the specially formulated, high fashion tint called a *blond* toner.

Prelightening

When you apply a prelightening mixture to the hair it does two things:
1 lightens the natural pigmentation of the hair;
2 makes the hair more porous.

For the application of blonde toners, the hair requires not only the right degree of prelightening but also the correct degree of porosity. Blonde toners are specially formulated tints, and they are not like usual tints. Nevertheless, they still require the precautionary patch test as they do contain para. They are very light and delicate and come in a range of colours, such as ash blonde, silver blonde, silver beige, champagne beige, platinum beige and silver platinum. They are sometimes iridescent. Manufacturers advise that these colours be mixed with a high volume of hydrogen peroxide, 30 or even 40 volume in strength. Be guided by the manufacturer's instructions as to how much prelightening is necessary. As a guide, the ash blonde range requires prelightening to either gold or yellow. Silver blondes need lightening to yellow and any platinum blondes (the lightest of them all) need lightening to the palest yellow or almost white.

Apply the lightener as previously described for a full-head application. The more porous the hair, the better the toners will take. Hair must be made sufficiently porous for the delicate toner result. Porosity can be achieved only by leaving the lightener on for long enough. If the hair is already naturally dark, say medium brown, then the length of time it takes to reach the gold yellow or pale yellow stage should also give the hair the required degree of porosity. If the hair is very dark, it may even need two applications of lightener. If the hair is naturally light, say dark or medium blonde, then it will reach the gold, yellow or pale yellow stage much more quickly. Often, while the hair is light enough for the delicate toners, it certainly may not be sufficiently porous. The lighteners should be left on the hair for approximately 50 minutes or one hour or more, not necessarily to make the hair lighter but to make it more porous.

You can now see how important it is to select the right lightening agent with the correct strength of hydrogen peroxide. Results can be disappointing if you lighten medium blonde hair with 30 volume hydrogen peroxide and a strong lightening agent as it may only take 20 to 30 minutes to reach the degree of prelightening necessary for the toner selected. While it may be light enough in colour, it will certainly not be sufficiently porous, so select a slow-acting lightener with a weaker hydrogen peroxide or the client will complain that the toner washes out and does not hold in the hair. As a guide, you can expect the hair to take less time to lighten than to reach the required degree of porosity. Oil lighteners are not recommended as they are not strong enough to lighten the hair properly or make it sufficiently porous. To determine if the hair is porous enough, you will need to give a preliminary strand test before applying the toner. If the hair is not porous enough, the colour will not be adsorbed.

Once you have achieved the desired amount of lightening and porosity, rinse and shampoo the lightener thoroughly from the hair. The hair should be towel dried. Don't apply conditioner (unless the hair has uneven porosity) as this will inhibit the toner action.

Figure 7.4

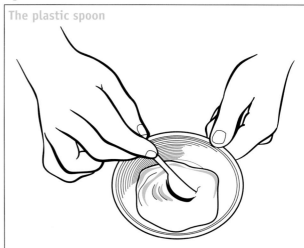

The plastic spoon

Always mix the formula with a plastic spoon. This will:
A ensure a good, thorough mixing;
B leave the tint brush clean to work with.

Figure 7.5

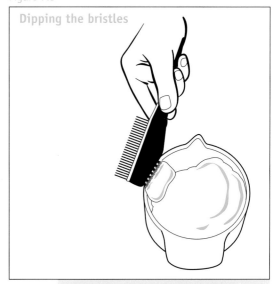

Dipping the bristles

Dip a third of the bristles of the tint brush into the formula. Wipe the mixture off one side of the brush against the rim of the bowl. The tint only needs to be on one side of the brush.

Preparing the blonde toners

Because of the many possible variations of the hair, you may not be able to tone it to the required shade. Very often there may be too many gold or warm reflects and ash shades may prove difficult to achieve. You, as the hairdresser, should have the final decision as to the choice of colour. It may even be difficult to lighten the hair to the required degree as some toners do need more prelightening than others. Remember, toners are para tints and still require the precautionary patch test.

Mixing

Read manufacturers' instructions. For a full head, one tube of blonde toner to 60 cc of hydrogen peroxide should be mixed thoroughly with a plastic spoon to a creamy consistency. Usually a stronger hydrogen peroxide is used to obtain the high-fashion iridescent effect.

Application

The lightener should be thoroughly removed from the hair and the hair left in a towel-dried state. Contrary to what you may assume, the toner is applied first to the roots of the hair, starting at the nape and working towards the front. The roots are done first because this is where the hair is going to be the most resistant, even though heat from the head will make the colour take more quickly. Once the toner has been applied to the roots, apply the remainder through the middle lengths to the ends. The ends of the hair are the most porous and therefore the toner will take more readily. Mulch through to the ends. Keep the partings small.

Don't pat the hair down but lift it. If the ends are porous, apply the toner to them only for the last 10 to 15 minutes. Check to ensure that no hair has been missed as this could cause patchiness in the final result. The toner will take in approximately 30 to 45 minutes. Strand test by drying a small strand in two or three areas of the head; re-apply the toner mixture if it has not reached the required colour. When the desired colour has been achieved, rinse and shampoo from the hair.

Retouch application for blonde toners

If there is a vast difference between the client's natural colour and the toner colour, regular retouches – every three to four weeks – are advisable. If the hair is left too long between retouches, it starts to build up resistance and the lightener needs to be left on the hair longer to obtain the required degree of porosity. If the client's hair is light in colour, retouches every four to six weeks should be advised.

Method

Lighten the new regrowth only, starting at the back. Don't overlap. This is important as the overlapped area will be more porous and will grab the toner; it could go dark if it has an ash base. Keep the partings as narrow as 0.5 cm. Check that no hair roots have been missed, especially around the front. Rinse the lightening agent out thoroughly and shampoo to make sure it is washed out of the hair. Towel dry.

Application of the toner

Patch tests should be given be fore the toner is applied.

Starting at the back, apply the toner to the prelightened regrowth only, with brush or applicator. Usually half a tube of toner to 30 cc of hydrogen peroxide is sufficient. For a good result, keep the partings narrow – 0.5 cm.

Check that all the roots have been adequately covered and leave the toner for between 20 and 30 minutes. If the mid-lengths and ends need freshening up, mulch the remaining mixture through the hair with the fingers. Shampoo can be added to form a colour bath. Don't comb the hair as this can pull and stretch it, especially while it's in a delicate, processed state.

Rinse, shampoo and condition when the desired colour has been reached.

Advice to the client on after-care

Hair which has been lightened and toned will need care and attention.

1 A general conditioner should be applied after each shampoo. A porosity filler will assist in hair combing.
2 The hair should be carefully combed from the ends after shampooing and conditioning and under no circumstances should it be brushed with a brittle brush while still wet.
3 Blow dryers should be used on a low or medium heat and, if the hair is set, rollers should not be the spike or brushed type but have smooth contours. Again the dryer must be moderate in temperature.
4 During the summer months, hair should be protected from sun and salt water. Wear a sun hat or, if swimming, a bathing cap.
5 Regular hair trimming will keep the porous ends from becoming frayed and damaged.

Removing unwanted colour tones from the hair – lightening problems

(Removing unwanted colour tones is further covered in Advanced Colour, Chapter 17)

As the hair is going through a considerable colour change, there may be times when some corrective work is needed.

Gold bands or spots

The hair is not porous enough and has not been sufficiently lightened in certain areas. These areas can be spotted with lightener before the application of the toner or, if time does not permit, it can be done at the next retouch. A double application of toner on these gold areas could temporarily overcome the problem. Apply the toner to the gold areas first and then again to the balance of the hair strands.

Ash bands or spots

The hair is overporous and the lightener has been left on too long or has been too strong. A porosity filler should be applied before the toner to make the hair uniformly porous. This will stop the toner grabbing and causing dark, drab areas. It can be difficult to assess overporous hair so a preliminary strand test may make these areas more noticeable.

Hair damage and breakage

This is caused by the hair becoming extremely porous and losing its elasticity to the extent that it feels very slimy and jelly-like when wet, and is easily broken when combed. It is the result of using a strong, lightening mixture with an excessive volume of hydrogen peroxide which reacts too quickly on hair which is fine and is perhaps naturally light. The mixture has been left on too long for the hair type. Don't continue to tone as this can cause more damage and breakage. Give protein conditioning treatments to revitalise the hair.

Figure 7.6

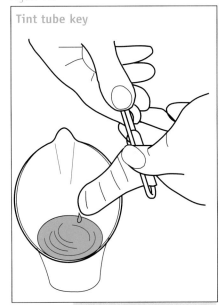

Tint tube key

Use a tint tube key to accurately measure the amount of tint required – a quarter, half or three-quarters of a tube. The key will ensure that no tint is wasted by being left inside the tube.

Tint back – colour fillers

If a client decides to tint back to his/her prelightened colour, a colour filler may need to be applied. As mentioned previously, when lightening, red, red gold and gold are removed from the hair. When returning to the client's natural hair colour you must put back the red, red gold or gold pigmentation. This is necessary in order to:

1 prevent the final result from looking khaki or matt;
2 help retain colour deposit;
3 maintain uniformity during development.

The intensity of the 'warmth' depends on the darkness of the client's natural colour. The lighter the natural colour, the less intense the warmth.

Apply directly over the prelightened hair from roots to ends. Do not be alarmed at the orange result (the client may be). Develop, then shampoo, rinse and dry. Now apply the natural colour in the conventional manner. The result will be deep, rich and natural. If the client has a lot of natural warmth this may just be added to the colour without the pre-application of a colour filler.

Figure 7.7

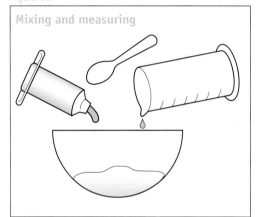

Mixing and measuring

Mix and measure all formulas accurately. A tint tube key and measuring the hydrogen peroxide with a cylinder will help. Mix the formula with a plastic spoon for a creamy consistency. Read the manufacturer's instructions.

Figure 7.8

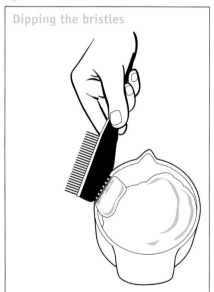

Dipping the bristles

Dip a third of the bristles of the tint brush into the formula. Wipe the mixture off one side of the brush against the rim of the bowl. The tint only needs to be on one side of the brush.

Questions

1 **a** Give three reasons why clients may ask for their hair to be lightened.

_____

_____

_____

   b Name two types of lighteners and the strength of hydrogen peroxide that is usually used with them.

_____

_____

2 Discuss the factors that determine the type of lightener and strength of hydrogen peroxide to be selected.

_____

_____

_____

3 **a** If you are in doubt as to what lightener and strength of hydrogen peroxide to select, what could help you decide?

_____

_____

   b List the changing stages that the hair will go through when a dark head of hair is lightened to a pale shade.

_____

_____

_____

4 **a** Give examples of when and why it may be necessary to shampoo the hair before the application of a lightener.

_____

_____

   b Describe the best way to mix the lightener formula.

_____

_____

5 **a** Describe the method of application used to lighten a virgin head of hair four or five shades from medium brown to dark blonde.

_____

_____

b Explain what lightening formula you would select.

6 **a** What factors will influence the length of time the lightener is left on?

b Give two reasons why it is important not to let the lightener dry out while it is on the hair.

7 **a** Describe how you would test to see if the hair has been sufficiently lightened.

b If you are slow in your application, what method can you adopt to ensure that the result is uniform?

8 Using diagrams, explain the chemical action of lightener on the hair shaft.

9 **a** What advice would you give to the client about the frequency of lightening retouches?

b Briefly explain your method of retouching, elaborating on two important considerations during the application.

10 Give an example of when it may be necessary to bring the lightener through to the mid-lengths and ends after a retouch application. Outline the method for this procedure.

11 a What is a blonde toner?

_____

b Name three factors on which blonde toners are completely dependent.

_____

_____

_____

c To what three stages does the hair require prelightening before the application of a blonde toner?

_____

_____

_____

d What stages of prelightening do the following blonde toners require:

i   ash blonde?

_____

ii silver blonde?

_____

iii platinum blonde?

_____

12 a What characteristic of the hair is important for the toner to take successfully?

_____

b How can this characteristic be reached on:

i   dark hair?

_____

ii light-coloured hair?

_____

13 a How are the blonde toners mixed?

_____

b What precautionary test should be given before their use?

_____

c Why does this test need to be given?

_____

14 How would you apply a silver blonde toner to hair which had been prelightened to Stage 5 (yellow)? Give your procedure and method.

_____

_____

_____

_____

15 Give your preparation and procedure for retouching a client's silver blonde hair if there is a 2 cm light brown regrowth.

_____

_____

_____

16 What advice would you offer clients in maintaining the health and condition of their lightened and toned hair?

_____

_____

17 What can cause the following problems when lightening or toning:

a gold spots or bands?

_____

b ash spots or bands?

_____

c loss of elasticity?

_____

d breakage?

_____

e overporosity?

_____

18 How can the following lightening and toning problems be either prevented, overcome or corrected:
a gold spots or bands?

_____

b ash spots or bands?

_____

c loss of elasticity?

_____

d overporosity?

19 What is the purpose of a 'colour filler'?

20 a What could be the final colour result if a dark brown colour were applied to yellow pre-lightened hair?

b What intensity of colour filler would be needed to prevent this result?

Highlighting and lowlighting using advanced techniques

Covering: frosting, naturalising, streaking, and multi-shading

Often a popular procedure, highlighting should give a natural, sun-streaked look to the hair and is particularly becoming on clients whose complexion is dark or tanned. Some clients want highlighting to give a lighter overall effect without having to have their hair retouched regularly.

Highlighting can take the form of:

- *streaking*: applying lightener to 6 to 10 specially selected areas, usually around the front;
- *frosting*: many fine strands lightened all over the head to give a lighter effect;
- *tipping*: similar to frosting but gives a lighter effect on the ends only;
- *naturalising*: a tortoiseshell effect, with high lightening and low lightening at one level with various reflects – chestnut, gold, auburn, ash, hazel, mahogany;
- *multi-shading*: using more than two shades in selected areas to enhance a cutting line or to emphasise a movement – a more marbled effect.

Apart from the fashion aspect, highlights can also be applied for practical purposes. If, for example, a client decides to grow out previously tinted or permanently coloured hair, highlights and low lights (darker streaks) can be used to blend in the regrowth. Streaking blends in with the natural hair colour and there is usually no noticeable regrowth line. Highlighting can be given two to four times a year without having to worry about overlapping.

Highlights are achieved by taking a mesh on a certain part of the hair and applying a lightener while allowing the remainder of the hair to keep its darker shade. It is not advisable to do exceptionally light highlights on dark hair.

The type of highlights required will influence what technique will be used. There are numerous ways to achieve highlighting effects but at this stage we will be using the cap method and the foil method.

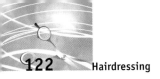

Cap method

The cap method of highlighting is used on short hair. Most salons have a frosting or streaking cap, which must be a snug, close fit. The cap is usually made of rubber and has prepunctured, self-sealing holes, so that the lightening mixture will not seep back through the hole when the mesh has been pulled through. There is also a lip around the perimeter of the cap to stop the lightener running underneath. You will have to determine the thickness of the hair strands – whether you are dealing with 'bold', strands or a fine subtle mesh. Be conscious of any discomfort you may cause the client when pulling the strands through the holes.

Preparation

Give a hair and scalp analysis. Protect the client with cape and towel. Dust the inside of the cap with talcum powder. This will help ease the cap on to the hair. Comb the hair into the desired style. A slight disadvantage with highlighting with a cap is that you limit the accuracy with which you can place the highlights.

Method

1 Pull the cap over the hair and secure it as firmly as possible. Try not to let the cap ride up on the hair.

2 With a fine crochet hook pull the hair through the holes (up to 100 strands can be pulled through). Take care not to push the crochet hook too far or you will puncture the scalp.

3 When all the selected areas have been pulled through the cap, comb the hair.

4 Mix the lightener into a firm smooth paste. A strong powder lightener is usually required with 20 or 30 volume H_2O_2. Apply liberally to the hair which has been pulled through the cap, mulching in with fingers. Don't comb the hair as this could damage it. Ensure that all the hair is covered sufficiently with the mixture.

5 Cover the cap with foil. This retains the heat and makes for uniform processing. (This retention of heat will be sufficient for processing.) Placing the client under an accelerator is not recommended. Although it will hasten the processing time, it may take the moisture out of the hair, causing dryness. Furthermore, it may cause the lightener to dry out. Remember – the faster the lightening action, the more damage it does to the hair. It's the speed of the action, not the action itself that does the damage. If you used 60 volume H_2O_2, the colour lightener may 'come down' in 10 to 15 minutes but at a cost to the hair condition. It is better to use 20 or 30 volume H_2O_2 where it takes 30 to 40 minutes to act but the hair is left in much better condition.

6 Once the desired lightening has been achieved, rinse off the lightener while the cap is still on. Then carefully remove the cap and wash the hair with shampoo formulated for lightened or tinted hair. Wash the cap thoroughly and dust it lightly with talcum powder. This will help preserve the cap and make it ready for use next time.

7 Create a hairstyle to complement the highlighted effect.

Foil method

The foil method involves covering the selected meshes in lightener and folding each one individually in a rectangular piece of foil. Precut tin foil for this technique is available from manufacturers. With this method you can be very selective as to where the meshes will be put; they can be put in the underneath sections as well as in the top layer. Foil meshes are also best suited to clients with long hair. There are various methods of taking the meshes but the most popular is the weave technique.

Preparation

Make sure that the client's hair is in good condition and discuss with the client the areas to be lightened. Usually, 20 to 60 meshes are taken and, as this is a lengthy and time-consuming process, the cost of the service should reflect this.

Method

1 Select your foil according to the hair's length. As a guide, the foil will need to be approximately 10 cm longer than the strand. The folded end is placed against the scalp. This folding helps to make the foil a little more secure and stable and reinforces it when handling. Stack neatly and don't crush. These small pointers are important for the success of the job.

2 Section the hair and trace a part across the back of the head, from ear to ear. Divide it into two and section the top. Ensure that sections are clearly divided so that the process is as accurate as possible.

3 Starting at the nape, weave approximately 6 to 10 fine meshes with your tail comb. Section 1 cm away from hairline and part this away. Stand in front of where you are working.

4 Take the aluminium foil strip (with the shiny side out). To assist you when you are learning, you can apply the lightener to the aluminium foil first as this will help the strand stick to the foil. Once you have mastered the foil technique, however, you will eventually be able to hold the foil flat against the scalp without applying the lightener to the foil first. Hold the strand down as far as your fingers will allow to control the foil and the hair.

5 Brush on the lightener, starting 1 cm from the roots (the depth of the prefolded end of the tin foil) and make sure all the strands are covered right to the end. Some methods allow for cottonwool to be placed at the roots to prevent the mixture from touching the scalp.

6 Now, using the ends of the tail comb, form a crease along the foil and fold it over across the foil. Try not to fold the hair inside the foil packet. Then fold the sides over, using the tail comb to make the creases; to ensure a neat packet, the end can be folded over once more.

7 Continue this method, working up from the nape, and complete the sides and top. If desired, small meshes can be left out in between the layers of aluminium foil

8 It may take up to 45 minutes to complete 40 to 60 meshes. During this time the meshes in the nape will have developed satisfactorily so these can be removed and rinsed once the top has been finished.

9 Don't use an accelerator on the meshes for the same reasons as previously outlined in describing the cap method. Also, if you used an accelerator, you would find that the meshes would expand as the lightener swells up and, if not packed correctly, could leak.

10 Shampoo and rinse, ensuring all the lightener is removed. A temporary rinse can also be applied to tone the hair. Dress to enhance the highlights.

With both the cap and foil methods, a permanent tint can be used instead of a lightener mixture. A wide variation of results can be achieved through highlighting – by applying the mixture to the ends or tips, or by applying to the hairline to create a halo effect which will emphasise the line of a cut. Other ways of multi-shading will be demonstrated and explained in Chapter 17.

Figure 7.9 (a–g)

Highlighting – the foil method

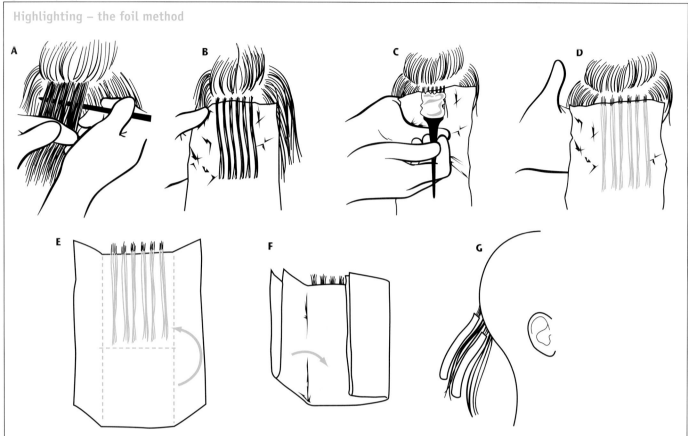

A Starting at the nape, weave approximately six fine meshes with the tail comb.

B Hold the aluminium foil and the hair strand as close to the scalp as possible.

C Apply the lightener to the strand 1 cm from the roots to the ends of the hair.

D Ensure that the whole strand is covered with the mixture.

E Using the end of the tail comb, form a crease along the tin foil and fold the sides and ends in.

F Form a neat packet. Avoid folding the hair inside the package.

G Depending on the individual head, take alternating sections of hair and packets.

Figure 7.10

Thorough mixing

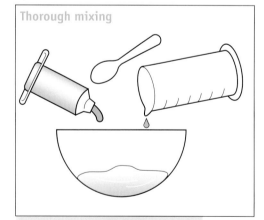

Mix the formula with a plastic spoon for a creamy consistency. Ensure that all the powder is mixed thoroughly with the hydrogen peroxide.

Figure 7.11

Dipping the bristles

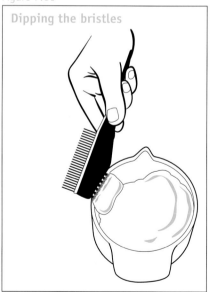

Dip a third of the bristles of the tint brush into the formula. Wipe off one side of the brush against the rim of the bowl. The tint only needs to be on one side of the tint brush.

Questions

1   To what does the term multi-shading refer?

_____

_____

2   Give two reasons why a client may ask to have his/her hair highlighted.

_____

_____

_____

3   a   What qualities should a highlighting cap have to ensure good results?

_____

_____

   b   What is the slight disadvantage in using a cap to produce highlights?

_____

_____

4   a   At what stage should the cap be removed from the head once the highlighting has been completed?

_____

   b   How should the cap be maintained to stop it deteriorating?

_____

5   Describe the method of highlighting using tin foil.

_____

_____

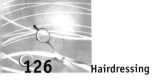

 # Removing unwanted additives from the hair – colour correction (colour stripping)

The standard method of removal of artificial colour (tints and rinses)

Sometimes clients will want artificial colour removed from their hair. This may be necessary for a number of reasons:

1 colour which has been applied repeatedly has built up and become dark;
2 the client wishes to lighten tinted hair a few shades;
3 there may also be times when you have selected colour which is too dark or when the wrong application technique has produced an unwanted dark result. You may even have read the colour label or colour chart incorrectly.

Sometimes shampoo will remove rinses, especially on grey hair. Three or four lathers of a concentrate shampoo should lift a temporary and semipermanent rinse. A temporary rinse on bleached hair may prove a little more stubborn as the bleached hair is more porous and accepts colour readily. If shampooing is unsuccessful, a useful tip is to try a bleach and water or bleach and shampoo solution. Some manufacturers offer 0 volume H_2O_2 and this can be used also. This can lift rinses that prove difficult to remove. It is not wise to use hydrogen peroxide by itself as it is difficult to control and will run down the hair strand.

Figure 7.12

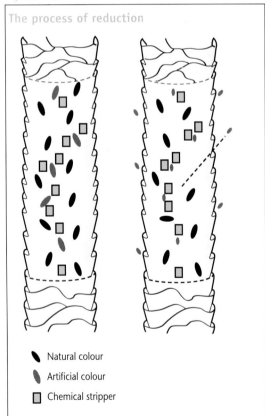

The process of reduction

- Natural colour
- Artificial colour
- Chemical stripper

The artificial pigment is reduced in size so that it can be washed out of the cortex.

Figure 7.13

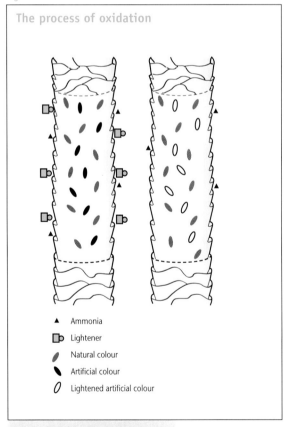

The process of oxidation

- ▲ Ammonia
- Lightener
- Natural colour
- Artificial colour
- Lightened artificial colour

The oxygen combined with the lightening agent gradually lightens the artificial pigment.

In most countries there are two methods available to remove artificial pigmentation in the hair. These are chemical colour stripping and bleaching.

Removing artificial colour requires skill and a careful analysis of the problem. It can be a difficult and time-consuming exercise for both the hairdresser and the client. Results may not always be predictable and this should be made quite clear to the client before the treatment begins. Analyse the hair and decide on the best method for the job. Be sure the hair is in good condition and not overporous. Check the scalp for scratches or abrasions. Determine what products have previously been applied to the hair. A decomposition test (1–20) will determine if a metallic dye has been used. If in doubt, do a preliminary strand test.

Chemical colour strippers – reduction

Most major hairdressing manufacturers produce chemical colour strippers. These products are especially manufactured to remove, either partially or completely, the unwanted artificial colour in the client's hair. Be sure to read carefully the manufacturer's instructions before using such products. Chemical strippers are usually mixed with water or hydrogen peroxide. Some have the slight disadvantage of leaving an unpleasant smell in the hair. This can be overcome by an after-rinse of 60 cc of warm water and a few drops of essence of lavender or peppermint. The chemical action involved in chemical stripping is called reduction. Reduction is the shrinking of the artificial colour molecules to such an extent that they can be washed out of the cortex and cuticle. It is the opposite chemical action to tinting where the artificial colour molecules swell. However, if a colour stripper is mixed with H_2O_2 the chemical process is by oxidation.

Bleaching (alkaline) oxidation

Oil and cream bleaches are generally used to remove artificial colour from the hair, as such bleaches are usually mild, slower in action and gentle on the hair. The stronger powder bleaches may be used where colour build-up is excessive and even then two applications may be necessary. Generally, 10 or 20 volume hydrogen peroxide is used with oil or powder bleaches. The chemical action involved is oxidation. Oxidation is the O_2 (oxygen) from the hydrogen peroxide combining with the bleach to gradually lighten the artificial colour.

Chemical colour strippers and bleaches which are mixed with hydrogen peroxide should be watched carefully because if they are left on too long or are mixed too strongly they not only lift the artificial pigment from the hair but also the natural pigment. These same formulas also have a tendency to leave warm or gold shades. Because of this it is difficult to obtain ash or cool colour results after using such products.

The product and technique you choose will be dependent on the problem you are facing. Choose one of the following:
- shampooing with a concentrated strong shampoo;
- using bleach and water (shampoo or 0 volume H_2O_2);
- chemical colour strip with water;
- chemical colour strip with 10 or 20 volume hydrogen peroxide;
- a mild oil or cream bleach and 10 or 20 volume hydrogen peroxide;
- stronger powder bleaches and 10, 20 or 30 volume hydrogen peroxide.

If you are in doubt as to what to use, give the client a preliminary strand test.

Figure 7.14

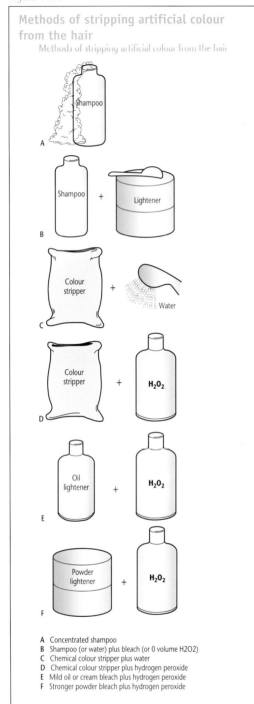

Methods of stripping artificial colour from the hair

A   Concentrated shampoo.
B   Shampoo (or water) plus bleach (or 0 volume H$_2$O$_2$).
C   Chemical colour stripper plus water.
D   Chemical colour stripper plus hydrogen peroxide.
E   Mild oil or cream bleach plus hydrogen peroxide.
F   Stronger powder bleach plus hydrogen peroxide.

Method and procedure for colour removal

1   On dry hair, apply the solution with a narrow fibre brush, to the darkest areas first. Allow to lighten before applying to the rest of the hair.

2   Leave the regrowth until last or leave it altogether if it does not require lightening.

3   Keep the sections small – 0.5 cm.

4   Once the application has been applied to all the hair strands, test frequently. The texture and degree of lightening will determine how long the solution is left on. This could be anything from 5 to 30 minutes.

5   Unless the client wants to change the natural colour, it's unnecessary to lighten beyond the red gold or gold stage.

6   If gold or warmth remains after the procedure, use an ash colour to tone down. Be aware that ash reflects do darken the final result.

Be sure to shampoo, rinse and dry the hair if a colour is to be applied after colour removal. Be aware that some manufacturers' instructions advise that after using a chemical stripper, recolouring should not be done for five to seven days. If the correct formula has been used and the application has been correct, it may not be necessary to recolour after the colour removal treatment. The hair will be porous after colour removal treatment, so condition it to maintain hair health. In some cases corrective work will be necessary, especially if the hair has patchy colour build-up on which spot lightening may be required.

Advise the client on hair care after colour removal and on the importance of going to a professional hairdresser for future hair colour treatments.

Practical exercises

1   Using a large cut strand of hair, tint the strand two shades darker. Divide the strand into three and try to determine the best method to return it to its original colour. Put the results of your exercise in your folder.

2   On a strand of bleached hair, apply a temporary fashion rinse and try:
   • shampooing;
   • bleach and water (or shampoo or 0 volume H$_2$O$_2$);
   • a chemical stripper
   to remove the rinse.
   Write the findings in your folder and attach the bleached strand.

Questions

1 Why may it be necessary to remove artificial colour?

_____

_____

_____

2 **a** Which two methods can be used to remove stubborn artificial pigmentation?

_____

_____

b What chemical action is involved in each of these two methods?

_____

_____

3 Hair can have unpleasant odours, especially after certain colour removals. How can these odours be eliminated?

_____

_____

_____

4 Name and describe the method of testing to establish whether a metallic colourant has been used on the hair.

_____

_____

_____

5 Using diagrams to illustrate your answer, explain what chemical action takes place when lightener is used to eliminate artificial pigmentation.

_____

_____

_____

_____

6 Describe the chemical action of the product which is especially formulated to remove artificial pigmentation only. Simple sketches should be used to illustrate your answer.

_____

_____

_____

7 Which two factors will influence the length of time the preparations (formulas) are left on?

_____

_____

8 What can be used if too many gold tones remain after colour removal? What important factors should be remembered when correcting this problem?

_____

_____

_____

_____

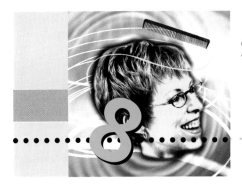

Straightening and relaxing the hair

In this chapter, you will learn about:

- relaxing a permanent wave;
- straightening the hair permanently.

Straightening and relaxing the hair

Relaxing and straightening over-curly hair is the reverse of permanent waving. There are a number of different ways to carry out this procedure and the techniques used will depend on the type of hair your client has, and the extent to which the hair needs to be relaxed or straightened.

Analysis

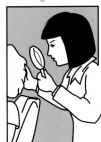

You must analyse:
- the texture of the hair – fine, medium, coarse;
- the porosity of the hair (poor on afro hair, good on permed hair!);
- the general condition of the hair, e.g. dry, fragile, weakened or processed;
- whether the hair is naturally curly or permanently waved;
- the scalp condition – abrasions, scratches or cuts;
- the hair's elasticity.

Generally, naturally curly, afro, coarse strong hair is the most difficult to straighten or relax. Fine-textured hair which has been permanently waved too curly is easier to relax, but requires extra care and attention. (Bear in mind that there will be some natural relaxation of the permed curl two or three shampoos later on.)

There are two methods.

1 Thioglycollic acid (permanent wave solution, approximately pH 7 to 8). Best for **relaxing** a permanent wave.
2 Sodium hydroxide (caustic soda, approximately pH 9 to 10) – a chemical hair straightener. Best for **straightening** strong curly or afro hair.

The techniques for the two methods involve combing the hair straight with a wide-tooth comb or winding the hair around large rollers.

The use of thioglycollic acids (thios) – relaxing

The method using thioglycollic acid is best suited for relaxing a permanent wave.

Thioglycollic acid can be mixed with fine powder (e.g. talcum powder, magnesium powder or cornflour) to form a loose paste. The paste physically aids the relaxing action. Mixed with a paste the hair may not need to be combed as the paste will hold the hair in a relaxed position.

As with the permanent wave procedure, relaxing involves the breaking of the di-sulphide bonds (reduction) and the rehardening of them by neutralising (oxidation).

Preparation

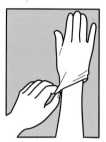

Determine the amount of curl to be relaxed. Ensure that the hair is in good condition and that the client does not have any cuts or scalp abrasions. Read the manufacturer's instructions. It is best not to try to relax a permanent wave which is over-processed. This hair is already fragile and may be damaged. Such hair may need treatments combed through to aid relaxation.

Figure 8.1

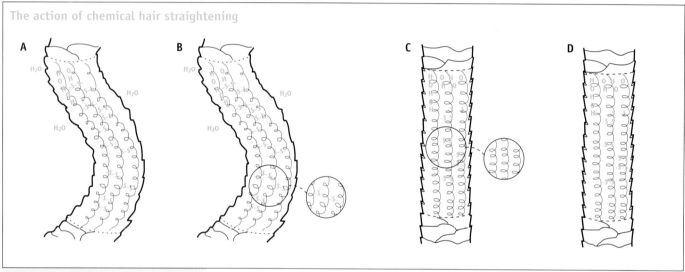

The action of chemical hair straightening

A Virgin curly hair

B The thios reduce the S bond from cystine to cysteine; that is, they break the di-sulphide (–SS–) link.

C The neutraliser is poured through the hair after it has been smoothed and straightened. This adds oxygen to the hydrogen atoms and rejoins the di-sulphide (–S–S–) links.

D Excess water and neutraliser are removed from the hair, leaving it straight.

Figure 8.2

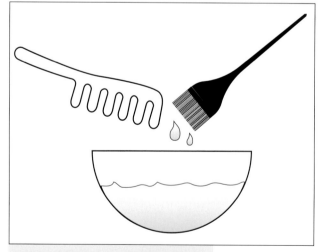

The straightener must be put into a non-metallic container – use a plastic bowl. Apply the straightener with a tint brush and comb it through with a wide-tooth comb.

Procedure

1 Shampoo the hair with a mild, soapless shampoo if the hair is dirty or greasy. Alternatively, the solution can be applied to dry hair. Comb the hair through and divide the hair from forehead to nape and across the nape. Starting at the nape, apply the solution to the hair strands from the roots to the ends, as shown in Figure 8.3. Gently comb through with a wide-tooth comb. Don't pull or stretch the hair from the roots.

2 Continue section by section, taking 1 cm partings up the back of the head and the sides. Don't get the solution onto the client's scalp. If a magnesium powder has been added to the solution, it will not be necessary to continuously comb the hair straight. This powder stiffens the solution, keeping the hair straight. If magnesium powder has not been added, it will be necessary to comb the hair gently during processing. Don't saturate the hair with solution or the solution will run onto the scalp and could burn it.

3 Once all the hair has been combed straight, leave it undisturbed. As a guide, the length of processing time will depend on the hair's texture and porosity. Normal to resistant hair will require 15 to 20 minutes of processing. Fine and porous hair may take from 5 to 15 minutes. Check to see if the hair is sufficiently straightened by wiping a strand with damp cotton wool. Reapply if the strand shows too much curl.

Neutralising

1 When the hair has been sufficiently straightened, rinse the solution out. Be extra careful not to disturb the straightened hair. Rinse thoroughly for five minutes. Ensure that all the solution is washed out. Blot dry carefully to remove the excess water, being careful not to disturb the straightened hair. Now apply the liquid neutraliser with the applicator nozzle, soaking the hair length thoroughly.

2 With a wide-tooth comb, comb the hair very carefully to distribute the neutraliser throughout the entire strand. Leave the neutraliser for the time indicated on the manufacturer's instructions (approximately five minutes) to ensure that the hair is completely neutralised.

3 Rinse the neutraliser from the hair with tepid water and apply an antioxidant conditioner or porosity filler.

4 Either set the hair on large metallic rollers with large sections, taking care to wrap the ends neatly and clip correctly, or blow-dry the hair. Dry set under a medium temperature dryer and comb or brush carefully into the desired style without stretching the hair. This technique of relaxing is suitable for hair with a natural curl which needs loosening, or hair which has been permanently waved too curly. A mild solution and a short processing time are usually required. Sometimes this type of hair can be relaxed sufficiently on extra large smooth rollers using a permanent wave solution. Don't use the plastic spike or brush type of roller. Remember also it is also important that you don't try to relax a permanent wave which has been over-processed as the hair will be damaged even more.

The use of sodium hydroxide – chemical hair straightener

For hair which is naturally very curly, strong or wiry, a chemical straightener incorporating sodium hydroxide can be used. This is usually called a cream straightener.

Background

Read the manufacturer's instructions carefully and follow them explicitly. Failure to do so can result in damaged or broken hair or the client being burned. If in any doubt, do a preliminary strand test or seek advice from the firm's technical representative. These chemical straighteners are usually strong alkali and should not touch the scalp or skin, especially the ears. Keep them well away from the eyes. It is not advisable to use this chemical straightener on fine, weak hair as this can cause damage and breakage. Damage can also result from misjudging the quality and texture of the hair or the processing time, or from stretching the hair unduly. The product straightens the hair by swelling the fibre and breaking the di-sulphide bond. This relaxes the polypeptide chain.

Preparation

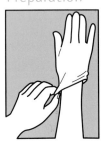

Check for cuts or abrasions and apply cream protection (such as vaseline) if necessary. The hair is not usually shampooed before a cream straightener is used. Part the hair into sections from forehead to nape and small 1 cm sections across the nape. Put the straightening cream into a plastic bowl (the bowl must be non-metallic). Apply the cream with a tint brush.

Method

Beginning at the nape, apply the cream with a tint brush to each 1 cm section at the roots, making sure no cream gets onto the scalp. Comb the hair through with a wide-tooth comb once or twice to distribute the cream. A wide-tooth comb is essential to ensure that the hair is not stretched. Proceed to the next section. Continue section by section, taking 1 cm parts, until all the hair is covered with the cream. Sections can be gently combed into each other. Once the head is covered with the cream, it is not advisable to comb or disturb the hair.

Some hairdressers comb the hair onto cardboard strips which physically assist the straightening procedure. As each mesh is taken, cardboard is placed underneath the mesh and the hair combed straight onto this. The cardboard strips can be left in place or taken out and used again on the next mesh. The cardboard may hold the hair in the straight position but it is difficult to comb the hair if the card is left in.

The processing time varies from 5 to approximately 20 minutes, depending upon the amount of relaxing required, the porosity and the hair texture. As a guide:
- resistant, strong, coarse hair – 20 to 30 minutes;
- porous, normal hair – 15 minutes;
- fine hair – 5 to 10 minutes.

Be guided by the strand test during the processing. Check the hair for curl reduction by the way the curl is being removed or relaxed.

Rinsing and neutralising

Rinse the cream out carefully with warm water, on a medium force, without stretching or disturbing the hair unduly. Shampoo the hair lightly with an acid shampoo. Remove excess water by towel blotting. With an applicator bottle, saturate the hair with neutraliser. Some manufacturers advise careful combing with a wide-tooth comb while applying the neutraliser. Leave on according to the manufacturer's instructions. Rinse all the neutraliser carefully from the hair and apply an antioxidant conditioner. Comb through carefully and set or blow-dry the hair. Advise the client how to care for the hair by regular conditioning and careful treatment.

General advice and precautions

1 Make sure the hair is correctly analysed and in good condition.
2 When using chemical straighteners, you must follow the instructions.
3 If in doubt, do a preliminary strand test on the client's hair at the central nape area.
4 Physically straightening the hair by setting it on large rollers without any form of relaxing chemical can relax the curl sufficiently, but this straightening is only temporary. This may be all that is necessary, however, on permanently waved hair which is slightly too curly.
5 Straightening retouches can be done by applying the cream only to the regrowth. Don't bring the product through to the mid-lengths of the hair.
6 With naturally 'afro' hair, it is difficult to get the hair extremely straight. This type of hair can benefit from perming on very large perm rods, to relax and soften the tight curl.

Note

If it is in good condition, afro hair may benefit from two straightening processes done in quick succession (perhaps in the same week). This may get the desired degree of straightening required by people who have afro hair.

After-care

Both services, relaxing and particularly straightening, can be harsh on the hair. The client will need to be advised on the best products to help maintain the condition and health of the hair. Manufacturers will have such products. The client should be advised on how to handle the hair; for example, to avoid excessively hot blow-drying, harsh or severe brushing, stretching the hair while combing and swimming in heavily chlorinated pools. The hair should be conditioned after every shampoo.

Figure 8.3

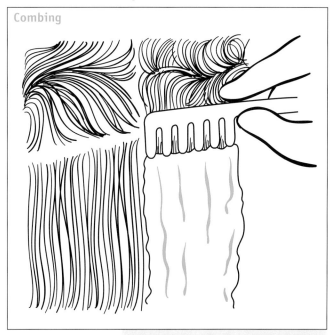

Combing

Gently comb the solution through the hair with a wide-tooth comb; don't pull or stretch the hair from the roots.

Questions

1 **a** What are the two chemical methods of curl reduction?

_____

_____

   b What points need to be analysed before their use?

_____

_____

2 How would you go about relaxing the curl on a head of hair that was permanent waved too curly? Outline your approach and procedure.

_____

_____

3 Using diagrams, explain the chemical action of hair straightening.

4 **a** Can you attempt curl relaxing on permed hair which has been overprocessed? Explain your answer.

_____

_____

_____

   b What advice would you give and what steps would you take to remedy this problem?

_____

_____

_____

5 What method of curl reduction would you attempt on the following types of hair:

   a Naturally curly 'afro' hair which is strong and wiry?

   _____

   b Permed hair which has been overprocessed?

   _____

   c Medium textured curly hair?

   _____

   d Hair which has been permed too curly?

   _____

   e Finer hair with a strong wave?

   _____

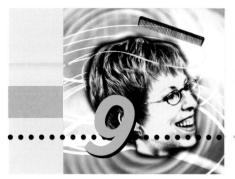

Diseases, disorders and conditions of the hair and scalp

In this chapter, you will learn about:

- contagious and non-contagious disorders of the scalp;
- dangerous infestations of the hair and scalp;
- male-pattern baldness.

Disorders and conditions of the scalp

Advise, don't treat

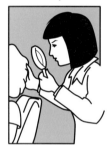

In your first year you were told that, as a hairdresser, you would inevitably come across scalp and hair disorders. You can advise on and suggest treatment for some of the more common hair and scalp complaints, such as dry and oily hair and simple dandruff. There are other, more serious disorders that you should be able to recognise, but in such cases you should tactfully recommend that your client visit a pharmacy or doctor. You are not expected to treat these more serious problems.

Dandruff (Pityriasis simplex)

This common and socially embarrassing condition results from a scaly accumulation on the scalp, caused by the massing of dead skin cells from the epidermis. These cells are not easily removed or shampooed out of the hair or scalp. Generally powdery, they flake onto the shoulders, and can make the hair become dull and unattractive. Do not confuse dandruff scales with the consequences of hard water or shampoo or sprays which may dry the hair. Dandruff can cause some clients embarrassment.

Having dandruff does not mean that the client is unclean. It is important to remember, however, that although dandruff is not contagious – you won't catch dandruff if you touch someone who has it – any pathogenic bacteria found in association with dandruff may be transferable. For that reason, you must wash all tools and implements after using them on the client. Seborrhoeic dermatitis and *pityriasis simplex* are closely associated and may even co-exist.

If there is a heavy coating of scaly accumulation on the scalp, advise the client to see a trichologist or dermatologist. In cases of mild scaling, you can brush the scalp and then use an antibacterial, medicated shampoo. These usually have a tar, zinc or sulphur smell and contain preparations which loosen the scales. They have a mild antiseptic action. Products such as Crisan, Kerastase, MDF, Selsun and ZP1 1 are effective, though for various reasons one may work for an individual whereas others in the range are of no help at all. The control of dandruff may only require more frequent shampooing to remove excess scales.

Ensure that the scalp does not become too inflamed as a result of using harsh medicated preparations. These can also destroy the skin's own antiseptic bacteria, and this, in turn, can cause other irritating problems.

If *pityriasis simplex* is allowed to develop and is not kept in check, then a more advanced waxy, greasy dandruff can occur. This is known as *pityriasis dermatitis*. The scales are yellow in colour, large (about the size of a little fingernail) and are quite firmly attached to the scalp. There may be an odour as the scales are so waxy. Don't attempt to treat this but recommend the client see a pharmacist, doctor or trichologist.

Psoriasis

Although this is a problem which requires attention, it is a non-contagious disorder. It is recognised in the early stage as a reddening of the skin, either on the scalp or even the face. Later on, scales which are silver-grey in colour develop. Eventually, these become thick, crusty and yellow, and quite hard. The scales tend to be firmly attached to the scalp, but some are so dense that they flake and get trapped in the hair. In its later stages, psoriasis is not a pleasant condition to handle or to look at.

Treatment is still at the research stage, and the disorder is thought to be brought about by a number of circumstances, such as nerves or stress. There is also evidence that the disease can be hereditary. Take a sympathetic attitude and be discreet and tactful. There is no reason to refuse clients service in the salon, although tools, towels and equipment should, as always, be adequately sanitised. Don't attempt to remove or interfere with the crusty scales in any way. Reassure the client and recommend that he/she visit a doctor. Psoriasis also occurs on the elbows and knees.

Seborrhoeic dermatitis

The boundaries between psoriasis, steatoide pityriasis and seborrhoeic dermatitis can often be vague.

Seborrhoeic dermatitis is one of the most common disorders of the scalp. As its name suggests, seborrhoeic dermatitis is the result of an overproduction of sebum. The condition usually appears as a fine, diffuse, dry, yellow scaling of the scalp. In more active cases, the symptoms may range from a greasy, scurfy scalp to a red, inflamed scalp with infecting bacteria. The condition can spread to the forehead, eyebrows and sides of the nose. This condition should not be treated in the salon; recommend that the client see a doctor.

Pityriasis steatoide

If simple seborrhoeic dermatitis is not treated effectively and the client does not maintain adequate scalp hygiene, *pityriasis steatoide* could develop. This is a more advanced greasy, waxy, scaly scalp condition. One area of the scalp may be particularly scaly – on the crown or behind the ears, for example. Quite thick, the scales are the size of a small fingernail, greasy and yellow in colour. They are attached to the scalp but also flake off in the comb. Although dandruff in itself is not contagious, the bacteria associated with this condition may be transferable. Clients can receive normal service but you must ensure that all tools and equipment are thoroughly cleaned afterwards.

Figure 9.1 (a–c)

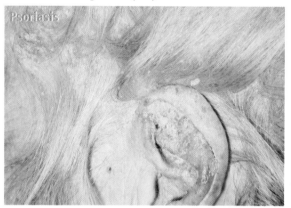

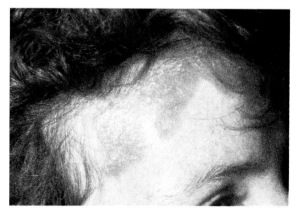

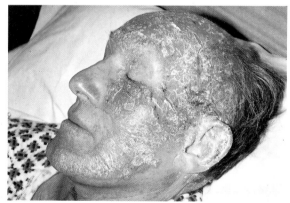

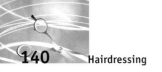

Figure 9.2

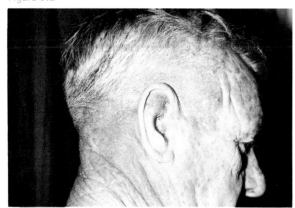

Impetigo

These are sores on the skin, primarily on the face, which start from broken skin or a bite. If hygiene is not practised, they erupt into blisters, forming scabs which prevent the poison (pus) or fluid escaping. The sores spread because of scratching and are easily transferred from person to person by contact.

Dangerous infestations of the hair and scalp

Animal and vegetable parasitic infestations

A parasite is a living creature which depends completely on its host – the person it is living on – for survival. Parasites on the skin or hair are referred to as infestations. They are all highly contagious, i.e. they can be transferred from one person to another either directly or indirectly, by means of contact or via infected tools and equipment.

You must be able to recognise parasitic infestations before the client receives any service, to prevent the disease from spreading from client to hairdresser and hairdresser to client.

Clients with parasitic infestations must be refused service of any description (as outlined in the Health (Hairdressers) Regulations). Be particularly discreet in your scalp analysis. Although you must not appear to be searching for infestations, you must bear in mind that all clients are susceptible. Tactfully recommend that any such client visit a doctor, pharmacist, or community health nurse. Don't attempt to treat the infestations yourself, although some hairdressing manufacturers do have shampoo treatments available. Ask the agents for more information.

Vegetable (fungal) parasitic infestation (*microsporum canis*)

Tinea capitis (*capitis* means 'of the head')

This highly contagious infection is commonly referred to as ringworm of the scalp. The sufferer will have isolated inflammatory sores in more than one area of the scalp. The affected areas will have broken stubs of hair causing round, balding patches of unclean appearance. The ringworm digests the keratin of the hair. The comb breaks the weakened hair which is then the carrier of the infestation. Other means of spreading the infestation are unclean towels, hats and brushes. Animals – cats, dogs, hedgehogs, cattle and guinea pigs can also carry and spread the ringworm; the new family kitten is often the culprit. Tinea is also seen in the nails. Advise the client to see a pharmacist, doctor or community health nurse.

Figure 9.3 (a and b)

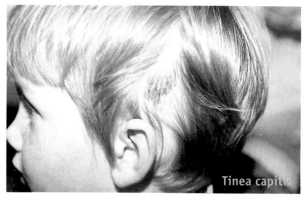

Tinea capitis

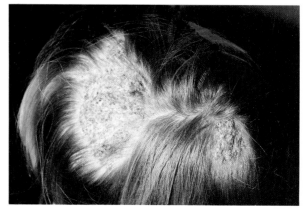

Animal parasitic infestations

Pediculosis capitis – infestation by the head louse

Head louse infestation (*pediculosis capitis*) is a common disease, which appears to be increasing; the head louse is, after all, a social creature, which loves to travel and loves a warm environment with human beings. During the Middle Ages social conditions sank to such low levels that infestation by insects and vermin became part of daily life. An indication of the deplorable state of personal hygiene is evident in some rules for the deportment of nobility which expressed disapproval of the habit of cracking lice or fleas in public. Lice have been parasitic on humans for a long time.

- *Appearance and life cycle.* Lice are wingless, blood-sucking insects with powerful legs. They vary in colour from an off-white to a greyish black, and inhabit that region of the hair nearest the scalp, within a centimetre of the scalp surface. They are usually found at the nape of the neck and behind the ears. The eggs are laid close to the roots of the hair, adhering to the hair shafts by a quantity of cement-like substance. It is the eggs' ability to stick firmly that helps us to identify the lice. Even when the shells are empty, they will grow on up with the hair. The eggs and shells are known as nits. They are 0.88 mm in length and white in colour. The nits take approximately eight days to hatch and the lice live for another ten days or so. The complete life cycle is approximately $2^{1}/_{2}$ weeks. Female lice lay approximately seven eggs per day. The lice feed on the blood of the scalp.

Figure 9.4

- *Preventing the spread of infestation.* The bite of the pediculosis causes inflammation and irritation. If it is scratched, this can cause secondary infection, such as impetigo.

All socio-economic groups can be susceptible to head lice infestation although community nurses find a higher incidence among schoolchildren from large families with poor hygiene standards, as compared with children from uncrowded areas with better hygiene, housing and income. Suggest that clients with head lice contact a community health nurse, pharmacist or doctor.

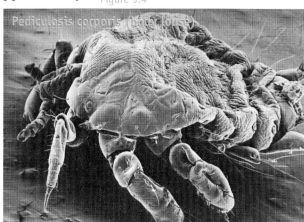

Pediculosis corporis (body louse)

Compare this to the head louse.

Scabies – the itch mite

Itch mites are very small insects which bury into the skin of the epidermis. They are noticed in the folds of the wrist or between the fingers; it is here that they lay their eggs. Small red blisters about the size of a pinhead appear under the skin, and when the eggs hatch they are seen as black spots under the skin. Because of the irritation it is impossible to avoid scratching, especially when the skin gets warm. This opens up the burrows and causes secondary skin infections such as impetigo or boils. Itch mites are spread by contact with an infected person or by using communal towels or other articles used by them. Advise the client to see a community health nurse, pharmacist or doctor.

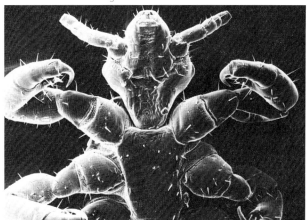

Figure 9.5

An 'awesome' creature which takes a meal of blood twice a day.

Figure 9.6

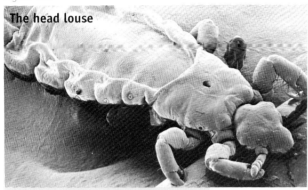

The head louse

'Those I catch, I throw away, Those I don't, I keep.' The holes along the side of the louse are called spiracles. They lead to breathing tubes (trachaea) which branch through the animal and carry oxygen directly to the cells. When the hair is washed these spiracles close – water and shampoo have no effect on the insect.

Figure 9.7

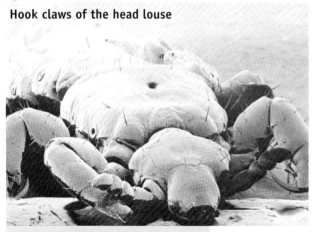

Hook claws of the head louse

Note the head louse's hook claws with which it attaches itself quite firmly to the hair and skin.

Hair disorders (non-contagious)

- *Trichoptilosis.* This is the technical term for split hair which is caused by drying hair in front of an electric heater, brushing it when wet with an incorrect brush or not having it cut.
- *Trichotillomania.* This is the pulling out of one's own hair. Young children have the habit of unconsciously twisting and pulling the hair around the fingers, and thus pulling it out.
- *Fragilitas crinium.* Fragile, brittle hair, easily broken, caused especially by overbleaching.
- *Concretion or plica neuropathica.* This is matted hair which cannot be untangled. Hair can become concreted after overbleaching or as a result of a lack of hair hygiene. Children's hair is particularly susceptible if it is not brushed.
- *Trichorrhexis nodosa.* In this defect affecting the hair shaft, nodules cause the hair to become split and frayed.
- *Pili torti.* The hair shaft is twisted on its axis at intervals and usually breaks off short.
- *Ringed hair.* A rare condition. The follicle produces pigmented or grey hair, intermittently.

Alopecia (hair loss)

- *Alopecia areata.* The loss of hair occurs in patches which are smooth, round and glossy.
- *Post-partum alopecia.* This is a temporary loss of a mother's hair after childbirth.
- *Diffuse alopecia.* This is loss of hair or a recession of the hairline found in women. The hair loss is usually diffused, i.e. it is not concentrated, it is spread out.
- *Alopecia totalis.* A more severe case of *alopecia areata*. Hair from the entire scalp is lost.
- *Traction alopecia (alopecia compressio).* Tight pigtails, braids and particularly cornrows can cause hair loss on the front hairline.
- *Alopecia universalis.* Total loss of hair from the head and body can be caused by medication (chemotherapy) or a disease of the follicles.

Male-pattern baldness (MPB)

Many, many products through the ages have claimed to prevent hair loss and to help replace lost hair – and all of them have been unsuccessful. There have also been countless theories as to why men go bald and women do not. Pressure caused by hats, mental stress, dietary habits and circulation problems are a few of the theories that have been put forward, but the question still remains: why men and not women?

Figure 9.8

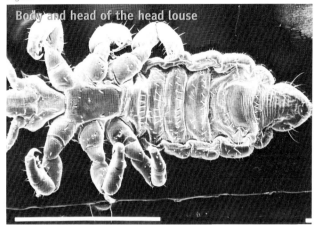

Body and head of the head louse

This photograph shows clearly the head louse's body and the claws by which it clings. The white line equals 1 mm.

Figure 9.9

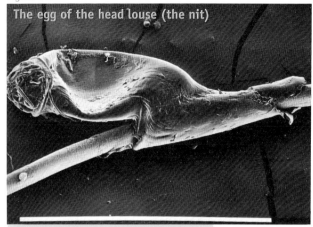

The egg of the head louse (the nit)

The white line equals 1 mm. Note the adhesive cement that keeps the nit firmly attached to the hair shaft.

Figure 9.10

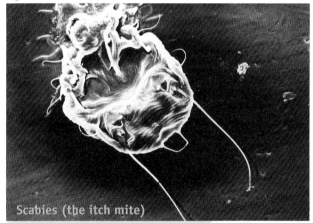

Scabies (the itch mite)

The adult mite buries into the skin where it lays its eggs.

Figure 9.11

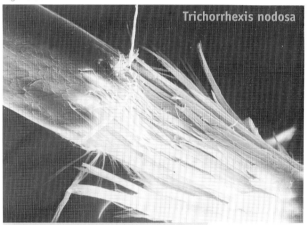

Trichorrhexis nodosa

This photo shows the broken nodules along the hair shaft.

In some Eastern (Arab) countries, men wear hats or turbans all the time, yet hair loss is not at all common. Women in the workforce are put under the same stress as males yet they don't lose their hair.

The dietary habit theory is interesting. Mexican, Inuit, Japanese and African people who live in their countries of birth don't have a high rate of baldness. This may be because of their dietary habits, since when they adopt Western eating habits, they become 'sleek' bald. What they eat may have an influence on their hair growth. However, there has been no conclusive research to prove a direct relationship between any of the above and MPB. The answer is that male pattern baldness is brought about by hereditary traits – it is inherited from either parent. This means that little can be done to prevent it. You only have to inherit the MPB gene from one of your parents to have this type of baldness. Although heredity is the main factor determining MPB, there is one other factor involved: this is the level of your male sex hormones which is also influenced by heredity. We all have both male and female sex hormones. The level of each differs from individual to individual, and is often determined by hereditary factors. Men produce a greater amount of the male sex hormone and women produce a greater amount of female sex hormones.

Figure 9.12

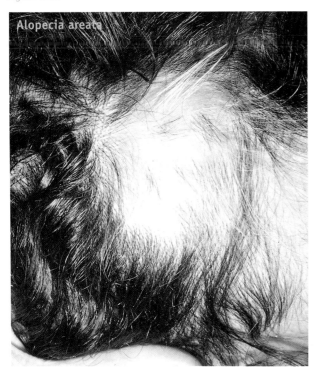

Alopecia areata

For MPB to occur in individuals who have inherited this trait, the hair follicles in question must be stimulated into regression – the hair becomes shorter and finer – by a particular level of male sex hormone. This level falls within the average range for men but well above the average range for women, which explains why MPB is rarely exhibited by women. Equally, male sex hormones are necessary for the development of female hirsutism, i.e. body and facial hair. Although little can be done to 'cure' MPB, the drug Minoxidil (Regaine) has been a recent treatment. This treatment is only prescribed through a doctor or dermatologist and is still at the research stage. There are also clinics which offer hair transplants.

Because of its hereditary origin, there is no cure for male pattern baldness.

Figure 9.14

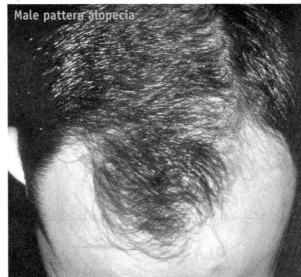

Male pattern alopecia

This client, although only in his early twenties, is already showing characteristic signs of male pattern baldness. There is a marked thinning of the hair at both the temples and the crown.

Figure 9.13

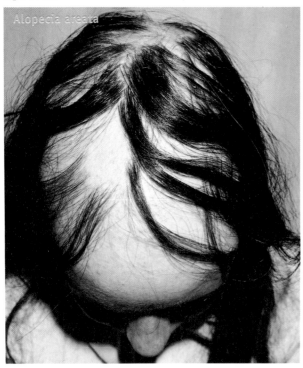

Alopecia areata

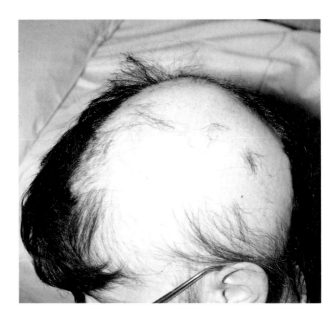

Figure 9.15

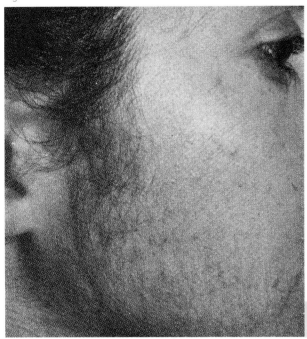

Hirsutism of the face and neck

Questions

1 **a** Briefly describe psoriasis.

_____

   b Is it contagious?

_____

   c Would you offer treatment?

_____

2 **a** What is seborrhoeic dermatitis?

_____

   b How is it recognised?

_____

3 **a** Is impetigo contagious?

_____

   b How is it recognised?

_____

4 Name two hair and scalp diseases where the sufferer must be refused salon service.

_____

_____

5   Name a scalp disease caused by:

a   a fungus;

_____

b   an insect.

_____

6   What is another term for:
a   ringworm?

_____

b   pediculosis?

_____

7   a   How would you identify ringworm?

_____

b   What advice would you offer a client suffering from ringworm infestation?

_____

8   Why is it important that the hairdresser should be able to recognise parasitic infestations?

_____

9   What is the first sign of the head louse before it becomes an infestation?

_____

10   Briefly describe the life cycle of the head louse.

_____

_____

11   Describe
a   _trichoptilosis;_

_____

b   _trichotillomania;_

_____

c   _fragilitas crinium._

_____

12   Name and describe three different types of alopecia.

_____

13   What is male pattern baldness (MPB)?

_____

14   What causes the tendency to have male pattern baldness?

_____

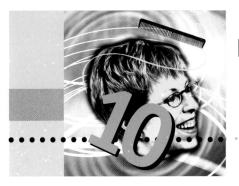

Physiology

In this chapter, you will learn about:

- nerves, and blood vessels of the head;
- the blood.

Nerves, and blood vessels of the head

Physiology is the study of the working functions of the body. Nervous activity and blood flow are physiological functions, and professional hairdressers need a fundamental understanding of the importance of nervous activity and blood flow in the face and scalp.

Although you may not use most of the terms associated with physiology in the hairdressing salon, you may read about them in other hairdressing books or hear them at demonstrations or seminars dealing with hair care.

A background knowledge of physiology will give you a better understanding of the functions performed by the body and will give you more confidence and proficiency in carrying out hairdressing services.

Nerves

One of the body's internal communication systems is the nervous system, made up of nerves which originate in the spinal cord and brain and are distributed throughout the body.

Nerves are important in the body because they transmit information from our senses. They are plentiful and they are found very close to the surface of the skin. Their endings finish in the papillary layer of the dermis, just under the epidermis. Some nerve endings, especially those concerned with sensation, are actually found in the epidermis. The brain receives and sends information along these nerves. As an example, touch – say the nerve endings at the fingertips – tells the brain that a surface is smooth, rough, hot, cold, and so on. Sight, hearing and smell are other senses which send impulses along nerves to inform the brain. Nerves are also involved when we move, i.e. they control the muscles that make us move our fingers to use scissors and perform other hairdressing skills. These nerves are found more deeply in the skin and inside the muscles. The spinal cord and brain core are important in controlling these muscles. If, for example, we cut or nick a finger with the scissors, two nerve pathways will be involved – a sensory nerve pathway and a motor nerve pathway.

1 The sensory nerve pathway informs the brain that a finger has been cut and that there is pain.
2 The brain (via the spinal cord) sends information along motor nerve pathways which control the muscle in the finger. This completes the circuit, and the finger is pulled away. This, understandably, happens very quickly.

The two types of nerve involved are:

1 sensory nerves, which send messages from the senses to the brain;
2 motor nerves, which send messages from the brain to the muscle.

The arrector-pili muscle is contracted using these two pathways. The body will inform the brain that it is cold (sense) and the brain will pass the message to the muscle (motor) to contract and try to retain the body's temperature. The skin gets goosebumps. All this is involuntary action; you can't control the arrector-pili muscle – you can't will it to contract and cause goosebumps. Unfortunately, the goosebumps are not sufficient to retain body heat as we are not hairy enough; the same principle works in a bird when it fluffs up its feathers to keep warm, by trapping insulating warm air.

All hair has nerves, which surround the base of the hair and are also attached to the hair root below the skin's surface. Pull out or stretch your hair and the sensory nerves tell the brain of feeling. A sensitive cat's whiskers operate in the same way. The hair is an extremely sensitive organ of touch; touch your hair with an object such as a comb and your scalp will feel the sensation.

All our nerves need food and energy to function. The sweat, or sudiferous, glands of the body are also controlled by nerves.

Massage to help nerve fatigue (tiredness)

We can become tired for a number of different reasons. Two of these are discussed below.

1 Physical tiredness – when the muscles (controlled by motor nerves) have been working hard because of manual activity. This activity burns up energy, because the nerves and muscle need energy to function. Fatigue-producing acids tend to linger in muscle tissue.
2 Mental tiredness – results from excessive mental activity, and from stress, worry or tension. Again, all this burns up energy. (Undue worry or mental stress can also cause other problems.)

Adequate dietary habits can help to maintain energy resources, but rest and relaxation can also help relieve tiredness. Scalp massage can assist greatly. It has a toning, soothing, relaxing effect on the nerves and muscles, and can relieve tension and sometimes even a headache. The blood flow to the nerves increases, which, in turn, supplies more energy. If food supplies nourishment to the blood, it is natural to assume that the blood nourishes all tissues, including nerves. Blood and lymph (mainly waste/fluid drainage) flow can be increased by hand or electric scalp massage. Some clients have even been known to fall asleep in the salon chair, because the massage has been so relaxing. Massaging the neck and top of the shoulders is also beneficial for tired nerves.

Nerves of the head and face

Concentrate your massaging on the sensory and muscular parts of the head and face.

Figure 10.1

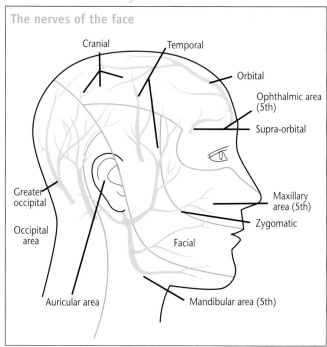

The nerves of the face

Figure 10.2

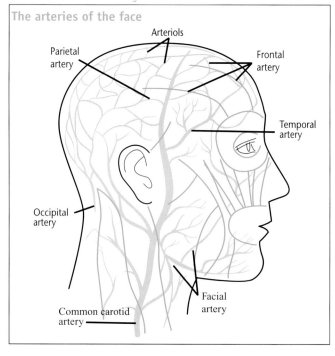

The arteries of the face

In this area the fifth cranial nerve – the senses – includes the eyes, eyelids, eyebrows and between the eyes (orbital), the side of the nose (nasal), and around the ears (auricular).

The seventh cranial nerve – the motor (muscles) – includes the base of the neck and shoulders, the muscles of the temple (temporal), the forehead (frontal) and the cheeks (zygomatic).

 ## The blood

The blood gives the body the nourishment it needs to perform the functions that are required for daily activity, mental and physical. The blood is circulated through the body by the pumping action of the heart.

The blood that reaches the head is necessary to feed the scalp hair, follicles, sebaceous glands and arrector-pili muscles as well as the nerves so that our senses can function. The blood reaches the head via large blood vessels called arteries.

The carotid arteries are the main source of oxygenated blood supply to the head. You can feel them on both sides of the neck, pumping blood to the head. The common carotid arteries on each side divide into the internal carotid and external carotid arteries, which divide again and supply certain areas of the head and face with blood nourishment, mainly the occipital, temporal and facial portions.

An adequate supply of blood helps to keep the hair and skin healthy and supple. This supply can be increased by scalp and face manipulation.

Once all the nourishment fluid has been used by the head and face, it must return to the heart so that it can be pumped to the lungs and digestive system to gather a fresh supply of nourishment and oxygen.

The blood returns to the heart from the head and face by means of the jugular vein. The jugular has two major branches – the internal and external jugulars – which run down each side of the neck alongside the carotid arteries. The jugular carries used, deoxygenated blood back to the heart.

Questions

1   a   From which two areas of the body do the nerves originate?

_____

_____

   b   What are the various branches that nerve endings divide into, called?

_____

2   Name and describe the two different types of nerve ending found in the skin.

_____

_____

3   a   Are any nerve endings found in the epidermis?

_____

   b   Give four examples of the types of sensation that nerves can register.

_____

_____

_____

   c   Where else are nerves found?

_____

_____

4   What is meant by nerve fatigue and how can it best be relieved?

_____

5   a   What organ is responsible for circulating the blood through the body?

_____

   b   Name the blood vessel that supplies blood to the head, neck and face.

_____

   c   Where does the blood collect fresh oxygen?

_____

d What are the differences in the types of blood that arteries and veins carry?

_____

_____

e Name the blood vessel that carries the blood from the head, neck and face back to the heart.

_____

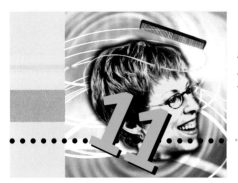

Advanced styling and setting
Introduces: 'Set the hair for complex styles'

In this chapter, you will learn about:

- directional setting;
- practical exercises;
- competition hairdressing.

Directional setting

In the first year of your apprenticeship, you were taught how to put rollers in the hair. In this chapter you will learn how to put the rollers in the hair to achieve a specific line or design. This type of roller control is called directional setting. The rollers (cylinder or conical) and pincurls are placed according to the way the style is finally to be dressed. Directional setting follows the contours of the head and the hair's natural growth pattern. It is used both in everyday salon styling and for more elaborate and sophisticated evening styles or competition styling. It should also be used in your end-of-apprenticeship practical examinations.

Directional setting involves the movement of lines throughout the hair, from the roots to the ends. These lines can move in two ways: straight lines and curved lines.

Straight lines

Straight lines are not bent or curved. Shapes made up of straight lines are: rectangles, triangles, squares and diamonds.

Cylinder rollers are placed in straight lines and shapes.

Curved lines

Curved lines are rounded or bent – no part of such a line is straight – so that they form a curve. Curved lines can move either clockwise or anti-clockwise. Shapes made up of curved lines are the various parts of a circle: a whole circle (eight sections), a half circle (four sections) or a quarter circle (two sections), ovals and oblongs.

The wet hair is curved around to form these shapes. Conical rollers, if available, are used in curved lines and shapes. The conical roller helps to force the finished line to become curved. Conical rollers are not, however, readily available in many salons so cylinder rollers will do, although they do not enforce the same degree of curved movement.

Roller control using straight lines – cylinder rollers

Straight volume rollers will give the hair bulk, fullness, height or lift. The hair is wound over the roller as it is being rolled towards you. The finished result depends on where the roller sits in relation to the size of the section or base. The different types of straight volume rollers are described below.

Straight volume – on base

This roller sits squarely on its base, which is the same depth and length as the strand being wound. It will give uniform fullness, height and lift, and is considered the perfect roller for volume. It can be used on any part of the head where fullness is desired. It is the roller control most frequently used in the salon.

Straight volume – overdirected

This roller is directed to sit high on its base and is usually wound at a 90° angle (or more) from the head to achieve the overdirection.

The overdirected roller will give the greatest amount of volume, height, lift and bulk. The degree of overdirection depends on how much volume is required; the more it is overdirected, the greater the amount of volume achieved. The base size is the minimum of the roller diameter and can be as much as $2\frac{1}{2}$ times the roller diameter. The angle at which the roller is wound and the size of the base both determine the degree of overdirection. Overdirected rollers are usually placed in the crown area. Avoid using them on the front hairline as they will leave gaps and parts.

The hair is wound over the roller and sits over or above its base. Overdirected rollers also collapse much more quickly because of the volume they produce.

Straight volume – underdirected

Straight volume underdirected rollers are the opposite of straight volume overdirected rollers; they reduce and give the least amount of volume, lift, height or bulk.

The roller is rolled and positioned sitting under its base although it can also sit half on its base or inside on the bottom of its base. The depth of the base and the angle at which the roller is wound from the head will influence the amount of volume. Again, base sizes can be as great as $2\frac{1}{2}$ times the diameter of the roller. The hair is generally wound less than 90° from the head form, so that the roller sits under its base. Don't be confused by the term under when underdirecting; the hair is still wound over the roller but sits under its base.

Straight indentation

Indentation is the opposite of volume. It doesn't give volume, lift, height or bulk but causes a 'dent' or recess in the hair – a hollow effect. To achieve the dent or hollow, the size of the base must be at least $1\frac{1}{2}$ times the diameter of the roller, although it can be more. The hair section is combed flat against the scalp and the roller is rolled away from where you are standing. If the hair is wound around the roller more than $1\frac{1}{2}$ times, the hair will come back on itself. If the hair has not been wound around the roller more than $1\frac{1}{2}$ times, the hair will roll up.

Figure 11.1

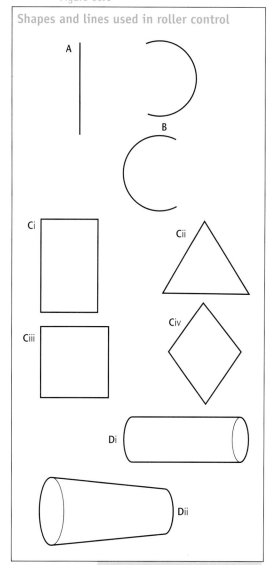

Shapes and lines used in roller control

A	straight lines
B	curved lines – clockwise and anti-clockwise
C	**(i)** oblong
	(ii) triangle
	(iii) square
	(iv) diamond
D	**(i)** cylinder roller
	(ii) conical roller

To summarise, the different types of straight line roller control are:

- straight volume on base;
- straight volume overdirected;
- straight volume underdirected;
- straight indentation.

Figure 11.2

Circle shapes

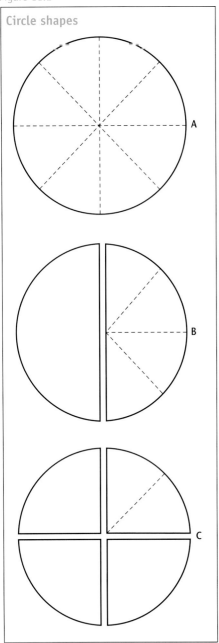

A The full circle – 8 rollers.
B The half circle – 4 rollers.
C The quarter circle – 2 rollers.

A Hold the hair slightly towards the starting point.
B Wind down with even tension. When finished, the narrow end of the roller will be one diameter away from the starting point.

Figure 11.3a

Roller control

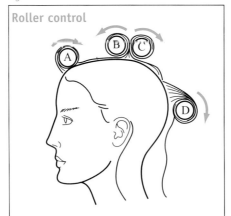

Note: Sections indicated by dotted lines.
A Straight volume – on base: for perfect volume.
B Straight indentation – base size $1\frac{1}{2}$ times the diameter of the roller: for a hollow effect.
C Straight volume – overdirected: for maximum volume.
D Straight volume – underdirected: for reduced volume.

Figure 11.3b

Roller control

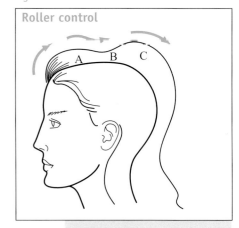

A Volume.
B Indentation.
C Volume.
Note: B (indentation) If the hair is wrapped at least $1\frac{1}{2}$ times around the roller it will roll back on itself.

Figure 11.4

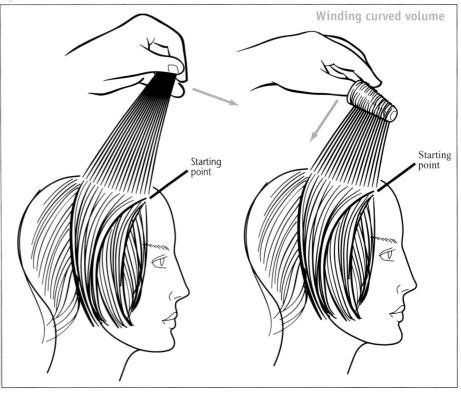

Winding curved volume

Starting point

Starting point

Roller control using curved line – conical rollers

When using conical rollers, always observe the following rules.

1 Place the clip at the narrow end. This will enforce the curved shape, like clipping a fingerwave in the same direction as the trough which enforces the wave.
2 The narrow end of the roller is always wound at least one diameter away from the starting point.
3 Overdirecting conical rollers, especially on the hairline, can leave parts and gaps. Don't overdirect conical rollers.
4 Hold the roller slightly forward of the starting point to spread the hair uniformly across the roller as it is being wound.
5 The roller should sit parallel to the parting.

Curved volume – on base

The base is triangular with curved end (one-eighth of a circle) and is the same length and diameter as the roller. It is wound on base. If the hair is wound around the roller more than $1\frac{1}{2}$ times, the hair will fall into an 'S' wave.

Curved volume – underdirected

The base size is generally larger than the diameter of the roller and is wound at a less-than-90° angle from the contours of the head. The hair is wound over the roller, towards you, but the roller sits under its base.

Curved indentation

The base size is a minimum of one times the diameter of the roller. The roller is wound with the narrow end of the roller facing toward the wide end of the base. It is wound up and away from where you are standing. It is still clipped at the narrow end. Indentation will give a hollow, dent or recess with a flare at the wide end of the roller.

Base sizes

In addition to being influenced by the roller type, the finished effect of a roller can be influenced by the size of the base and where the roller sits in relation to the base. Base sizes can be (a) one, (b) one-and-a-half, or (c) two times the diameter of the roller. The roller can be positioned:

a within its base parting;
b half off base;
c completely off base.

You can see that if base sizes, roller position and roller type are taken into account, there are many different roller control variations possible. For example, let's take *straight volume underdirected*. This roller control type can also be:

i one diameter base size – half off base;
ii one diameter base size – completely off base;
iii one-and-a-half diameter base size – positioned within the base partings;
iv one-and-a-half diameter base size – half off base;
v one-and-a-half diameter base size – completely off base;
vi two diameter base size – positioned within the base partings;
vii two diameter base size – half off base;
viii two diameter base size – completely off base.

The general principle in the result of these roller positions is that the bigger the base, the less the volume; the further off its base, the less the strength.

The same situation as set out above exists in the case of many of the other roller types.

> **To summarise, the different types of curved line roller control are:**
>
> - curved volume on base;
> - curved volume underdirected;
> - curved indentation.

Figure 11.5

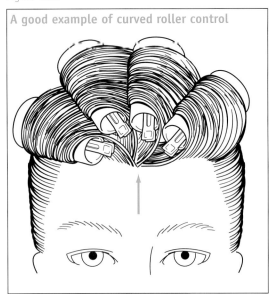

A good example of curved roller control

A All the rollers come from the arrowed starting point.

B The rollers are clipped at the narrow end.

C The rollers are one diameter from the starting point.

D The four rollers are in a half circle.

Never overdirect curved volume or an unavoidable break or part in the hair will occur.

Designing a style using straight and curved lines

When designing a hairstyle, the aim is to develop a working plan, so you need to draft a pattern. This pattern is the arrangement of shapes which is to become the artistic construction. You must build the design using the various shapes associated with straight and curved lines.

Try to make up patterns out of shapes on the head into which you put the rollers. Shapes such as squares, rectangles, triangles, diamonds and the various parts of a circle (half circles or circles) need to be scaled out on the head and the rollers must be put in to fit these shapes.

When you change the design of a hairstyle, you must change the shapes which make up the design. If you change the parting from left to right or flick the hair around at the front instead of under, this changes only the arrangement or ornamentation, not the pattern (design). Changing the pattern (design) means changing the shapes into which the rollers must be put.

How the rollers are put into the straight and curved shapes

Any of the four straight line rollers can be placed in the straight shapes.
- *Square shapes*: one length cylinder rollers in either volume or indentation.
- *Rectangular shapes*: one length cylinder in either volume or indentation.
- *Triangular shapes*: cylinder roller one quarter and one half and full size in either volume or indentation.
- *Diamond shapes*: two triangles put together – one quarter and one half and full-length rollers in either volume or indentation.
- *Curved lines*: conical rollers if possible.

Any of the three curved rollers can be placed in curved shapes, but in the diagram (Figure 11.6) curved volume on base rollers have been used.

Comb the hair around to form the curved shape. Take the sections from the starting point with the tail comb. Ensure that there is only one starting point.

If the hair is wrapped around the roller more than $1^1/_2$ times, the hair will come back on itself and form an 'S' wave. If it is not, it will form a curl.

Figure 11.6

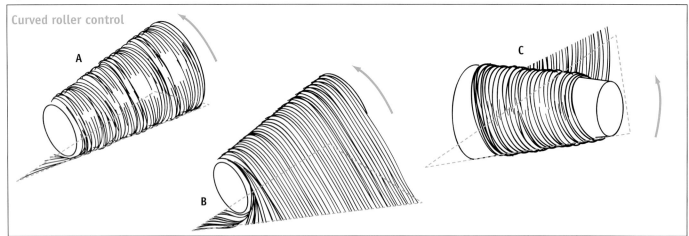

Curved roller control

A Curved volume on base.
B Curved volume underdirected.
C Curved indentation.

Practical exercises

Setting the hair in various shapes

This section deals with putting rollers in shapes that are a little more difficult than the elementary 'straight shapes' you were taught in your first year. We will deal here with mainly curved shapes (i.e. half circles, large and small ovals, and oblongs). Conical rollers should be used for these shapes but if your salon has not got this type of roller then cylinder rollers will do.

To help enforce the shape of the curved lines, always secure or pin the roller at the end closest to the starting point. Once you have mastered putting the rollers into these shapes, the next step is to learn how to combine these shapes. For example, you can combine a large half oval with a rectangle, or a diamond with two triangles.

There are many combinations but in this section we will discuss two variations – you can do your own if you wish.

Do the exercises on different parts of the head and vary the size of the rollers you use. Observe the effects you get when you brush out the shapes.

Putting rollers into shapes – I

Large oval shape

This exercise requires the positioning of eight rollers in an oval shape. All roller bases are one diameter base size.

Rollers one, two, three and four can be positioned on base; rollers five, six and seven can be positioned half off base, and roller eight (half length roller) can be positioned off base.

Note the dots (Figure 11.7) which represent where the partings are taken from. All rollers are at least one diameter away from their starting point.

This large oval shape takes up a good proportion of the side and top of the head. Remember, if the hair has been wrapped more than $1^1/2$ times around the roller, it will form a wave.

Oblong shape

The rollers in the oblong shape are 'edged'. That is, the rollers are only placed in the second direction of the oblong shape. The first part of the 'C' formation is left untouched and the roller is positioned on the lower portion of the 'C' motion.

Note where the conical end of the roller goes (if you are using conical rollers) (Figure 11.9). Also, note the angle of the roller. This correlates with the sectioning for the roller position.

Ensure the hair is wrapped a minimum of $1^1/2$ times around the roller if you want a wave formation.

Half-circle workshop

This half circle (Figure 11.10) is positioned at the side of the head.

Distribute, mould and scale the half circle. Place five rollers into the shape: the first two rollers on the base; the third underdirected, the fourth half off the base, and the last roller off the base.

Set one half-circle with rollers around which the hair is wrapped more than $1^1/2$ times, and a half circle with large rollers around which the hair is wrapped less than $1^1/2$ times.

Include an indentation roller as another exercise. Place the indentation roller on a base at least $1^1/2$ times the roller diameter and place it where the half-off base roller and off-base roller are positioned. This indentation roller will

Figure 11.7

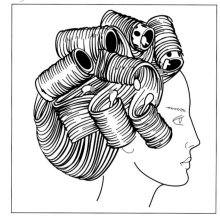

Figure 11.8

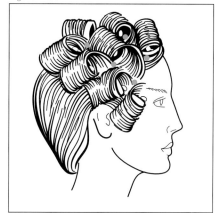

Figure 11.9

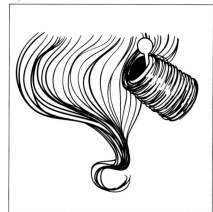

produce a hollow or depth effect. Remember to place the narrow end of the conical roller (if you have used one) away from the starting point.

This type of setting pattern is used frequently in setting the hair over to the side. You need to determine how much hair comes onto the forehead and how much comes back off the face. This will influence where the starting point will be.

Small oval shape

Set two small half ovals, one at the top of the head and one at the side. The small oval is set in rollers that are of different lengths. This enforces the shape. Half rollers are placed at the 'tight' end of the small oval.

- Side-small oval: start at the larger end and work toward the tighter end. As in the half circle shape, place the first two full length rollers on base, the third roller underdirected. The fourth roller should be half off base, and the last half length roller should be completely off base.
- Top-small oval: start at the tight end and work toward the larger end. Place two half length rollers on base. Then place a full length roller underdirected, half off and off base.

Figure 11.10

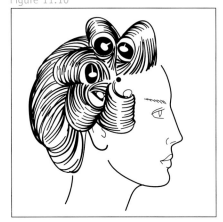

Figure 11.11

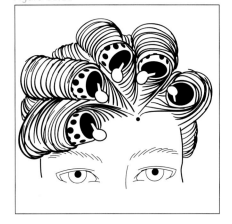

Figure 11.12

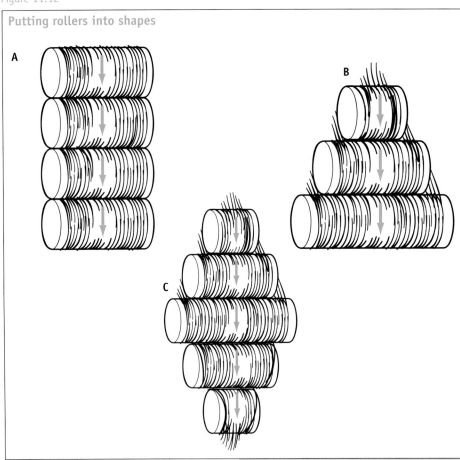

Putting rollers into shapes

A rectangle shape – same size rollers
B triangle shape – half, three-quarter and full size rollers
C diamond shape – half, three-quarter and full size rollers

Practical setting exercises

1 Practise putting the following roller control in the hair on either a manikin or a model.

 a Triangle shape – three straight volume on base rollers in a triangle.

 b Rectangle shape – three straight volume overdirected rollers in a rectangle.

 c Square shape – three straight volume underdirected rollers in a square.

 d Rectangle shape – three straight indentation rollers.

 e Half circle – two curved volume and the third a curved indentation roller in a half circle.

Place under a dryer; when the hair is dry and the rollers are removed, you will see more clearly the differences between the various patterns. Note how they sit, how much volume each produces. Observe the difference between indentation and volume, and the direction in which the curved lines move in relation to the straight lines.

2 Scale off the head contour into shapes. Set the hair in rollers, incorporating 15 pincurls into the shapes.

Dressing out

When the rollers have been set precisely, using volume and indentation, you will be assured of ease in the final combing out.

Using a half-round or flat bristle brush, brush in the same direction as the rollers have been set. Move the hair from the roots, lifting and brushing it firmly in the final direction that the hair is to be dressed. To create finish, use a small dressing-out brush.

Hold the hair strand firmly at the starting point of the shape and direct the hand and hair strand in the direction it is to be dressed. At the same time, force the brush underneath the section and push to form a cushion of hair at the base. This will give volume at the roots and establish some direction. This technique is called *directional back-brushing*.

Figure 11.13 (a and b)

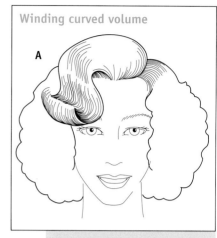

Winding curved volume

A

When winding curved volume, if the hair is wrapped $1\frac{1}{2}$ times around the roller, the result will be a wave movement (A). If this is not done, a curl movement will result (B).

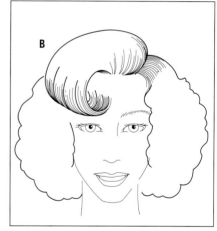

B

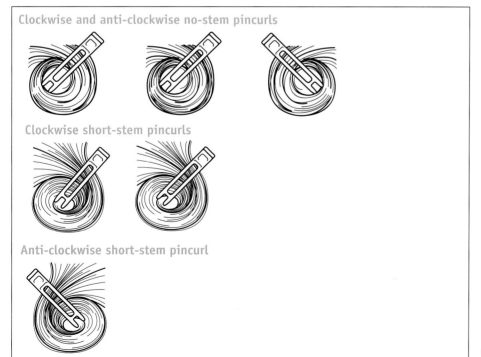

Clockwise and anti-clockwise no-stem pincurls

Clockwise short-stem pincurls

Anti-clockwise short-stem pincurl

Figure 11.14 (a-f)

Figure 11.14 (g-k)

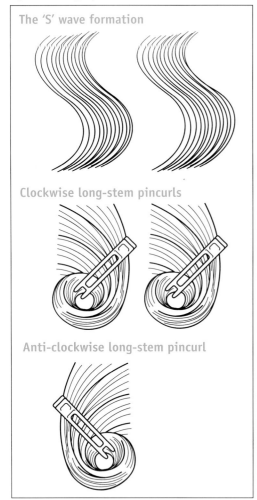

The 'S' wave formation

Clockwise long-stem pincurls

Anti-clockwise long-stem pincurl

Figure 11.15 (a–c)

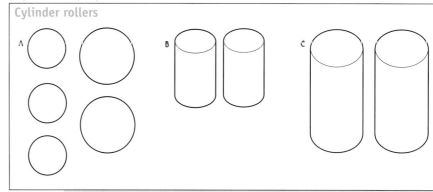

Cylinder rollers

A Circumference of the rollers
B Half size
C Full size
Copy and place these shapes and the pincurls on pp. 159–160 onto the head forms on pp. 162–165 to create a style. Get your art tutor to check your work. Now practise the styles on your manikin or 'client'.

Figure 11.16 (a–c)

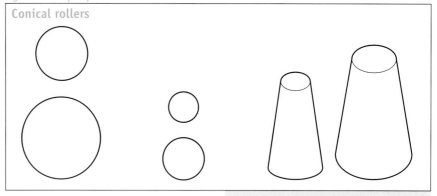

Conical rollers

These are full and half size, showing circumference.

If more volume is needed, hold the hair further away from the head while forcing the roots away with the dressing-out brush. Ensure that all the hair strands are both interlocked at the roots and combined at the ends. Once sufficient directional back-brushing has been done, brush the top surface of the hair. Again, see that all the hair strands are both interlocked at the roots and combined at the ends. Follow the direction and pattern that the rollers have been placed in.

If the first pli has been well directed and planned, a minimum of back brushing and combing will be necessary. Brushing the style will achieve most of the final dressing.

Putting rollers into shapes – II

Completing the set

Now let's put the whole head in rollers using the combinations of patterns and shapes that you have been practising. The two sets are fundamental, everyday classic styles – nothing fancy! One style is straight back off the face and the other is over to the side with a small fringe. These are not complicated styles but they may be set a little differently than you would do normally – instead of just 'putting the hair in rollers', we will 'design' the set – and of course they are excellent examples for you to practise for a practical examination. At first, you will be referring to the diagrams frequently but if you keep on practising, you will eventually be able to do the style without looking at the picture, and much faster.

Style 1 (straight back off the face)

Distribute, mould and scale off the whole head using the following shapes:

- diamond;
- quarter circles;
- half circles;
- rectangles.

Set the diamond in half, three-quarter and full length rollers (to further emphasise the diamond shape, the rollers can vary in size so the diamond shape has a three-dimensional effect).

If your salon uses conical rollers, place two of these in the quarter circle – two on each side of the diamond. The narrow end is toward the face and it is secured closest to the starting point.

Now place four conical rollers (or cylinder rollers) in the half circles at the sides of the head. Finish off the lower sides in pincurls. Toward the back, place barrel curls or stand-up pincurls with flat-reverse pattern pincurls (with no or short stems). Place these in a rectangle shape.

Tips

1 Make sure the hair is wet (the wetter the better). Use a setting lotion to assist the roller positioning and placement.

2 If you wrap the hair around the side rollers more than $1\frac{1}{2}$ times, the result will be a wave. If you have not wrapped the hair around the roller more than $1\frac{1}{2}$ times, you will get a curl.

3 Position the pincurls accurately and secure them carefully.

4 Secure all rollers that are placed in curved shapes at the narrow end of the roller section. This will enforce the roller direction (even if you have used a cylinder roller you must do this).

5 Make sure no pins or clips will cause marks on the skin or leave marks or kinks in the hair. Clips may get hot while under the dryer and if these are positioned against the skin, they could burn the client.

It is important to get all the rollers and pincurls technically correct before the hair is dried. Once the hair has been dried, you cannot change the setting pattern.

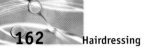

Figure 11.17 (a–d)

The lines of a hairstyle
The right profile

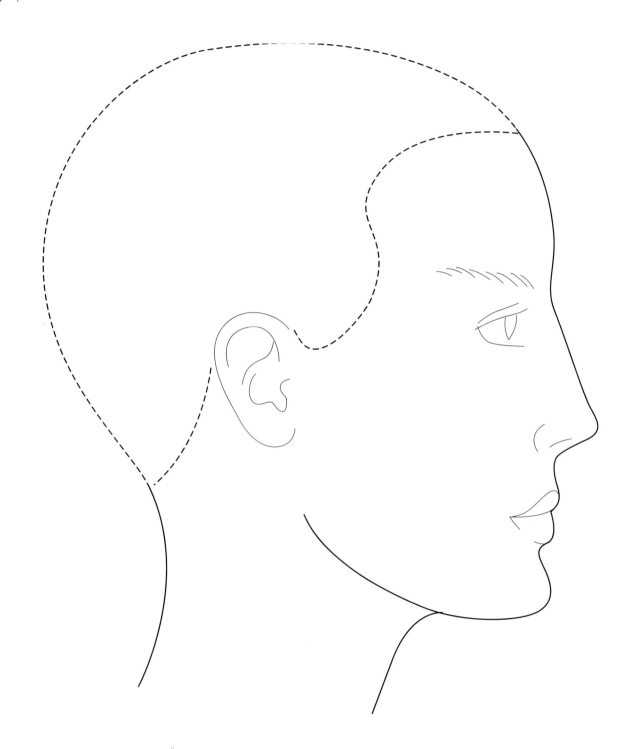

The back

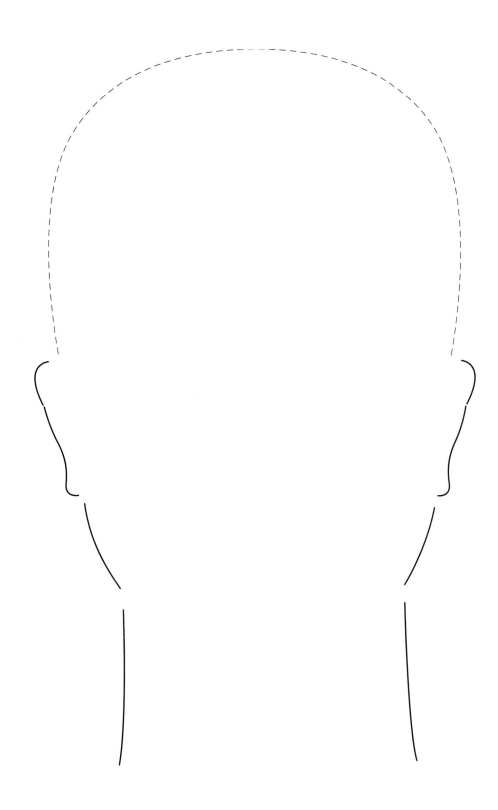

The front

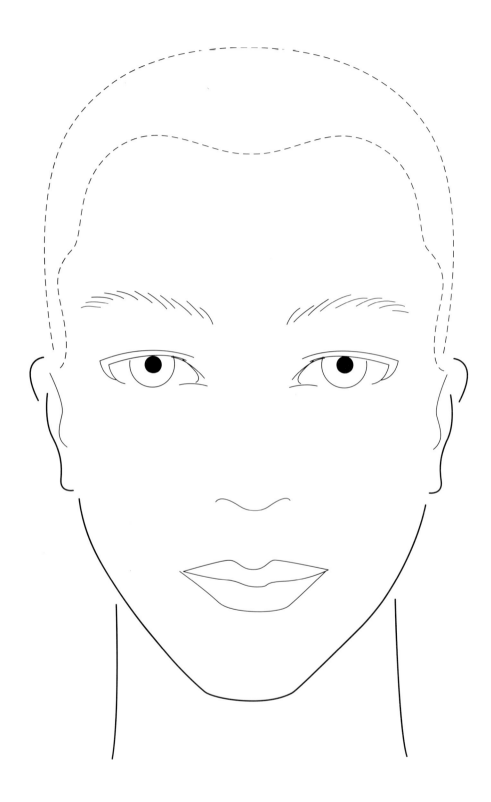

The left profile

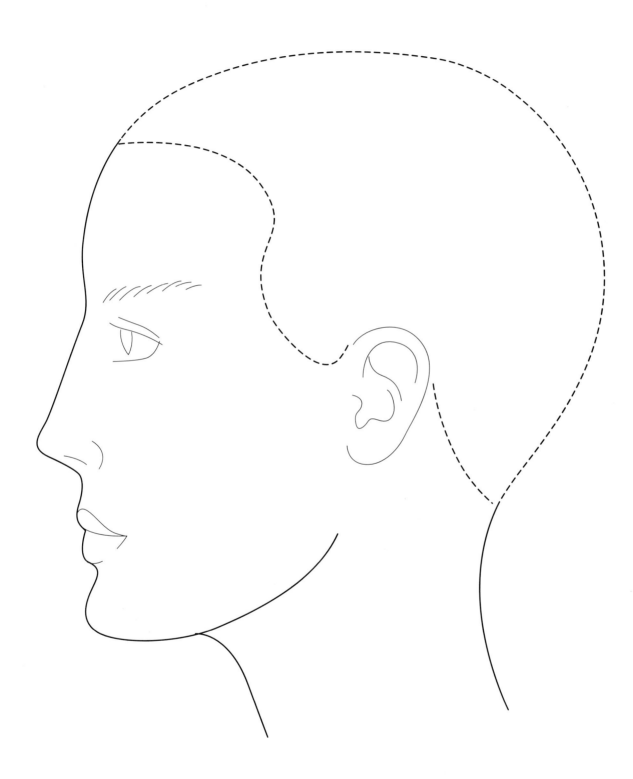

Figure 11.18 (a–d)

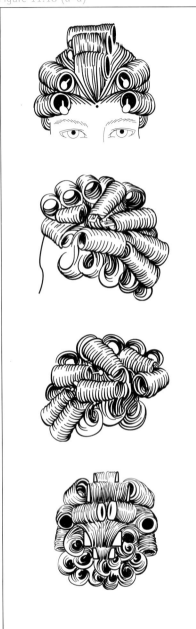

Dressing out

Once the rollers have been removed, relax the set with a Mason Pearson nylon/ bristle (Popular) brush. Brush the hair for two to four minutes, in the same direction as the placement of the rollers. You will begin to see the movement and the shape of the style as you brush. The majority of the work is in the relaxing of the style with the brush. Now take a large dressing comb or postiche brush and back-comb gently underneath the hair. Do not disturb the brushed shape more than required.

Now smooth and define the movement and finish the style with the comb or postiche brush. Make sure no back-combing is visible and gently spray. Don't 'fiddle' – be confident in your approach. Check the shape from the profile and front. Make sure the shape looks good.

Style 2 (dressed over to the side)

This style is also a classic look and a popular starting design to practise. The style is made up mainly of curved shapes. Half circles, large ovals and oblongs dominate the style. A rectangle is positioned on the crown.

Set a half circle at the front. Calculate how much hair you want coming onto the face (i.e. fringe), or how little hair should be positioned on the face. This will influence where the starting point will be. As an example, a style with a large amount of hair coming onto the face will require one roller positioned off the face while the second, third and fourth rollers are directed onto the face within a half circle shape. A small amount of hair coming onto the face would require the first three rollers positioned off the face while the fourth roller is positioned coming onto the face.

Set the rectangle on the crown in equal length cylinder rollers. The large oval shapes at the side are set with variable starting points. Finish off the shape with reverse pattern pincurls.

Remember, if you want the side rollers to dress out into a wave ('S' movement), then you must wrap the hair around the roller more than $1^{1}/_{2}$ times. If you do not do this then the result will be a curl.

Dressing out

Dress out using the Mason Pearson Popular brush to 'relax' the set. Use the large dressing comb or postiche brush to define the shape. Follow the setting pattern in the dress out. Notice how the curved lines move from the roots of the hair to the ends. It is this type of movement (roots to ends) that ensures the style is long lasting. If the hair is set in straight lines, this root-to-end movement is not possible.

These two styles are classic, simple, popular and practical salon styles. Practise them until you have reduced the time they take you, then move on to something a little more advanced. Make up some designs yourself from the shapes that have been discussed.

Figure 11.19 (a–c)

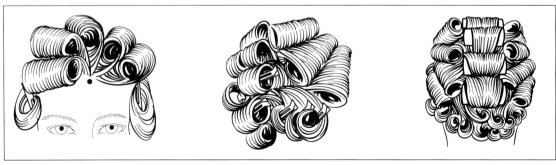

Questions

1 Explain the term *directional setting*.

_____

_____

_____

2 **a** What are the two ways lines move in directional setting?

_____

_____

   b Name two shapes in which each of these lines can be placed.

_____

3 **a** Name three types of roller control using straight lines.

_____

_____

_____

   b What will the finished results of each of these three types of roller control achieve?

_____

_____

_____

4 What is the minimum size base for a roller placed in straight indentation?

_____

_____

5 What is characteristic about a roller placed in curved indentation?

_____

_____

_____

6   Name five shapes that make up a design pattern for first pli setting.

_____

_____

_____

7   State:

    a   where the clip is placed on a conical roller;

_____

    b   how far the conical roller is wound from its starting point;

_____

_____

    c   an important 'don't' concerned with curved volume.

_____

_____

8   What is the result when:

    a   the hair is wound $1\frac{1}{2}$ times around the roller?

_____

_____

    b   the hair is wound less than $1\frac{1}{2}$ times around the roller?

_____

_____

Competition hairdressing

Competition rules are always changing so ask your local Association member or representative for a copy of the competition rules booklet. Most competitions include cutting, setting and blow-drying.

Competition hairdressing provides the extension or test that some hairdressers feel is necessary to give added stimulus and challenge to their work. It is an opportunity to test yourself against others and your expertise against theirs. In competition hairdressing, you are putting into practice the fundamental skills you have been taught, such as fingerwaving, pincurling, roller control, balance, movement, rhythm, harmony and suitability of style.

Figure 11.20
Competition hairdressing is of benefit to your practical work in the salon.

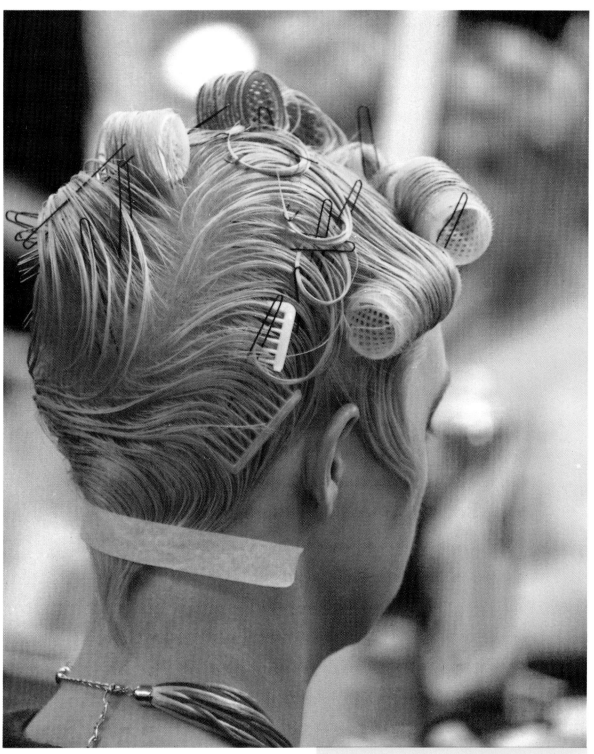

Conical rollers emphasise the movement and direction.

Figure 11.21
First pli

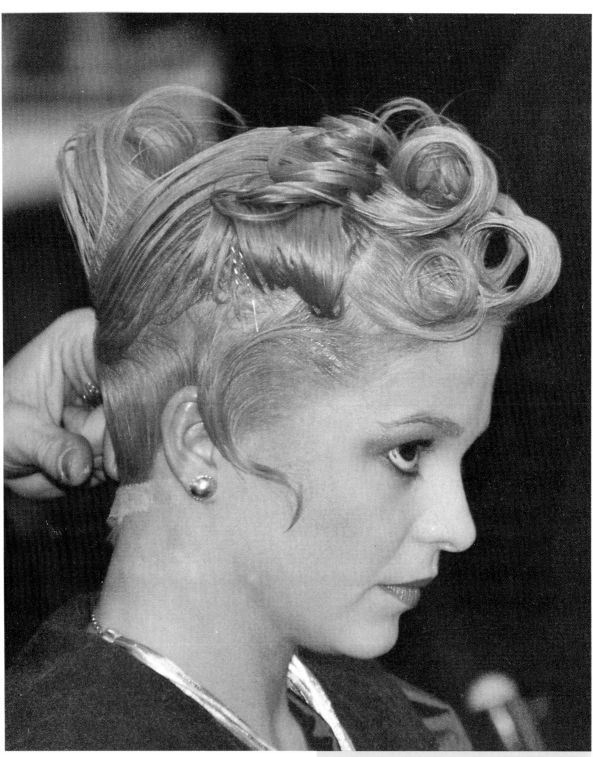

Incorporates conical roller control, pincurls, grade lines and waves.

Figure 11.22
Second pli

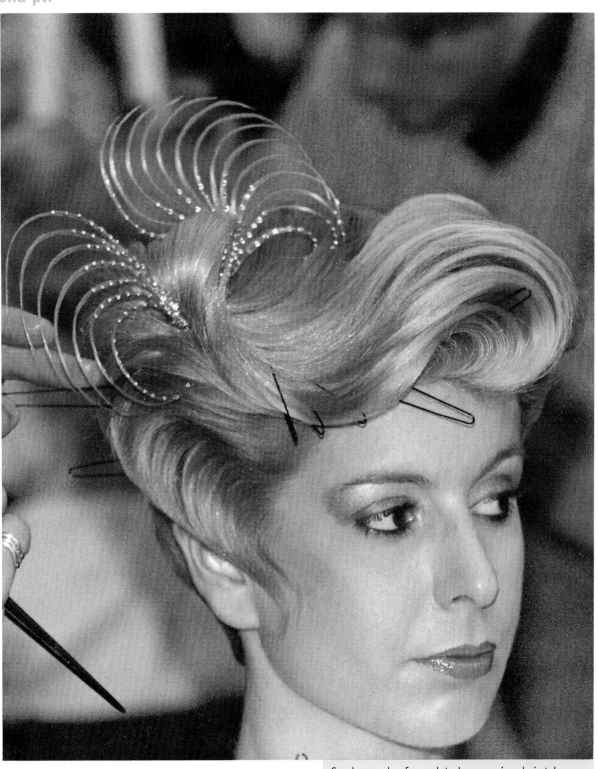

Good example of complete harmony in a hairstyle.

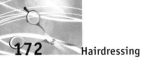
Figure 11.23

Harmony

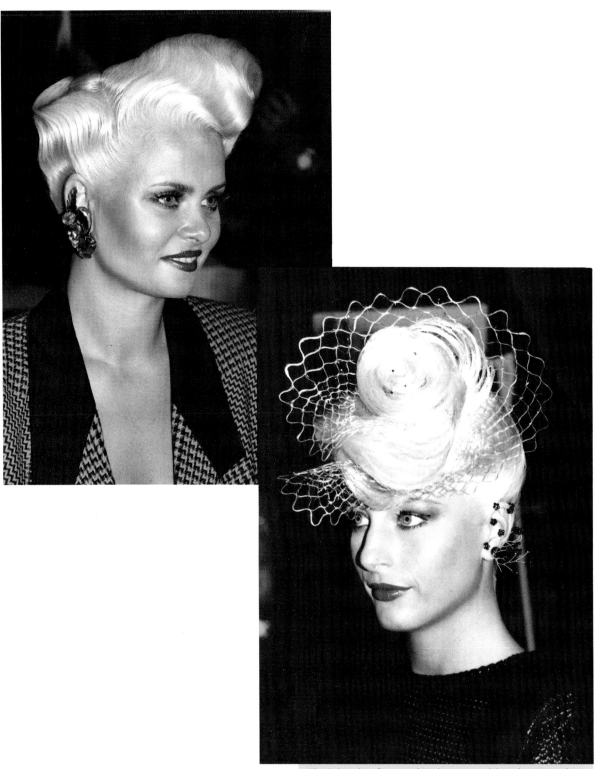

Final dressing for creative day competition, incorporating emphasis, rhythm, balance and proportion to give total harmony. Note the use of accessories and make-up.

First pli for a creative day competition line

The model

The model is said to account for up to 80% of the result, although the style must still be good.

The model does not have to be glamorous, but should be tall, with good posture (no round shoulders), skin and bone structure. The hair should be fine – but there should be lots of it – and strong, with a light base colour, either blonde, gold or red. Don't be put off by natural hair tendencies.

The judges are looking for a total look which includes make-up, dress, accessories and suitability of hairstyle.

Creative day style

An individual interpretation of current practical fashion trends, this style should be fresh and, if possible, have a certain newness about it. The line should be developed with a competition flair which makes use of the control in the setting technique (which should be technically correct). The dressed-out line is achieved in seven to ten minutes.

Gala

This refers to a high-fashion gala hairstyle in line with European concepts and incorporating current fashion trends, combined with creativity and total look of the model.

Hair design

This is the interpretation of the newest practical line with a strong emphasis on the cut. The line should be developed with individual flair, making full use of colour and perm techniques. Implements pertaining to blow-drying are used to achieve the final dressing. Hair must be shortened by at least 3 cm to create a new shape.

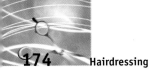

Figure 14.1 (a–h)

See Chapter 14, pp. 213 – 214 for explanation of Figure 14.1 (a – h).

Lightening

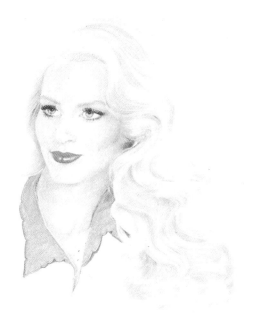

Changing tone

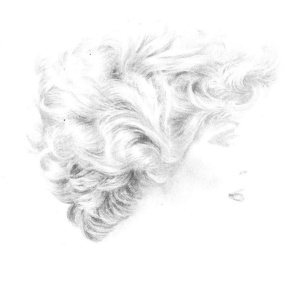

Darkening

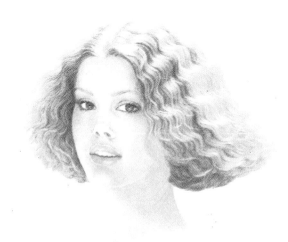

Halo colouring

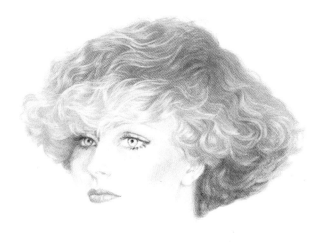

Block colouring

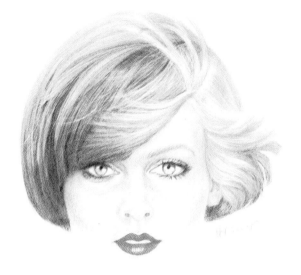

Touch colouring

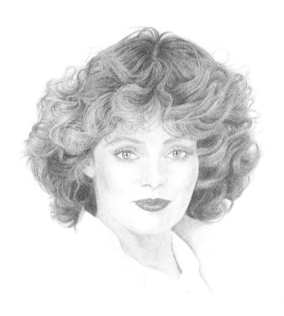

Shimmering

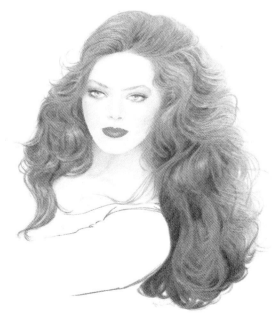

Naturalising

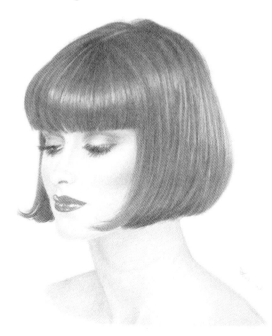

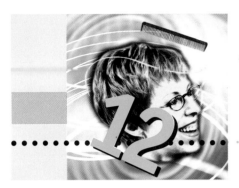

Advanced trichology

In this chapter, you will learn about:

- the molecular structure of the hair;
- nutrition – how diet affects the hair and skin;
- the composition of hairdressing products.

 ## The molecular structure of the hair

Protein structure

Keratin proteins are complex organic compounds (substances made up of two or more elements derived from living organisms, the smaller of which is an atom) and contain the following elements: carbon, hydrogen, oxygen, nitrogen and sulphur.

The hair and skin are both constructed from proteins. The skin's own antibodies in the blood are made from proteins; they help fight invading bacteria. Enzymes, the substances which break down the food we digest, are also proteins. The red blood cells that carry oxygen to the body's tissue and muscle are protein. Fundamentally, proteins are the building blocks of the body.

The basic structure of amino acids

The proteins of the hair are made up of many molecular blocks called amino acids. Hair protein is constructed of approximately 18 different amino acids which make up the hard protein, keratin.

The amino acids consist of the elements which are found in proteins, but in various arrangements. It is this arrangement of the elements that makes each amino acid different. Cystine, cysteine, glycine and lysine are some of the amino acids.

Of the 18 measurable amino acids, each has a side chain, R, by which it is described or characterised. The R side chains can be described as:

- basic side chain;
- sulphur side chain;
- acid side chain.

There are others but these three are the R side chains that are important to us. For example, it is the sulphur side chain that is affected in permanent waving. Cystine is a well-known example of the amino acid that has the sulphur side chain. The side chains are responsible for up to 50% of the hair's weight.

The amino acids are obtained from the foods containing protein that are eaten and digested by the body's enzymes. Certain foods which are richer than others in amino acids and sulphur content are called A-grade proteins. These include meat, fish and dairy products.

All the amino acids that make up the keratin protein of the hair are constructed of a carboxyl group (COOH), composed of:

- 1 carbon atom;
- 1 hydrogen atom;

- 2 oxygen atoms.

Amino acids also have an amino group (NH_2), that is composed of:

- 1 nitrogen;
- 2 hydrogen atoms.

These are linked together by the same carbon atom. They therefore show both basic and acidic properties. What makes each amino acid different are the other atoms that attach themselves to this carbon atom. This is called the R side chain. As an example, the basic side chain has an extra amino group (NH_3, positive), while the acid side chain has an extra carboxyl group (COOH, negative). It is these positive and negative charges that form the salt bonds in the hair fibre.

A simple amino acid is:

Glycine (NH_2) CH_2 – COOH.

Another is cystine:

$$S-CH_2 \underline{\hspace{6em}} CH\ COOH \quad (NH_2)$$
$$S-CH_2 \underline{\hspace{6em}} CHCOOH \quad (NH_2)$$

Note: This is the amino group NH_2, the carboxyl group COOH, with the two sulphur atoms linked to the carbon (this is the side chain). In science, R represents any form of side chain.

It is this side chain which accounts for the different proteins in the chain. It could join with another carboxyl group from a second molecule and so on, until a chain has been built up.

The various amino acids (made up of different arrangements of elements) are linked together end-on-end by a peptide bond. The amino acids are also joined together in a particular sequence. This sequence of amino acids, linked by the peptide bond, is called a polypeptide chain. The polypeptide chain is found in the protofibrils of the cortex layer and its formation is a spiral. This spiralling effect of the polypeptide chain is called a helix coil. In its natural state, the helix coil is in a state of alpha keratin (a-keratin). Cross-linkages or bonds help to keep the helix coil (or polypeptide chain) in its state of a-keratin. Hair is an intensely cross-linked structure. The cross-linkages or bonds are:

- hydrogen bonds;
- salt bonds;
- di-sulphide bonds;
- end bonds;
- Van der Waals forces.

Hydrogen bonds

The hydrogen (H_2) bonds are the most numerous on the helix coil (polypeptide chain). They are responsible for holding the coil in shape and for maintaining the hair's elasticity, especially when it is dry. They are relatively weak and are easily broken by physical or mechanical changes such as wetting with water, setting or applying heat (such as tongs or crimping).

Figure 12.1

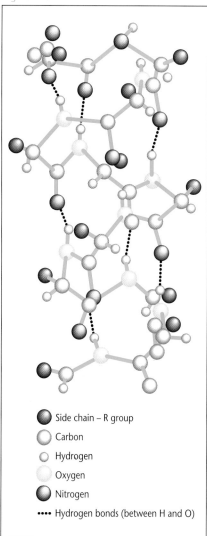

- ● Side chain – R group
- ○ Carbon
- ○ Hydrogen
- ○ Oxygen
- ◐ Nitrogen
- •••• Hydrogen bonds (between H and O)

Amino acids combine by means of peptide bonds to form a polypeptide chain. The dotted lines are hydrogen bonds; the dark circles indicate the side chain R.

The H_2 bonds occur between the helix coil (polypeptide chain) and also above and below each turn of the spiral coil.

They are formed between a hydrogen atom in one amino acid and an oxygen atom in the opposite amino acid. The hydrogen bonds contain some water which they have adsorbed (from the air (approximately 5% in average conditions) The breaking of hydrogen bonds causes the hair to swell. The H_2 bonds are broken during most salon services.

Figure 12.2

The protein chain

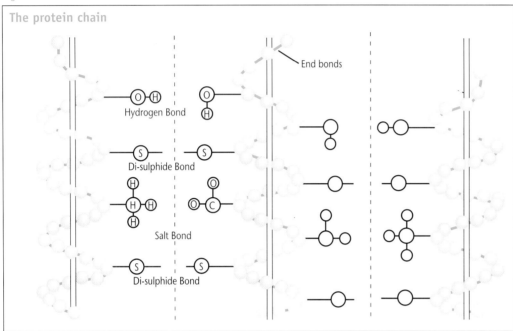

The spiralling shape of a polypeptide chain (helix coil) linked with chemical bonds.

Salt bonds

These are also called ionic bonds and are established between the amino acids by the attraction of unlike positive and negative electric charges, usually between an acid and a basic side chain. For example, a positively charged molecule is attracted to a negatively charged molecule. A salt bond is relatively strong but can be broken by water.

Di-sulphide bonds

The amino acid which contains the di-sulphide bond is called cystine. This is an essential bond in giving the helix coil (polypeptide chain) its alignment and it shape. Cystine is the dominant amino acid found in the hair and constitutes approximately 17% of the hair's amino acid content.

The di-sulphide bonds are very strong and are the important ones that are broken and reformed during permanent waving or straightening of the hair.

End bonds or peptide bonds

The peptide bonds that join the amino acids together are the strongest bonds in the molecule structure. They are responsible for the hair's strength. If they become damaged or broken, the hair will be irreversibly damaged and nothing will repair it. It is the end bonds that are broken when hair removal creams are applied.

Van der Waals forces

Attractive forces which are quite independent of the links previously mentioned also exist between the molecules. These are called Van der Waal forces and occur when the molecules are in close proximity. The attraction is very weak in the protein chain.

Keratinisation

The development of hair in the follicle

Hair grows by cell multiplication – the division of cells (mitosis). The nucleus of the cell plays an important part in the division. In the early stages, cell look alike and are a soft jelly-like mass found in the germinating matrix of the hair bulb. The cells' cytoplasm contains all the nutrients necessary for the hair's growth and reproduction. The germinating matrix is similar to the germinating layer within the epidermis, except that the skin's keratinised cycle produces softer keratin. The cells are nourished by amino acids which seep in by osmotic action (a seeping through of the capillary wall) from the minute blood capillaries (arteriols). As the cells divide, they are pushed up and begin to move slowly up the follicle, becoming harder (keratinised) and dying as they do so. They also take on the shape of the follicle. As the cells move upward, they begin to take on the layers of the hair, the cuticle cortex fibres and the medullary canal (if medullated).

The cells containing amino acids join together. They form three parallel spiral coils (polypeptides) and these are linked crossways by di-sulphide, hydrogen and salt bonds to become a strong, hard, interlocking fibre called *keratin*. These three coiled spirals form a *protofibril* – the smallest of the cortex fibres. Seven of these protofibrils wrap around two more protofibrils to form a *microfibril* – at this stage the hair fibre is becoming quite strong.

Note: Some authorities are of the opinion that nine protofibrils wrap around two *protofibrils*.

Seven microfibrils wrap around two more microfibrils to make a macrofibril. Seven macrofibrils wrap around two other macrofibrils to form an even stronger fibre called a *cortical cable* – this is the largest fibre in the cortex and can be seen with the aid of a transmission electron microscope. These cortical cables lie parallel to the shaft and wrap around each other – seven wrap around two. This is the cortex of the hair and makes up the bulk of the shaft (approximately 80%).

Between the fibres is a much more randomly distributed protein called the matrix protein. The *matrix protein* is also hard keratin and is even stronger than the fibrous protein.

A hair strand is formed by the amino acids taking on a spiral shape, like a coiled spring (a helix). Three twisted helix coils form a protofibril. These entwine to form microfibrils which twist together to make macrofibrils. These in turn spiral to form the cortical fibrils (cortex). The twisted spiral construction is why the hair is able to stretch.

Cuticle

The cuticle is made entirely of maxtrix protein. It consists of several layers of overlapping scales (containing a high degree of sulphur) which encompass the hair shaft. These overlapping scales trap sebum, hair spray, setting agents, conditioners, and protein revitalisers. Any dead cells or scales from the scalp, dirt and debris also lodge in these scales. The scales are very hard and flat, providing protection for the cortical cables and fibrils in the cortex.

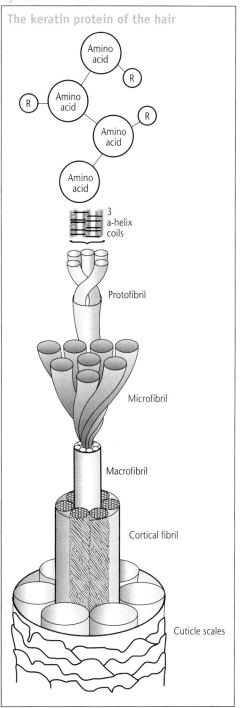

Figure 12.3

The keratin protein of the hair

- Amino acid
- R
- Amino acid
- R
- R
- Amino acid
- Amino acid
- 3 a-helix coils
- Protofibril
- Microfibril
- Macrofibril
- Cortical fibril
- Cuticle scales

The cuticle can encompass the hair shaft many times – approximately three to six times on average textured hair. In any case, the cuticle has two major cellular layers – the external or *exocuticle* and the internal or *endocuticle*.

The cuticle cells interlock and stick to one another as they harden. Matrix protein is also present between the cells and helps to hold the cuticle together.

The hair's various physical properties (its tensility, strength and elasticity) are due to the nature of the cuticle and cortex structure.

Figure 12.4

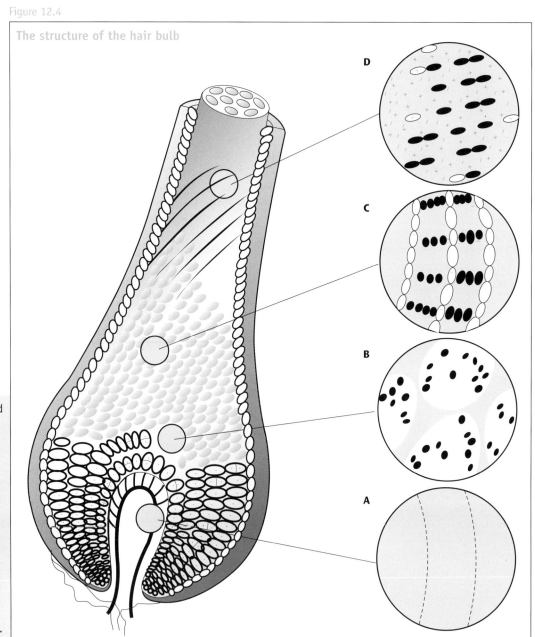

The structure of the hair bulb

A Amino acids from the blood leave the arteriols through minute cracks in the vessels' wall (osmosis).

B Cortex cells begin to form.

C As each cell hardens, the amino acids are joined by peptide (end) bonds, creating a chain.

D The keratin is now hard as sulphur and hydrogen bonds form a complex cross-linked structure.

Fibres twist around each other and become strong, hard, and interlocking. This is the cortex.

The hair structure – summary

1 The protein in food is broken by the digestive system into amino acids.
2 The amino acids are the building blocks for the hair.
3 The amino acids enter the bloodstream and reach the hair's matrix where they nourish the cells.
4 The amino acid cells are linked end-to-end by a peptide bond to form a polypeptide.
5 The polypeptide is twisted (like a rope) to form a helix coil.
6 The helix coil is held in place by cross-bonds – hydrogen, salt and sulphur.
7 The helix coil (polypeptide) groups into a protofibril.
8 These protofibrils twist and wind around each other to form other fibrils and cables which are held by adhesive protein to form a strong fibre.
9 The cuticle encapsulates the cortex fibres many time to protect and secure the fibre completely.
10 Matrix protein (hard protein) surrounds the cuticle and is important to the strength of the fibre. This is the first part of the hair to suffer any damage.

Figure 12.5

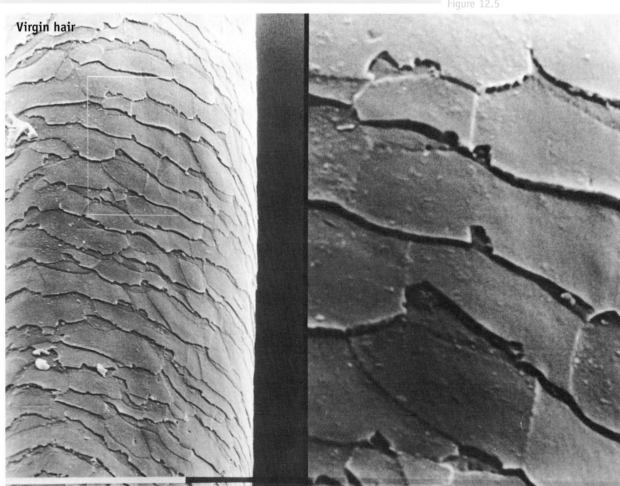

Virgin hair

This hair fibre has had no chemical treatment, just natural weathering. The cuticle scales are well aligned and the hair is in good condition. Compare this fibre with the other micrographs of damaged cuticle structure.

Follicle and fibre type

Hair follicles produce a great variety of fibre types. Variations in the diameter, length, medullation and waviness of the fibres are often of considerable importance. Some of these features are associated with the type of follicle producing the fibre and some with the arrangement of follicles in the skin. Hair follicles are classified as:

- terminal – long, soft, mature hair and short, bristly hair;
- vellus – fine, unpigmented, unmedullated hair covering most of the body;
- lanugo – hair which is present before, and sometimes at, birth.

As hairdressers, we are concerned primarily with the hair of the scalp, which is terminal hair.

Terminal hair (long, soft, mature hair)

This is the type of hair found on the scalp, in the beard (of the male) and in the armpits. This hair is longer, thicker and stronger than most other hair. Its chief purposes are to protect against injury and to conserve heat. Men who lose their hair usually need to take some steps to prevent injury to the scalp as a result of the sun's ultraviolet radiation. This type of hair also functions as adornment. It usually grows faster than other hair, particularly in females and younger people. It does, however, tend to grow a little more slowly as we get older. It has a long growing cycle and a short resting stage. The hairs may grow in clusters from the follicle 3 mm deep, perhaps two or three from the same follicle.

Short, bristly hair includes the eyelashes and eyebrows which don't contain arrector-pili muscles. In an adult male, the nostril hairs and ear hairs also fall into this category. The function of this hair is protection; the eyebrows prevent sweat from entering the eye (they shouldn't be removed entirely by plucking) and the lashes stop dust from getting into the eye. These hairs are usually quite thick and taper toward the end, and they are well supplied with nerves which makes them very sensitive. They have long resting periods and short growing cycles.

Vellus hair (usually unmedullated hair)

This is the baby-fine hair which is found over most of the body. These hairs have no medullary canal as they are so fine in texture. Vellus hair is found on the faces, arms and body of most women and men who have smooth skins. The hairs are usually very short and usually unpigmented. Vellus hair is replaced by terminal hair in the axillary and pubic areas and, in males, in the beard regions.

Follicle structure

The molecular and cellular processes occurring during fibre formation result in differences in properties and types of hair fibre. Fibre formation is the main function of the active or anagen follicle. The active follicle is a rod-like epithelium-derived downgrowth into the dermis. It is enclosed in a connective tissue sheath, associated with a network of blood vessels. The dermis supplies the follicle, at its base, with the dermal papilla, which is also supplied with blood vessels. The dermal papilla is necessary for normal fibre production.

Hair follicles are divided into zones or areas which are used to describe the follicle.

Hair bulb

Bulb cells surround the dermal papilla and are generally mitotically (multiplication of cells) active. The diameter and length of fibre grown are determined to a large extent in this area by the number of dividing cells present and the rate of cell division. In follicles producing non-medullated fibres, the mitotic zone ends at the level of the top of the dermal papilla.

Inner root sheath (IRS) – the follicle lining

The follicle lining is composed of a surface which is in close contact with the hair. The inner root sheath interlocks with the overlapping cells of the cuticle of the growing hair and moves with it, but the keratinizing cells are desquamated as the hair emerges from the skin. Thus the outer surface of the inner root sheath glides against the stationary outer root sheath which is the inner most part of the folliclular wall. There are two distinct layers of cells which slough off into the follicle – Huxley's layer and Henle's layer. These disappear towards the opening of the skin's surface. If the hair is forcibly removed from the scalp, the IRS and some of the follicle is removed, and can be identified as a white, thickened end.

Outer root sheath (ORS)

Surrounding the IRS is the ORS which is a downgrowth of the epithelium into the dermis, usually sloping at an angle. This is a protective covering for the follicle.

Figure 12.6

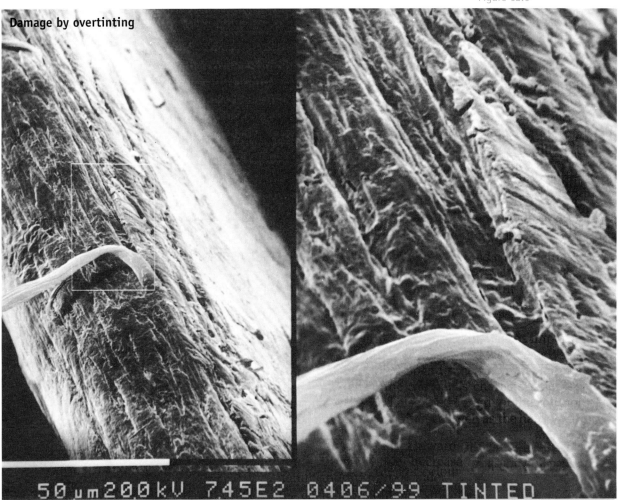

Damage by overtinting

50 um 200 kV 745E2 0406/99 TINTED

Overtinting has caused the cuticle of this hair fibre to become completely stripped. This has exposed the cortical fibre which although strong, is completely dependent on the cuticle for protection. Here, the fibre is already starting to fall apart. This hair is extremely damaged.

Pigmentation of the hair

The pigment of the hair is carried in the cortex layer. The melanocytes are situated in the matrix of the hair root just above the dermal papilla and produce coloured pigment granules called *eumelanin* (black and brown) and *phaeomelanin* (red and yellow). The presence of air space in the medulla or cortex can also affect the colour of the hail These four pigments can be intermixed in a full head of hair or even in a single hair.

The melanocytes inject the hair with melanin or phenomelanin granules where the cells divide at the germinating matrix. The *tentrical arms* of the melanocytes extend into the passing stream of dividing cells. The concentration of pigmentation in the cells will influence the final level light or dark. If the granules are openly distributed, the colour will be light; if there is a much greater concentration – more of them packed closely – then the colour will be darker. The cuticle of the hair, however, can sometimes contain melanin pigment.

If the hair becomes grey, the melanocytes have simply stopped producing melanin or phaeomelanin pigment. If there is a complete lack of pigment, the hair is said to be white. Genetic factors, aging and a lack of certain vitamins can affect the greying process. Darker hairs scattered among the white hairs give the illusion of grey hair. People deficient in pigment in skin and hair from birth are albino.

Figure 12.7

Cross-section of hair

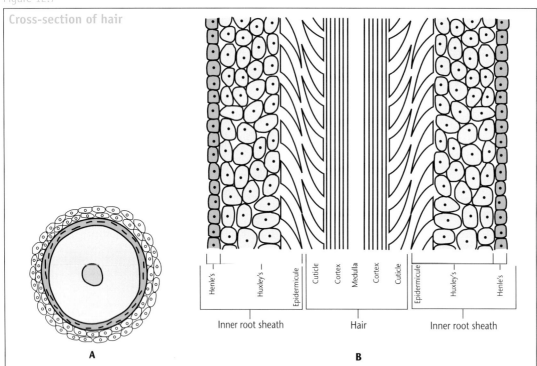

A   A cross-section of the hair and the inner root sheath.

B   The follicle lining, the cell layers of the inner root sheath. The follicle lining is composed of a surface which is in close contact with the hair. Distinct layers of cells make up the inner root sheath. These layers are known as *Henle's layer, Huxley's layer* and the *epidermicule*. Henle's layer is composed of non-nucleated cells. Huxley's layer is composed of coarsely granulated cells derived from the papilla. The cell layer of the root sheath known as the epidermicule moves up alongside the cuticle to the level of the sebaceous gland where it is decomposed.

Figure 12.8

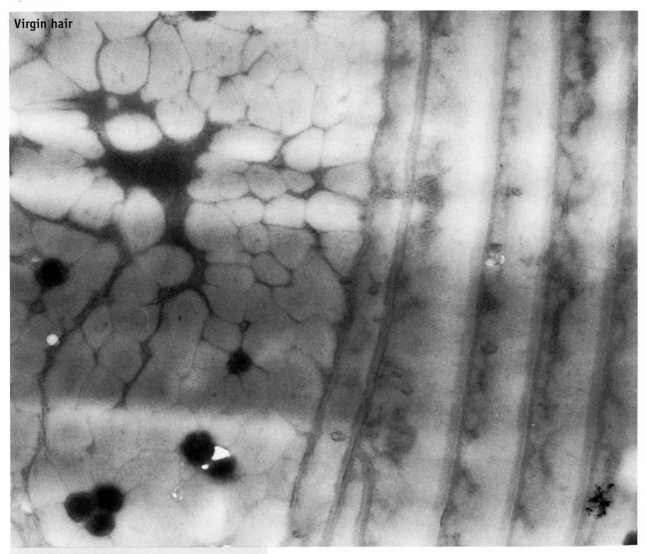

Virgin hair

This cross-section of a virgin hair shows (arrowed):
A the layers of cuticle scales;
B the macrofibrils;
C the melanin pigment of this virgin hair.

Nutrition – how diet affects the hair and skin

The blood feeds the hair and skin, and what we eat (our dietary habits) in turn supplies the blood.

Food

Skin, and hair roots, because they are living, depend on blood for their nourishment, so it must contain all the required nutrients.

Most people today are aware of the need for proper nutrition and realise that healthy skin and hair thrive on a well-balanced diet. Let us discuss diet and food.

The food that we eat should be fresh and unprocessed. Dried foods, however, can maintain their goodness and some good food sources can be successfully dried. Canned and refined foods (sugar, sweets, canned drinks) should be kept to a minimum. Vitamins should be taken in their natural food sources as the required ones are available in a variety of foods. Be aware that many foods that are white – white sugar, salt, bread, white rice and flour – have had a lot of nutrients taken out of them; often, these have been replaced by synthetic chemicals.

Ideally, the food we eat should be of good quality and quantity. We should avoid excess fats; although they give the body energy and warmth, any surplus fat is stored in the subcutaneous tissue.

A well-balanced diet should supply the necessary 'fuel' needed for normal hair growth, skin health and nourishment. A diet which is unbalanced and lacking in certain nutrients can be responsible for poor health, tiredness and hair and skin problems.

Stressing that a balanced diet is essential is just as important a piece of advice to your client as any other beauty tip. A balanced diet will include the following.

Protein

The body's building blocks, proteins are rich in sulphur and nitrogen and are needed for building and repairing body tissue. The digestion of the proteins starts in the stomach where the walls of the stomach secrete gastric juices. These juices contain enzymes which act as catalysts upon the protein foods. The enzymes break the proteins down into amino acids so that, eventually, they can be absorbed into the blood and used by the body. The protein keratin is used for hair and skin growth.

Carbohydrates

Carbohydrates play a major role in the diet as they supply energy for physical and mental activity. Carbohydrates are of three main types:

* sugars (sucrose, lactose);
* starch;
* cellulose.

The digestion of sugars and starch begins in the mouth, since the saliva contains enzymes. The intestinal juices then break these nutrients down further into secondary sugars, such as:

* sucrose (cane sugar);
* maltose (malt sugar);
* lactose (milk sugar);
* fructose (fruit sugar).

These are broken down into glucose for energy and can be readily absorbed into the blood. Energy is produced when the air we breathe reacts chemically with the glucose. The energy helps to divide the hair cells in the matrix and skin cells in the germinating layer.

Figure 12.9

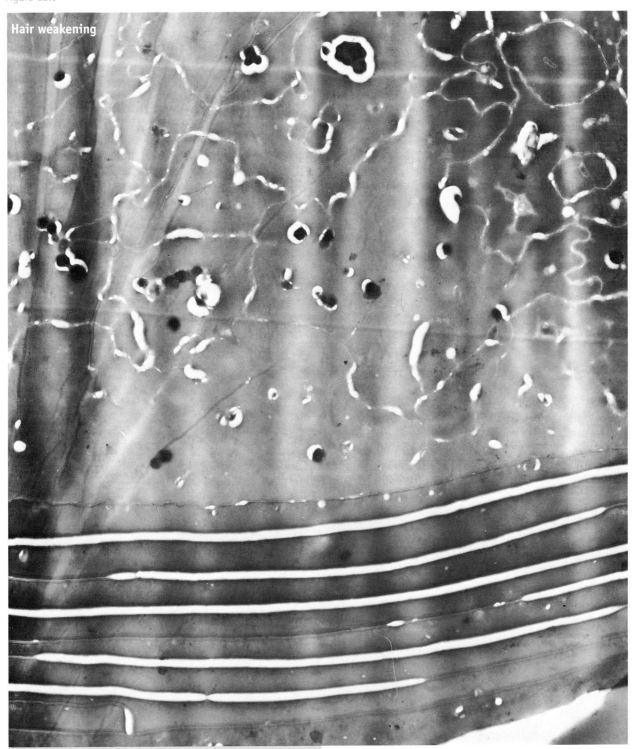

Hair weakening

This hair has been lightened and tinted. The intercellular cuticle cement has been removed and the cuticle is weakened. Channels are starting to open up in between the cortical fibrils and around the melanin pigment. The fibre is becoming weakened. (X 8200)

Cellulose is another form of carbohydrate that is present in fruits and vegetables; it provides fibre or roughage in the diet and is not digested. Cellulose is necessary for the regular functioning of the bowel.

Excess carbohydrate is converted to, and stored as, fat.

Figure 12.10

Macrofibrils

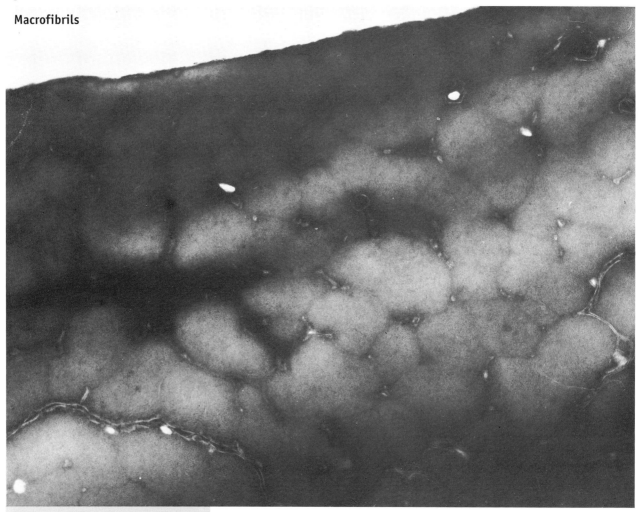

The transmission electron microscope shows a cross-section of fibre with the macrofibrils arrowed and the pattern of minute microfibrils arrowed. There is no cuticle layer. (X 23 000)

Fats

Fats are similar to carbohydrates in that they, too, are rich in energy-giving value. Fats also supply the body with heat. Fats are classified as either saturated, which come mainly from animal sources, or unsaturated, which are the vegetable variety. Fish is also an important source of unsaturated fats. Animal fats are said to contain a high cholesterol content and are best kept to a minimum in the diet.

The digestion of fats occurs in the duodenum where bile, which is secreted by the liver, and pancreatic juices, which are secreted by the pancreas, act upon the fat. These juices break the fat down into fatty acids and glycerol which can then be absorbed by the blood and used, when necessary, by the body. Fats are beneficial to the skin.

Overcooking can destroy a lot of the goodness in food. To avoid destroying the vitamin content of foods:

1 cook vegetables with the minimum of water, and as quickly as possible;

2 use vegetable oils for cooking rather than butter or animal fats;

3 avoid adding extra chemicals, e.g. large quantities of salt, sugar or artificial sugar;

4 use sugar substitutes (honey) and whole-grain flours.

Sources of nutrients

Proteins	Animal: all meats; dairy products.
	Vegetable: soya beans, grains, nuts.
Carbohydrates	Sugars: honey, fruit, fruit juice, syrup, molasses.
	Starch: potatoes, bread.
	Cellulose: fruit, vegetables, raisins, cereals, grain flour.
Fats	Saturated: animal, fatty meats, butter.
	Unsaturated: vegetables, nuts, oils such as olive, sunflower, peanut, corn, avocado.

Figure 12.11

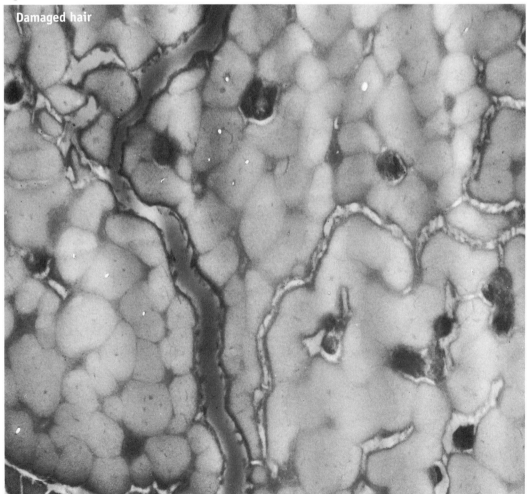

Damaged hair

The transmission electron microscope shows that this permed hair fibre is completely devoid of cuticle protection. The cortical fibrils and macrofibrils are falling apart. Large channels have opened up, severely weakening the hair. This hair is extremely damaged.

Figure 12.12

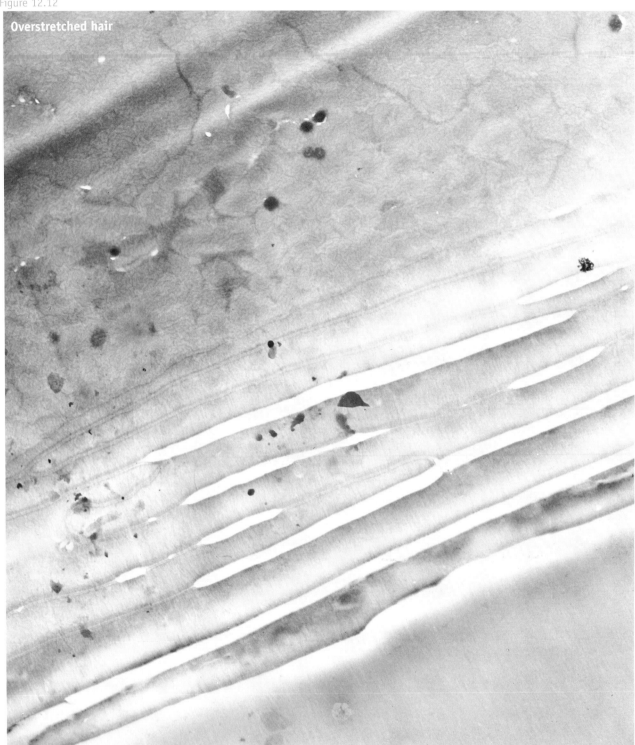

Overstretched hair

This cross-section of hair shows that it has been overstretched. The outside layers of the cuticle may indicate little damage, but the cuticle layers are becoming detached. The cellular cement holding the cuticle scales in place has become loose, weakening the cuticle.

Vitamins

Vitamins regulate the body's metabolism (the rate of energy expenditure), and help to convert fat and carbohydrates to achieve this. As they are only needed in small amounts, it is difficult to detect any vitamin deficiency, but ill health can occur if vitamins are lacking. A lack of a certain vitamin can upset the efficiency of other vitamins in the body, because vitamins work as a team to perform many vital body functions.

All vitamins are considered essential for the best possible health and some are linked particularly to hair and skin health.

Vitamin B complex

There are 13 vitamins in this range which need to be taken daily as they are not stored by the body. Those directly concerned with hair and skin are listed in the table below.

Vitamin	Food and other sources	Benefit
Vitamin A	carrots, fish, liver, green vegetables, tomatoes	Maintains a healthy complexion; prevents dry, lifeless hair.
Vitamin B_1: thiamine	green vegetables, liver, kidneys,	Prevents rough and reddened skin and scalp dandruff; improves hair quality; strengthens fingernails.
Vitamin B_2: riboflavin	eggs, meat	
Vitamin B_{13}: niacin		
Vitamin B_3: pantothenic acid	brewer's yeast, liver, mushrooms	May prevent premature greying; helps maintain natural hair colour.
Vitamin B_{12}: folic acid folacin	liver, green vegetables, kidneys	May prevent premature greying; necessary for cell multiplication.
Vitamin C:	citrus fruit	Needed for a healthy skin.
Vitamin D:	eggs, milk, fish, sunshine	Helps the body absorb calcium and digest food.
Vitamin E:	eggs, green vegetables, bread, wheatgerm	Thought to improve blood circulation and promote hair growth; also said to prevent aging of skin.
Vitamin K:	made by intestinal bacteria; green vegetables, e.g. Brussels sprouts, cabbage, broccoli and puha	Helps with blood circulation and blood clotting, and maintains a healthy skin.

Minerals

Minerals occur in very small quantities in the body and all are necessary for the general health of the hair and skin. A well-balanced diet will provide the essential minerals. Of the 16 minerals required by the body, cobalt, copper, iodine, iron and zinc are particularly beneficial for hair and skin.

Mineral	Food source	Benefit
Cobalt (as part of B_{12})	green vegetables, broccoli, fruit.	Lack of cobalt leads to dry, scaly skin.
Copper	nuts, liver cereals, scallops	Lack of copper can cause premature greying and hair loss.
Iodine	seafood, shellfish, kelp	Deficiency can cause dryness, thinning and poor hair growth.
Iron	kidneys, liver, egg yolk, puha	Lack of iron may cause brittle hair and nails and premature greying.
Zinc	oysters, gelatine, wheatgerm, bran	Deficiency is known to cause hair loss and is associated with dry hair and oily skin.

Water

Water is an essential part of the diet as both the hair and skin retain moisture. There are different types of water available for drinking and for washing the hair.

1 *Hard water.* This type of water contains dissolved salts such as calcium and magnesium. These are picked up as water flows on the earth and finds its way into the water reservoir. In addition, community water may have added chlorine for purification and even fluoride to help prevent tooth decay. Hard water has the slight advantage of adding calcium and magnesium to the diet.

2 *Soft water.* This contains less dissolved salts but may contain sodium, copper, iron and zinc. Some people believe soft water does not taste quite as pleasant as hard water.

Conclusion

There is little danger that a client's diet will be lacking in the required nutrients, except perhaps in cases of extreme starvation. However, dieting is a common practice and while it is important to cut back on calories, it is important not to cut back on essential vitamins, minerals and adequate amounts of complete protein. You should appreciate that correct dietary habits form the basis for an effective programme of skin and hair health.

The growth and nourishment of the skin and hair depends upon the nutrients carried by the blood. The nutrients are broken down by the digestive system. Oxygen levels are maintained by the respiratory system and the end result is the type of nourishment necessary for the body to function.

All you have to do is to tell the client the best possible foods to eat.

The composition of hairdressing products – shampoos, conditioners, setting agents and fixatives

Many chemical formulas can be used in manufacturing hairdressing products, and manufacturers use sophisticated equipment and technical knowledge to formulate their particular products.

Shampoos

The primary function of a shampoo is to cleanse the hair of accumulated oil, sweat, dead skin cells, cigarette smoke and any hair fixatives. Shampooing is mainly a matter of removing grease; if this is removed, dirt will be removed too. Most detergents will do this job, but some have undesirable side effects such as overdrying, which leaves the hair dull, difficult to comb, harsh and unmanageable. It is also hard on the hands. A detergent can also remove substantial amounts of oil but still leave the hair in good condition. Removing natural oil does not necessarily harm the hair.

Detergent action

Use of a detergent involves a number of physical processes: wetting, emulsifying, foaming and rinsing.

- *Wetting and emulsifying*. The detergent must 'wet' the hair's surface rather than forming droplets which will not spread over the hair's surface. This quality of wetting is known as a surfactant – a surface acting agent. If grease or sebum is present on the hair fibre it will not become wetted by water. For the hair to become wet, the surface tension must be reduced by a surfactant.
- A detergent molecule has a *hydrophobic* ('water hating') portion and a *hydrophilic* ('water loving') portion. The hydrophobic property gives the affinity to grease and the hydrophilic the affinity to water. The hydrophilic portion has a negatively charged (anionic) water attraction which will wet the surface of the hair. The other hydrophobic (lipophilic) portion is attracted to the grease which it lifts from the hair fibre in the form of an emulsion. The shampoo should rid the hair of all dirt and debris in either soft or hard water without causing irritation or excessive dryness (to hair or hands).
- *Foaming*. Many detergents' cleansing actions are judged on their foaming capabilities. Foam is not, however, an essential characteristic, though it may be of psychological importance as the majority of clients have come to evaluate a shampoo by its foaming action. There are shampoos available with a limited foaming action that work equally well.
- Rinsing. The detergent should rinse easily from the hair rather than continuing its foaming action while it is being rinsed. This continued action is frustrating for the shampooist at the basin.

Materials used in shampoos

- *Soap*. Soaps are made from vegetable oils such as coconut, palm, olive, or from animal wax and fats such as lanoline or tallow. These are saponified, i.e. converted to soap by hydrolising and boiling with bases such as potassium hydroxide. This saponified liquid soap is diluted with distilled water and used as a shampoo.

  A common soap shampoo is green soft soap which is diluted with distilled water. The two are heated together until the soap dissolves. On cooling, sediment will form at the bottom. The clear liquid above is carefully poured into a bottle and used as shampoo.
- *Soapless shampoo*. Soapless shampoos are also made from vegetable oils and animal wax and fats but are sulphonated, i.e. mixed with sulphated lauryl alcohols. The most common lauryl sulphate salts are triethanolamine, ammonium and sodium. Although good for cleansing and foaming, these chemicals have a tendency to be potential irritants.

In addition, soapless detergents will contain other ingredients such as:

1 salts – either calcium or magnesium salts, used as thickeners and opacifiers;
2 conditioners – lanolin, proteins, egg derivatives or lemon to improve hair quality;
3 preservatives – formaldehyde stops the growth of mould and bacteria which will impair the colour and performance (allergen);

4   perfumes – essential oils, floral, rose, lavender, herbs or fruit extract produce a psychologically pleasing fragrance;

5   water – usually distilled, to make up the volume.

Soapless shampoos are formulated in various combinations.

1   Liquid cream shampoos – most shampoos fall into this category and examples are egg, lemon, cream, protein.

2   Clear liquid shampoos – various formulae produce transparent or translucent liquids. These are popular shampoos. The main difference between these and liquid cream shampoos is that the clear liquid shampoos don't include any opacifier or thickening agent.

3   Conditioning shampoos – include oil, such as mineral or olive, to improve the quality of the hair.

4   Baby shampoos – non-irritating shampoos, especially to the skin and eyes (can even be swallowed); these have a limited cleansing action.

5   Anti-dandruff shampoos (medicated) – contain a germicide, e.g. zinc pyrithione, coal tar, selenium sulphide.

Conditioners (cationic detergents)

Conditioners are recommended as post-shampoo treatments for clients who have had some form of chemical treatment. They can also be used as preconditioning treatments for hair which has become weathered or is overporous, harsh or brittle. They make the hair feel smoother and softer, give it a shine and more manageability. Conditioners also generate less static charges.

The early conditioners formulated in the late 1940s were based on lanolin and vegetable oils, waxes and mild acids, such as citric acid. Because of the hair's anionic negative charge, it has an attraction or affinity toward cationic (positive) substances. This is why conditioners still have an action on the hair even though they have been thoroughly rinsed. It is important that conditioners are rinsed away, as they tend to dull the hair when they dry.

Conditioners are usually an oil-in-water emulsion and contain derivatives of ammonia such as cetrimide BP or a quaternary ammonium compound. Also included, to repair hair damage, will be hydrolysed protein, collagen and liquid keratin (from horn or horse hair). Oily derivatives are another ingredient used to improve the condition of the hair and to add lustre by coating the fibre so that it reflects the light. Lanolin derivatives, beeswax, fatty acids, lanette wax, lecithins, olive oil, cholesterol and silicone oils are used for their softening and oily qualities which replace the beneficial effect of sebum. The chemicals act as emulsifiers, allowing the oil and water to mix. The mixture is heated until the waxes and oils form an emulsion; perfume is then added.

Setting agents

Setting lotions, in general, do not greatly affect the internal structure of the hair fibre except for breaking a few hydrogen and salt links. The aim of a setting lotion is to coat the hair in a lotion which prevents the hair drying out too quickly. The set is held by preventing moisture and humidity from entering the hair fibre, thus ensuring the cohesiveness of the style. Setting lotions based on mucilages are now seldom used.

Most setting agents now are of the synthetic variety and are based on polyvinylpyrrolidone (PVP). Gels, setting lotions and mousse foams encapsulate the hair fibre in a flexible plastic film and adhere to the hair even through the dressing out. Good setting agents should not flake or make the hair sticky or water soluble, and should maintain adhesion even during blow-drying. They should remain flexible and be easily shampooed out. These types of agent incorporate plastifiers which help to maintain the good qualities of a setting lotion. They also contain film-forming polymers, silicone, alcohol, proteins, water and perfume. While the hair is drying, the alcohol and water evaporate, leaving the plastifier to coat the fibre.

Other products

Foams (mousses)

These contain many of the above ingredients but will also contain a propellant (and sometimes colour).

Gels

These control the hair well and are good fixatives. They are based on aqueous polyethylene glycols combined with a cellulose thickener such as isopropyl cellulose.

Hairsprays

Hairsprays need similar qualities to setting agents to deposit a fine film on the hair fibre to protect it against moisture and humidity and help hold the style in place.

The earlier lacquers used natural resins such as shellac, but nowadays synthetic resins such as polyvinylpyrrolidone (PVP) are used as a base.

A good hairspray should have a number of qualities. It should:

- have good holding properties;
- be water soluble;
- be non-sticky when touched and non-flaking when brushed, and should not cause lack of natural shine;
- dry quickly;
- readily coat the hair;

A typical hairspray will include:

- plastifiers (PVP) – to coat the hair;
- lubricating, softening and shining agents – lanolin, silicones;
- solvents – alcohol, ethanol, isopropyl mysistate to spread the spray;
- propellants – freon or butane (50% approximately);
- perfumes – a minimum is necessary to enhance only.

No water is added to hairspray as it makes the can go rusty inside.

Questions

1   The protein keratin is made up of many amino acids.

   a   How is each amino acid identified?

   _____

   _____

   b   Give three examples of how amino acids differ, using this identification.

   _____

   _____

   c   Give an example of the amino acid that is affected by permanent waving.

   _____

   _____

   d   Of what elements are amino acids constructed?

   _____

   _____

2   a   What is meant by:
       i   a carboxyl group?

   _____

       ii   an amino group?

   _____

   b   Which is the positive charge?

   _____

3   Using simple diagrams, show how the amino acid cystine is constructed.

4 Match the words in Column A with those in Column B.

COLUMN A		COLUMN B	
i	helix coil	a	positive and negative charge
ii	carboxyl	b	COOH
iii	salt bonds	c	digestion of proteins
iv	enzymes	d	hydrogen bonds
v	amino group	e	positive charge
		f	spiral polypeptide

5 The polypeptide chain is linked by numerous bonds and cross-chains. Name four of these bonds and their function in helping the coil keep its shape.

_____

_____

_____

_____

6 Using diagrams, explain the process of keratinisation and the development of the fibrils.

7 a Describe the three hair follicle types found on the body.

_____

_____

b How is the follicle structured?

_____

_____

8 Discuss how the hair fibre is pigmented.

_____

_____

_____

9 Describe the digestion and breakdown of:
a proteins;

_____

b carbohydrates.

_____

10 **a** Name the vitamins that are necessary for:

    i preventing scalp dandruff and strengthening fingernails;

_____

    ii preventing premature greying;

_____

    iii promoting hair growth and slowing down the aging process of the skin.

_____

  b Name the food sources that are rich in these vitamins.

_____

_____

_____

11 What food source is rich in the following minerals:

  a iodine?

_____

  b iron?

_____

12 **a** Explain, using diagrams, the action of the shampoo molecule in removing dirt from the hair fibre.

  b What are the physical processes involved, and what properties should shampoo have to carry out these processes?

_____

_____

13 Discuss the qualities involved in the formulation of soap and soapless shampoos.

_____

_____

_____

14 Explain why the 'feel' of conditioner still remains in the hair fibre even after copious rinsing.

_____

_____

_____

15 Give a typical formulation of a hair conditioner.

_____

_____

16 a What is the function of a setting agent?

_____

   b Name the synthetic chemical used in most setting agents.

_____

   c What does 'water soluble' mean?

_____

_____

17 a Name five qualities of a good hairspray.

_____

_____

_____

   b Give a typical formula for a hairspray.

_____

_____

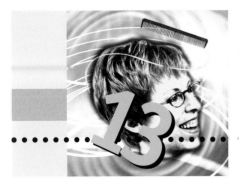

Advanced permanent waving

In this chapter, you will learn about:

- the chemistry of permanent wave lotion;
- typical permanent wave problems and correct advice;
- combined permanent waving and colouring.

Introduction

Many chemicals can be used as effective reducing agents for permanent waving. The most commonly used permanent wave reducing agents are based on thioglycollic acids (thios) in various forms. The thio reducing agent reduces one double sulphur keratin molecule (cystine) to two single keratin molecules (cysteine).

The percentage of reducing agent in the permanent wave solution will determine its strength – 10% thio for strong difficult coarse hair; 7 to 8% for medium/normal hair; and below 5% for processed/tinted hair. In the alkaline form, the thioglycollic acid ($HSCH_2COOH$) will be combined with excess ammonium hydroxide to form ammonium thioglycollate.

Even in acidic permanent waving (pH 5.5 to 7) thioglycollic acid is used. Unlike alkaline wave formulations, however, acid waves contain no excess ammonia. They are not compounded with ammonia, although the thioglycollic acid is made more alkaline. These chemicals may include: thiolactic acids, glycol thioglycollate, glycerol thioglycollate, or thioglycollamides.

A low pH is maintained throughout the waving process because excess ammonia is not present to swell the hair. Heat is usually applied to assist penetration of the solution during the processing time, either with a dryer, a clamp or with chemical heat (exothermic) reaction. Acid permanent waves are gentle on the hair and produce good results.

Permanent wave solutions may also contain:

1 boosters – urea which helps break the hydrogen bonds;
2 alcohols – ethanol to strengthen the lotion;
3 softening agents – animal oils, lanolin derivatives or vegetable oils and hydrolised proteins (these additives improve the aesthetic properties of the waved hair);
4 colouring agents – chemicals which make the solution opaque (opacifiers) to give the impression of a gentler, milky lotion;
5 cationic compounds – to improve the waved hair's condition (elasticity).

The reduction of di-sulphide links

These solutions are among the best reducing agents available. The reduction is accomplished by the addition of the hydrogen which comes in contact with the di-sulphide (–S–S–) links in cystine. The reducing agent by no means reduces all the di-sulphide links. During a typical permanent wave, between 15 and 45% of the cystine links will be broken. The ideal level of reduction is 25% of the di-sulphide bonds with a 5% thio content.

The hydrogen then becomes attached to the sulphur atoms between the polypeptide chain. This breaks the link between each molecule, forming sulphydryl group (–SH HS–) bonds or two molecules of an amino acid called kerato-cysteine. The hair can now undergo relaxation and conform to the shape of the perm rod.

Once the hair has been reduced by the addition of the hydrogen atoms, it must be rebonded again to form cystine.

The neutraliser

Most permanent waves are neutralised using hydrogen peroxide as it is easy to use and relatively inexpensive. It is acidified by adding citric or lactic acid for stability and usually contains cationic compounds to improve its wetting capability, together with foaming agents. Softening agents such as lanolin derivatives or waxes are also used. These agents may help to reduce the possibility of decolouring or lightening the hair during the neutralising stage.

During this restoration, the di-sulphide bonds are formed by an oxidising agent (H_2O_2). This can be done using hydrogen peroxide, sodium bromate or sodium perborate (the latter being richer in oxygen). The neutraliser also performs a second function – to neutralise any excess permanent wave solution (the citric or lactic acid) and to restore the hair's strength. There may be small amounts of alkali solution left in the cortex and the neutraliser can remove these traces because of its acidic nature. This will stop the slow weakening of the fibre by the possible continuation of the permanent wave solution on the end or peptide bonds.

This rapid rate of rehardening or reformation which alters the pH of the hair fibre does not always allow for the fibre's complete restoration. It is not so much the overprocessing of the permanent wave solution that does the damage as the overneutralising or rehardening process.

Oxidation must be carried out carefully and timing is critical, especially in the case of sodium bromate or sodium perborate neutralisers. If the neutraliser is left on longer than the instructions indicate, then the oxidation action will continue, and will start to lighten the hair fibre. Cysteic acid is also formed, which reduces the number of cystine links to be reformed; it also destroys the matrix protein and weakens the fibre. Hair which has been lightened also has many of the sulphur molecules changed into cysteic acid, which explains why this type of hair is difficult to permanently wave. As up to 45% of the di-sulphide links are reduced, this means that over 50% of the links are unchanged. The neutraliser, however, will account only for a majority rebonding, that is, not all the links are rejoined. There is, therefore, some initial relaxation of all permanent waves in the first few days following the service.

The neutraliser contains oxygen which combines with the two sulphydral groups containing the hydrogen atoms. The extra oxygen atom from the neutraliser plus the hydrogen from the sulphydryl group form water. This allows the sulphur link to rejoin and form cystine again. This formation of water in the hair fibre during neutralising is the reason why the hair is so wet after a permanent wave, and therefore takes longer to dry.

Interestingly enough, the cuticle – both the exocuticle and endocuticle but particularly the exocuticle (external) – has great levels of di-sulphide cross-links which suggests that this layer is the most resistant to damage. In this case, approximately half the links are broken during permanent waving.

Permanent wave precautions – points to remember

What is important about the permanent wave process is not so much what the finished curl looks like as the condition that the hair is left in after the service.

1   It is easier to damage hair if it is already weak as a result of tinting or lightening.

2   Select the chemical best suited for the job and, in any case, don't leave solution on the hair longer than necessary.

Acid permanent wave is best for: delicate hair, i.e. frosted, lightened, coloured; soft and limp hair; previously permed hair; hair which lacks moisture and tends to dryness; frequent permanent wave client.

Alkaline permanent wave stronger solutions are best for: thick, coarse, wiry hair; fine resistant hair; directional permanent wave winds; hair which tends to oiliness.

3   Alkali permanent waves can break peptide or end bonds if left on the hair too long. (Acid permanent waves are usually self-timing.)

4   Most damage can occur within the first 15 minutes of the application of the solution.

5   The size of the permanent wave curl is due to the altered position of the di-sulphide links. This is controlled by the circumference of the perm rod.

6   The percentage of reducing agent (thio) content will determine the strength of the solution (10% for stronger difficult hair, 7 to 8% for normal medium hair and below 5% for lightened or tinted hair). This affects pH value. Highly lightened hair needs only 1 or 2% thio content.

7   Don't overneutralise the hair as this could overharden it, remove too much intercellular cement (soft amorphous protein) and weaken the fibre.

8   Not all the di-sulphide links are rejoined and there may be some relaxation of the curl in the six days following the treatment.

9   Don't put alkaline permanent waves under any heat source to speed up the process as they are formulated to work within certain temperature ranges and acceleration can cause scalp burns and irreversible hair damage.

10 It takes longer to rinse out an acidic solution than it does to rinse out an alkaline one because the hair fibre is less swollen.

 ## Typical perm waving problems and correct advice

Question 1: What precautions should I observe if I decide to cut the hair after a permanent wave?

Bear in mind that when the hair is cut after a permanent wave the wave itself will appear looser, especially if long lengths are cut off. If there is a large amount to cut, it is better to take the majority off before the perm.

Avoid excessive pulling, stretching or tugging of the hair by the comb as this can collapse the curl formation and cause damage.

You should also consider the psychological aspect, where the client feels the permanent wave is being cut out. Some hairdressers may take the attitude that by cutting after the permanent wave they can hide a multitude of sins! The permanent wave may be wound unprofessionally, with the thought that the ends are being cut anyway; this attitude is not suitable for good hairdressing.

Question 2: Can I permanent wave hair which has previously had a henna treatment?

If in doubt, do a prewave test curl, but it is not recommended to permanent wave hair which has been treated with henna. Although a vegetable colour, henna still enters the fibre and so can inhibit the chemical action of the permanent wave. Loss of colour or discolouring can also occur. If a permanent wave must be given, wait at least a month, and treat the hair as though it has been tinted, i.e. select the solution accordingly.

Question 3: What solution should be used on hair which has been streaked or frosted?

Hair which has been lightened has lost a good deal of its cross-links and will swell much more rapidly than normal hair and adsorb the waving solution more completely. This does present a problem, as there are two types of hair to consider, one being more porous than the other. The problem area is the lightened streaks which will process far more quickly. Apply a porosity filler to the hair generally, especially to the areas streaked. Use solution for normal hair, wind carefully and check regularly, i.e. every three minutes. The filler will retard the action of the permanent wave lotion and slow the processing time, particularly on the streaked areas. Follow all precautions and treat hair as though it has been tinted.

Question 4: How can colour loss be prevented on tinted or coloured hair?

The type of colour will influence the amount of loss. Temporary and semipermanents will, understandably, be easily removed by the permanent wave procedure; a temporary rinse may be added to the neutraliser during this process. Tinted hair may incur some fading, because of:
1 The permanent wave lotion.
2 The neutraliser.

The permanent wave lotion acts as a reducing agent and decreases the artificial colour molecule size so that it washes out more readily through the cuticle. This can be partially prevented by using the recommended solution for coloured hair. Leave it on the hair for no longer than necessary and ensure that the solution is thoroughly rinsed from the hair. Also, the swelling of the hair shaft by the permanent wave lotion can increase the porosity and allow some colour molecules to wash out.

The neutraliser, being an oxidising agent, may lighten the colour if it is left on for an extended period. Read the instructions carefully and rinse the neutraliser off completely, after the time indicated has elapsed.

It is advisable to allow a week or two to go by between a colour application and a permanent wave.

Remedies: A bromate-based neutraliser may help to avoid excessive colour loss. Temporary colours or a semipermanent colour bath can be used to recolour the faded hair. Remember, however, that the hair will be porous and so the final colour may be too dark.

Question 5: What causes the unpleasant smell (ammonia) in the hair after permanent waving and how can it be eliminated?

This odour is solely the result of insufficient rinsing of the permanent wave lotion. It can be eliminated in two ways. First, it can be treated by applying equal portions – 30 cc of each – of 20 volume hydrogen peroxide, shampoo and conditioner. This will neutralise the excess thio left in the hair. Second, a rinse of essence of lavender or peppermint will mask the smell: 1 to 5 drops to half a litre (500 cc) of warm water. Pour through the hair; don't rinse.

Question 6: What is the problem when the permanent wave does not last as long as expected?

This will generally be the result of an incorrect pre-analysis and can happen for a number of reasons. Underprocessing and insufficient neutralising of the permanent wave is usually the reason why the curl will collapse, so watch development carefully. Common mistakes are:
1 mistiming – the solution is removed before it is processed;

2 incorrect solution selected for hair type (too weak) – give a prewave test curl if there is any doubt;

3 solution diluted because the hair is too wet;

4 insufficient dampening of the solution;

5 too large a perm rod for the curl desired;

6 mesh size too big – too much hair wound around each rod;

7 buckling and uneven winding (tension);

8 failure to follow manufacturer's instructions.

The neutraliser application may not have rejoined as many of the di-sulphide links and the wave will become gradually looser. This process should not be skimped; it is as important as any other step in the permanent waving procedure.

Question 7: What causes the hair to become dry and difficult to comb through?

If the solution is an alkali wave, it could be due to applying heat either by dryer or lamps. Although this reduces processing time, you lose control, and the hair is damaged. Other reasons can be:

1 too strong a solution;

2 incorrect timing (too long);

(Note: Prewave test curls will assist in determining these factors.)

3 insufficient rinsing of the permanent wave solution;

4 hair stretched during winding.

Nowadays neutralisers are fast-acting ones. Some are instant and work within about 60 seconds. Others need to be left on for 5 minutes. If the neutraliser is sodium bromate perborate, it must not be left on the hair for any longer than the maximum time indicated in the manufacturer's instructions. This will convert the di-sulphide link to cysteic acid which makes the hair difficult to comb. Ensure the neutraliser is thoroughly removed.

Question 8: After a permanent wave the crown area collapses but the back and sides hold the curl. Why is this?

The hairdresser tends to wind larger perm wave rods on the top as a matter of routine, assuming that the hair is longer or needs to be looser. In actual fact, the hair may be shorter than the back and sides and the larger rod collapses the wave curl. You need to concentrate and envisage the finished look throughout the entire procedure. Too large meshes on the crown with a slight underdirection can cause a premature collapse of the curl. Hairdressers who dampen the rods with solution may skimp on the top because they are running short of solution in the bottle. Because the top is more porous, dampening should begin at the nape area. The same procedure may happen when it comes to the neutraliser solution.

Wind the top with even tension, ensuring that the rods sit neatly on the base or section. Don't take too large a mesh and create buckling along the perm rod. Remember, the top is the area that the client sees easily, so make sure that this area looks good; take extra time and pay attention to detail.

Figure 13.1

Reverse stack wind variation

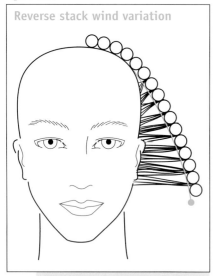

The perm rods can be held with a large knitting needle. The reverse stack allows the perm rods to be progressively dropped from the crown.

Figure 13.2

Stack winding variation

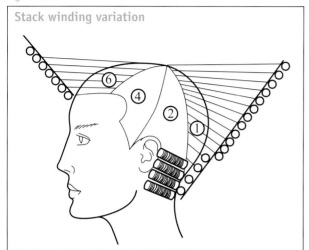

In this stack winding variation, each section is wound separately, starting at the bottom. Sections 3 and 5 are on the other side of the head.

Figure 13.3

Root perming

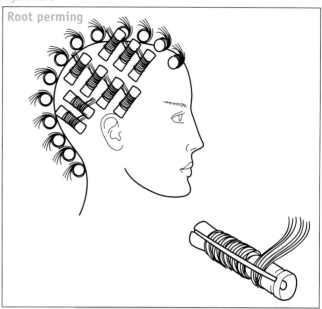

The perm rod is wound similarly to the piggy-back style except that the last 4 to 6 cm of hair is left free from the perm rod. This technique also allows for alternating sections of hair not to be permed. The finished style has an uncontrived, spiked look.

A Roll up a perm rod as usual and insert a second rod.
B Wrap hair around both rods.
C Wind and secure with a perm rod rubber. Ensure that the perm rod rubbers don't leave marks. The rubber on the inserted perm rod can even be left off and both rods secured by the first perm rod rubber. The result is a firmer end curl with volume only at the roots.

Figure 13.4

Double perm rod wind

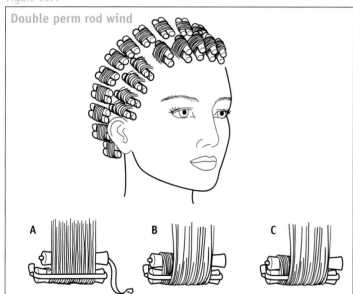

Figure 13.5

Piggy-back wind

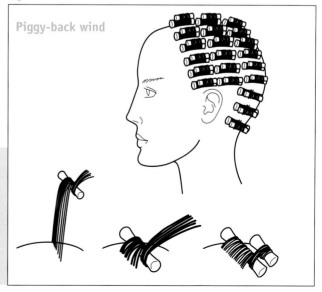

A Start to wind the perm rod in the middle of the strand of hair.
B Wind the rod towards the scalp, leaving the ends of the strand free.
C Wind the ends onto another perm rod.
This technique allows for alternating sections of the hair not to be permed. The result is a firmer end curl with volume at the roots.

Figure 13.6

Spiral winding

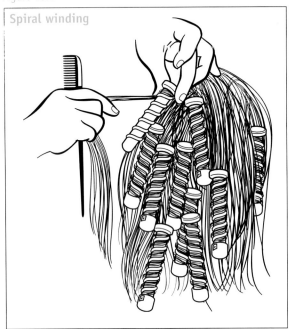

This winding technique uses spiral rods. A 2 cm² (approximately) section is taken and the hair is wound down the spiral rod, leaving the ends to be secured last with a simple clasp. This technique is ideal for long hair where a spiralled, ringlet effect is required. The spiral rods can be dampened down by immersing the rods, individually, in a test tube.

Figure 13.8

Alternating rod sizes with a high/ low variation

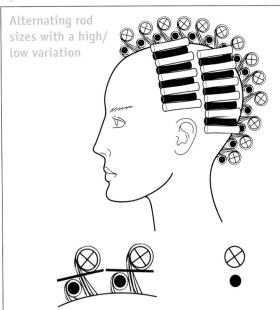

Figure 13.7

Weave winding (rick-rack)

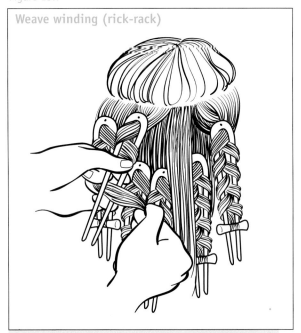

Weave the hair in and out of the sticks. Secure the end with a perm rod, which is also used for test curling. The finished effect is similar to a brushed-out plait.

Figure 13.9

Ponytail wind

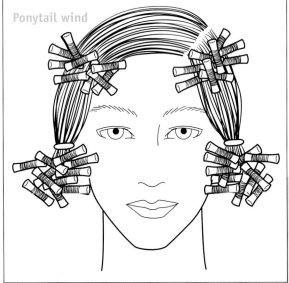

The hair is held in elastic bands. Don't dampen with the perm wave lotion above these.

The hair is wound on large and small perm rods, alternating a high and low variation. The result is a firmer curl at the roots with a larger, looser end curl.

Question 9: Why is the finished curl uneven?

Because the hair is not uniformly porous, this can affect the look of the finished result. The front, especially the hairline, is more porous and finer in texture and so it will process quicker. This area should be left until last when dampening. Improper dampening and dilution of the solution can also cause uneven curl development.

The rod size should be correctly determined and wound with even tension. Make sure that your elbows are at an even angle while winding. Inconsistency during winding will cause uneven curl development.

Question 10: Is it wise to relax a permanent wave which is too curly?

Do this only if, in your opinion, the hair is in good enough condition. Care should be taken. The problem is remedied by winding the hair, using large rods. Wind the hair after a filler type conditioner has been applied and a mild solution used. Check progress at two-minute intervals. Rinse and neutralise. Some manufacturers may offer a protein conditioning formula to relax an overtight curl. This is usually left on the hair for 15 to 20 minutes. Two or three treatments may relax a curl sufficiently.

Figure 13.10

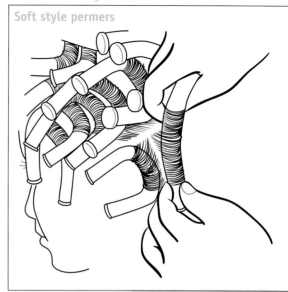

Soft style permers

These are made from foam rubber. The hair is wound around the foam and secured with a simple twist on the final turn. The wound look resembles small antennae. There are no pins or perm rod rubbers to hold the foam rods in place. These permers are available in different diameters and lengths. The finished look is soft and natural. Soft stylers are fun to use.

Fashion and directional permanent waving winding techniques

- Reverse stack wind variation.
- Stack winding variation.
- Root perming.
- Piggy-back wind.
- Double perm rod wind.
- Spiral winding.
- Weave winding (rick-rack).
- Ponytail wind.
- Alternating rod sizes with a high/low variation.
- Soft style permers.

Combined permanent waving and colouring

There may be times when a client requests both a permanent wave and a colour on the same day. Generally, it is not recommended that these two processes be done on the same day, but if it is necessary, perhaps for travel reasons or because time is short and the client's hair must look good, then there are some guidelines to follow to ensure that results are good and that the hair is left in the best possible condition.

A preliminary strand test and pretest curl will help you, especially if the hair is lightened. You must determine whether to do the colour or the permanent wave first.

Factors to consider
- The length of regrowth.
- The porosity of the hair.
- The depth or level of colour and the reflect of colour.

When to apply the colour first

- On a regrowth which is longer than 3 cm (approximately).
- When the porosity is uneven or of extreme variations.
- On dark colours which have little or no warmth.

Advantages of applying the colour first

If the regrowth is longer than 3 cm (approximately), you will not be sure which permanent wave solution to use – one for tinted hair or one for normal hair. If the colour is applied first, you can choose a solution for tinted hair because the hair is now all one type and therefore of even porosity. Permanent wave solutions can be selected according to hair type, but colours cannot. For example, you can't choose a colour for permed hair.

Disadvantages of applying the colour first

If you apply the colour first, the application of the perm wave lotion can result in some colour loss, thereby decreasing the intensity of the colour. This is common when permanently waving tinted hair; you may have noticed staining on the end papers which is the same colour reflect as the tinted hair. This is because permanent waving lotions are reducing agents, that is, they actually decrease the size of the artificial colour molecules in much the same way as the action of a chemical colour stripper, causing the artificial colour to be washed out of the cortex.

The decrease in colour intensity will not be as noticeable on dark ash colours because these colours can stand a loss of half a shade or so whereas a delicate, light, warm colour can go brassy and a half shade lighter can reflect a different shade altogether. Careful neutralising will be necessary to overcome this slight disadvantage. The oxygen in the neutraliser will re-swell the artificial colour molecule and lock the colour in the cortex, thereby preventing colour loss. Permanent wave lotion and neutraliser should not be left on the hair for any longer than necessary. Any differences in the colour loss can be put back into the hair using a temporary rinse of the same shade. Ensure that the hair is well conditioned if hair has been coloured and permanently waved.

When to do the permanent wave first

- On light, delicate fashion colours, especially those with gold or warm reflects.
- If the regrowth is shorter than 3 cm.
- On a head of hair not previously coloured (a virgin head of hair).

Advantages of doing the permanent wave first

The advantage of doing the permanent wave first, especially on lighter shades, is that you will obtain a better colour result because the permanent wave lotion will not have such an influence on lightening the more delicate, light reflect colours. A half shade or so lighter on a light colour will be more noticeable than a half shade on a dark head of hair. On previously tinted hair, the difference in the varying porosity is not enough to cause an uneven curl in the finished permanent wave if the regrowth is shorter than 3 cm.

Disadvantages of doing the permanent wave first

Because of the procedure involved in applying the colour, there can be some relaxation in the strength of the permanent wave curl. Anticipate this and wind a slightly smaller perm wave rod. The porosity of the hair will also increase because of the two chemical processes being carried out. This is easily overcome by applying a porosity filler to the hair after the treatment, to reduce porosity.

When you have decided to give both a permanent wave and colour on the same day, for best possible results make sure of the correct preliminary analysis. As an extra safeguard, water wind the permanent wave, regardless of whether it is done before or after the colouring.

Practical exercise

On a weft of natural hair, strand test a permanent wave and then a colour. Note the following (a) condition; (b) porosity, and (c) any variation in the result of the permanent wave or colour. Keep the test and clip it in your folder.

Questions

1 **a** Give examples of how the percentage of thioglycollic content in permanent wave solution will affect its strength.

_____

_____

b What is meant in acidic permanent waving when the label states it contains 'no excess ammonia'?

_____

_____

c What other factors do acidic permanent waves rely on to do the job of the ammonia?

_____

_____

d Name two chemicals which may be included in acidic waves to keep the pH acidic.

_____

_____

2 What else may permanent wave lotions contain in addition to ammonia and thios?

_____

_____

_____

3 Using diagrams, show:
   a the reducing effect that thioglycollic acid has on the sulphur amino acid side chain;
   b how the restoration of the amino acid takes place.

4   Explain what the following refer to
    a   sodium bromate?

    b   cysteic acid?

    c   cationic compounds?

5   Give examples of factors which will influence whether you need to use either an acid or alkali permanent wave solution.

6   Explain the considerations when selecting a permanent wave solution for streaked or lightened hair.

7   Discuss the possibilities of colour loss during a permanent wave. How can this problem be overcome or remedied?

8   What are the reasons for the curl collapsing in the crown area but holding well at the back and sides of the head?

9   List 10 reasons why a permanent wave may not last as long as desired.

10 Explain the following fashion permanent wave winding techniques:

a root perming;

_____

_____

b spiral winding;

_____

_____

c rick-rack;

_____

_____

d piggy-back winding;

_____

_____

e reverse stack.

_____

_____

11 A client requests both a permanent wave and colour on the same day.

a Name three considerations which will determine whether you should do the colour or the permanent wave first.

_____

_____

b What is the name of the tests that can be given if there is any doubt about the procedure?

_____

c Explain why you might decide to apply the colour first.

_____

_____

_____

d List two advantages and two disadvantages of applying the colour first.

_____

_____

e   Why would you decide that the permanent wave should be started first?

_____

_____

f   List two advantages and two disadvantages of doing the permanent wave first.

_____

_____

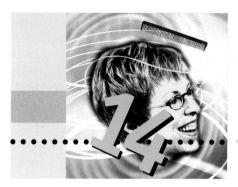

Advanced colour

In this chapter, you will learn about:

- the chemistry of artificial pigments;
- fashion colouring;
- typical colour and lightening problems – causes and remedies;
- ultraviolet radiation in New Zealand.

The chemistry of artificial pigments (dyes) or intermediates

Permanent artificial hair colourants can be called:

- colour intermediates;
- synthetic tints;
- mineral dyes (tints);
- para dyes (tints);
- analine derivatives;
- oxidation dyes (tints).

The terms *dye* and *tint* are both used to mean permanent colour. *Dye* is a little old fashioned and has connotations of the old metal dyes. It also can be associated with dyeing clothes, so the term *tinting* is more commonly used.

Most tints are able to parallel the way natural hair colour reflects and absorbs light, the only difference being in the way the colour is formed. Natural hair colour pigment is injected into the growing cells at the germinal matrix of the hair root by melanocytes. Artificial colour intermediates are produced by oxidation of the minute colour molecules which diffuse easily into the hair fibre. They form a chemical reaction with hydrogen peroxide and develop their final colour.

Manufacturers use the terms *colour intermediates* or *analine derivatives* when referring to tints, which are derived from the mineral benzine (a distillation of coal tar). The molecule can be illustrated as a six-sided (hexagonal) structure.

Most tints nowadays contain para. The earlier products contained para phenylene diamine which coloured the hair quite deeply but was likely to cause allergic reactions. Most manufacturers now use para toluene (tolyene) diamine, meta toluene diamine or para amino phenol, which does not colour quite as deeply but is less likely to cause an allergic reaction.

Oxidation of tints into stable colour pigment

The action of these tints on the hair shaft is one of oxidation, hydrogen peroxide being the oxidant. Hydrogen peroxide lightens the natural pigmentation of the hair so that the introduced pigments will overpower the original hair colour. Oxidation involves the release of oxygen. When the oxygen is given off, the para converts to quinone di-imine. At this stage the quinone di-imine molecules are still small and colourless and can pass easily into the cortex.

Once they are left to develop, the quinone di-imine molecules combine into a large giant chain of colour pigment called a polymer. Once these large coloured polymers are produced in the hair fibre, it is difficult to remove them completely. The colour is stable and therefore considered permanent; it either has to be cut out, bleached out or grown out. The tint molecules become chemically attached to the keratin of the hair. It is understandable that these tints should not be mixed until ready to use as once the large polymers have formed, they will not be able to enter the hair fibre.

The formulation of a tint will include the following.

1 Ammonia to open the cuticle scale and allow easy penetration of the tint molecules, and to liberate the oxygen for oxidising purposes.
2 Conditioners – to maintain the quality of the hair while it is being treated. Conditioners also provide an emulsion base to bind all the ingredients together.
3 Buffers – to prevent premature oxidation which will retard the tint action; sodium sulphite is sometime used.
4 Wetting agents – to overcome the surface tension of the emulsion, to assist adhesion of the tint and to facilitate rinsing. The wetting agents may be lauryl sulphates – soapless detergents.
5 Colour intermediates – to be oxidised into synthetic colour.
6 Perfume – to eliminate unpleasant odours.

The mixture is prepared as a thick liquid or cream. It may cause serious inflammation of the skin, so use with care.

Semipermanent colourants

Colouring materials based on nitro dyes such as nitro-amino benzines or nitro-amino phenols penetrate the hair fibre. The molecules are small enough to enter the cortex where they combine with the hydrogen bonds in the keratin. Nitro dyes do not, however, normally become fixed in the hair fibre and the dye gradually washes out.

More recent semipermanent colourants are mixtures of the oxidation tints, which contain ammonia to aid their penetration. They give a wider range of colour choice but regrowth is more apparent. Treat them in a similar manner to permanent tints and take any necessary precautions. They may also contain soapless detergents to form a cream which allows the hair fibre to swell and gives better penetration. Soapless detergents can also make them foam.

Temporary colourants

These are acid and only stain and harden the cuticle. The molecules are too large to enter the cortex and therefore usually wash out readily. They are formulated with acid dyes also known as azo dyes and sodium salts or organic acids such as citric acids which improve the colour's adhesion to the cuticle.

Lightening

This involves the removal of the natural pigment, melanin, by a chemical action. When a lightening agent is applied to the hair, the fibre is first swelled to allow the agent to lighten the natural colour in the cortex. This action also breaks down the melanin pigment and causes it to dissipate. This is a true 'bleaching out' of the hair's natural pigment. The chemical action is one of oxidation, usually with hydrogen peroxide. Hydrogen peroxide is combined with magnesium carbonate or ammonia carbonate and mixed into a thick paste. These types of lightening agents are usually the strongest but can cause the hair to become porous and dry if incorrectly used. Milder lightening agents contain sulphonated oils and do not lighten the pigment as completely.

Fashion colouring

(see Figure 14.1(a–h) on pp. 174–175)

Changing tone

Changing tone is a simple process, provided you are familiar with the fundamental principles of colour. A slight change of hair colour can often be achieved by adjusting the tone.

Darkening

Darkening can be an ideal way of adding weight and volume to finer areas of the style. It can cover grey hair. You should, however, consider your client's age and skin tones when choosing a darker shade, bearing in mind that the final result should look natural.

Darkening natural hair

If the natural base colour does not contain enough pigment for the chosen shade, the colour will be too light and bright and this can result in a rapid fade. Adding extra base colour and a weaker hydrogen peroxide can avoid this.

Darkening hair that has been previously lightened

When the hair is lightened, warm pigments are removed from the hair; when going darker, this pigment must be replaced. If the client is a light blonde, to achieve a darker blonde or brown the colour formula must contain extra warmth to replace the missing pigment.

Halo colouring (multi-shading)

Halo colouring is an ideal technique for precision-cut hair as it emphasises and enhances the line of the style. By using a foil-covered cardboard cut-out on medium layered hair, you can create a flattering individual look.

Technique

Comb the hair into the finished style. Use the centre of the head as a guideline and take a circle of hair approximately 2 to 3 cm around this centre point. Twist and secure. Place the 'halo' on the head, keeping the twist as the centre point, and lift out approximately 1 cm of hair and place on top of the halo. Colour (using varying shades) or prelighten the ends of the hair. About 5 minutes before the end of the development, merge the colour or prelightener further up the hair to remove a definite line. The hair can be toned if prelightened or left natural.

Block colouring (multi-shading)

Block colouring offers personalised colour to the more adventurous client, as well as giving you a chance to create your own design. By applying a number of shades to different sections of the hair, you can define the cut and style of the hair, giving either dramatic or subtle results, depending on the colours chosen.

Preparation

Ensure that the hair is carefully cut and styled before applying the colour. Choose a variation of colours following the design line of the style.

Technique 1

Section areas using zigzag partings to avoid hard lines. Prelighten or colour sections as desired to emphasise the weight or strength of the design lines.

Technique 2

Divide hair into three sections and prelighten the two front sections (A and B) to different prelightened bases. Apply the same colour shade to the whole head to give three variations of depth and reflect or tone.

Touch colouring (multi-shading)

A creative technique for the professional colourist, touch colouring recreates the sun's effects on the hair, lightening the ends and adding interest to the style.

Preparation

Hold the hair away from the head, spraying the roots, lengths and ends liberally with hairspray. Continue until all the hair is held away from the head. If the hair is long, back comb gently before applying hairspray.

Technique

Mix lightener to a creamy consistency. Apply with gloved fingers to the tips of the hair, and leave and develop until the desired prelightened base is achieved. Shampoo the hair and either:

1 leave hair as it is;
2 apply a semipermanent rinse; or
3 apply a tint to the hair – all over.

Naturalising

Naturalising is an ideal technique for introducing clients to hair colour. It easily overcomes objections to a regrowth with a full head of colour. When choosing shades for naturalising (for the most natural look), choose subtle colours to blend with the natural hair colour. Ensure two depths' difference between each colour to avoid colour merging.

Preparation

Use perforated cling film or hairdressing tin foil. Use 30 volume hydrogen peroxide when lightening and 10 or 20 volume hydrogen peroxide when darkening.

Technique

Section the hair, leaving 1 cm around the hair line and, if light colours are being used, along the parting line also. Weave sections of hair with a tail comb. Ensure woven sections are slightly larger than for highlighting.

Apply the chosen colours to alternating sections, emphasising the cut and style of the hair. Wrap each individual woven section in cling film and leave to develop normally.

Typical colour and lightening problems – causes and remedies

Problem 1: Colour result is too dark

Causes

1 Hydrogen peroxide too low in strength, therefore not giving sufficient lift.
2 Colour chosen with too much ash or drabbing reflect. Ash colours always make colour appear darker.
3 Hair texture is fine, and it accepted too much colour pigmentation.
4 Natural base too dark for colour selected.
5 Hair has good porosity and grabs colour.

Remedies

1 Check strength of hydrogen peroxide using a hydroxometer. Store the chemical so that it does not lose its oxygen strength.
2 Because ash colours contain silvers, greens or blues, this creates the illusion of a darker colour. Select a shade lighter to compensate for this.

3   Manufacturers' instructions may indicate the need to use a shade or two lighter for hair which is fine in texture. It will accept the colour pigment readily.

4   If a direct application has been given, the base colour may be so dark that the new colour will have no effect on the darker natural colour. Use a higher strength hydrogen peroxide or prelighten with a mild lightener.

5   Porous hair will grab the colour and go darker. Apply a porosity filler before the colour application or select a shade one or two levels lighter.

Hair which has gone darker can present a difficulty as it is usually only a shade or so too dark. A lightening shampoo – using lightening agent and shampoo only – can be mulched through for 10 to 15 minutes. There is a danger, if hydrogen peroxide is used, of imparting red tones – particularly at the roots. This reddish cast may be undesirable. Continuous shampooing using concentrate shampoo can lighten to the same degree.

Colour reduction can also be considered if the treatment involves lightening of more than one shade.

Finally, you can wait a few days to see if the dark result fades. If in doubt, give a preliminary strand test.

Problem 2: Colour result is too light or fair and lacks enough depth

Causes

1   Hydrogen peroxide too high in strength, giving too much lift.
2   Insufficient development.
3   Hair has resistance and is strong, wiry, coarse.
4   Incorrect application.
5   Colour selection too light in reflect.

Remedies

1   The higher the volume strength, the more oxygen is liberated and the lighter the natural pigmentation becomes. Follow manufacturer's instructions for special lightening tints and the strength of hydrogen peroxide recommended.

2   If the maximum time indicated by the manufacturer's instructions is not followed during the development period, then the full oxidation process may not be complete, resulting in colour loss and a less intense depth of final colour. Always develop as per instructions to ensure the full development of the colour polymer in the cortex.

3   Resistant hair will not accept colour readily and will throw off the mixture, thereby not allowing full penetration for colour development. Resistant formulas can be applied or the hair can be presoftened.

4   Certain areas of the hair will develop more readily than others, thereby giving a lighter result. The heat from the scalp will usually develop the root area of the hair strand more quickly.

5   Gold reflects make the colour appear lighter and possibly too brassy.

Hair should be able to take a recolour to give it more depth. Bear in mind, however, that the first colour application will make the hair more porous and the colour can become too dark. Finally, suggest a shampoo especially formulated for coloured hair to reduce the possibility of further colour loss or fading.

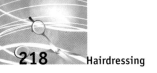

Problem 3: Final hair colour lacks any warmth and appears too ashen (matt)

Causes

Hair which has been lightened to pale yellow has lost the warm pigmentation. Colour applied which lacks in warmth will reflect ash, drab, khaki shades.

Remedy

If the red pigment has been taken out of the hair during lightening, it must be replaced when returning to a darker shade. This is called prepigmentation.

Prepigmentation usually takes the form of a warm (auburn, chestnut, mahogany) semipermanent colourant (given full development time). Some manufacturers may market products which are designed as colour fillers. A permanent colour with an abundance of warmth in the reflect may also be suitable.

The prepigmentation maintains an even development of the colour molecules, helps prevent colour fading as a result of shampooing, and prevents green discolouration (a fading to green) in the final result.

A greenish cast may sometimes become apparent after a colour has been applied to white hair, especially after four or five shampoos. This again is due to insufficient red pigment in cases where a matt, ash or cendre colour has been applied. A green cast can be noticeable, owing to the ready penetration of the reflect colour. In both cases, the remedy is to apply a complementary colour in a warm shade, either a temporary rinse or a semipermanent colourant.

Problem 4: Colour result too red, warm or brassy

Causes

1 A colour has been applied which has too much warmth in the reflect.
2 Excessive use of steamer, heat source or colour accelerator.
3 Hydrogen peroxide too strong.
4 Incorrect application technique.
5 Natural base colour of the client's hair too light.

Remedies

1 Become familiar with manufacturers' colour charts and be aware of the intensity of these warm colours. The traditional chestnuts, hazelnuts, mahoganies, auburns, burgundies and golds all contain varying amounts of warmth. All will produce a different effect on various natural base colours. If in doubt, do a preliminary strand test.
2 Heat, especially from lamps or steamers, tends to impart excessive warm reflects. It is better to process naturally if the client doesn't want any warm reflects.
3 The higher the volume strength, the more colour lift and the more obvious the warm reflect. The hydrogen peroxide will also impart the red/gold natural melanin pigmentation if it is too strong.
4 Certain areas of the hair strand will be more porous than others and will 'grab' the warm reflect. The front hairline, especially the temples, will do this. Apply colour to the more porous areas last or apply a porosity filler to slow the penetration of the colour. The ends of the hair can also be more porous and require special care.
5 The lighter the natural base colour, the more apparent the reflect. Select a colour with more subtle warmth.

Applying a complementary colour will tone down any excess warmth or brassiness. Ash, matt or cendre colours will be effective. Remember, the hair will be already porous and these colours naturally appear darker, so there is a double likelihood of the final result being too dark. Select a colour one shade lighter. The client may have to forsake a lighter result to compensate for the elimination of the warm reflects.

Red colours are the most stubborn colours to remove, especially if they are the result of lightening or if the client has a naturally warm colour. If full development of the complementary colour is not given, then the warmth may return gradually with each subsequent shampooing.

Problem 5: Coloured hair feels harsh and dry, lacks bounce and body and feels fragile

Causes

1 Overcolouring, too frequent colour application, build-up of colour.
2 Too high a volume of hydrogen peroxide.
3 Hair badly treated during and after colour process.
4 Colour build-up as a result of overlap.
5 Hair not in good condition before colour application.

Remedies

1 Permanent colour tint need only be applied on a monthly basis; if it is more often than this, it can create an encapsulated feeling to the hair structure. The colour does not need to be brought through to the ends at each application. Ensure that the hair is adequately conditioned between colour processes.

2 The higher the volume strength, the quicker the chemical action and the more damaged the result. Follow manufacturers' instructions but generally no stronger than 30 volume hydrogen peroxide is recommended.

3 Combing the colour through with a narrow comb or tint brush causes damage and loss of elasticity. It is better to mulch the mixture through when you need to bring it through to the mid-lengths and ends. Processing under a dryer or lamp or allowing the mixture to dry on the hair is not advocated. You should advise the client on how to maintain the coloured hair. It should be protected from sun and salt water in summer and conditioning agents should be used after shampooing. This usually involves selecting a shampoo formulated for coloured hair. Explain the correct use of brushes, tongs, blow-dryers or heated rollers, to ensure the minimum amount of damage to the coloured hair.

4 If a regular client has a tint, don't apply colour to the previously coloured hair. A line of demarcation will occur which will result in a harsh band of colour. This is called a tint overlap. Colour the regrowth only up to the previously coloured hair. Be precise and accurate in your application and only mulch through the mid-lengths and ends if the colour goes muddy after two or three retouches.

5 Don't suggest a colour treatment if the hair is not in good enough condition. This attitude is good professional hairdressing. Advise the client to have a series of preconditioning treatments so that the hair is in the best possible condition. Unless the hair is in good condition, you can't expect good results, no matter how good a colourist you are.

Figure 14.1
Damage by overtinting

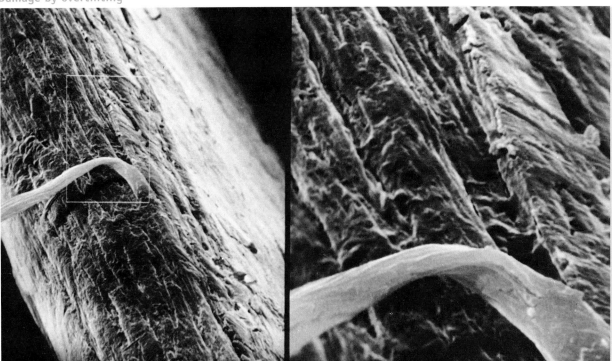

Overtinting has caused the cuticle of this hair fibre to become completely stripped. This has exposed the cortical fibre which, although strong, is completely dependent on the cuticle for protection. Here, the fibre is already starting to fall apart. This hair is extremely damaged.

Problem 6: Uneven lightening

Causes

1 Uneven application of lightener.
2 Differences in hair porosity.
3 Differences in the natural base colour.

Remedies

1 Prelightening the areas that have not lightened sufficiently. Spot lighten if necessary.
2 It is always wise to take a preliminary strand test to establish whether any uneven porosity exists. Hair is seldom completely uniform in porosity and, even with the correct application, there may still be areas that require decolouring.

Problem 7: Colour loss on fashion toners following lightening

Cause

Hair not receptive enough to the delicate toner colour. The hair is not porous enough and therefore the colour deposited is not sufficient and the hair loses colour with each shampoo.

Remedy

Toners are light, delicate tints and are successful only with the preliminary prelightening. The hair should be sufficiently light and porous to take the application. It is important to select the correct lightening agent, combined with the correct strength of hydrogen peroxide, so that the hair becomes porous for the toner to deposit the colour properly.

Apply a mild lightener and decolour the hair strand further. If the hair is sufficiently light, but not porous enough, then a presoftener should be used.

A diluted lightening solution is mixed and mulched through the hair for 10 to 15 minutes. This should give the hair extra porosity, without a great deal of extra colour lift. Alternatively, a double toner application can be made, in which the first application merely softens the hair in preparation for the second application.

A higher strength hydrogen peroxide mixed with the toner may also help to deposit and give the required colour lift.

Problem 8: After lightening the hair is too brassy (too yellow)

Causes

1 Mixing the lightener and leaving it to stand before application.
2 Lightening mixture/formula not strong enough.
3 Hydrogen peroxide too weak.
4 Incorrect application procedure.
5 Coating covering the hair strand.

Remedies

One of the problems when lightening is the tendency of the yellow melanin pigments to persist in the hair, leaving brassy tones. This can be counteracted by applying temporary, semipermanent or permanent tones, the most effective being the permanent lightening toner. These are generally used with higher strength hydrogen peroxide to give extra lift to the final colour.

Timing is important, since the lightening becomes active from the moment the mixture is prepared. (Application should therefore be as quick as possible.) On a full-head application, it may be advisable to mix only enough formula for half the head and to mix a further quantity for lightening the balance of the hair.

If the hair or scalp is excessively oily, dirty or coated with hairspray, then give the hair a shampoo. Dry under a cool dryer.

Problem 9: Unable to reach required lightening lift at the roots during retouches

Causes

1 A resistant regrowth.
2 The mid-lengths and ends have become lighter due to atmospheric oxygen reacting with the sunlight, residue oxygen left in the hair fibre after application, or loss of natural pigmentation because of extreme porosity.

Remedy

Generally, overcome this problem by carefully repeating the lightening application until a good match is obtained.

If the regrowth is allowed to grow too long, resistance will develop. A 1-cm regrowth will be easier to match than a 3-cm regrowth.

Problem 10: Client wishes to grow out his/her permanent colour. What advice should you offer?

Reasons

In recent years, the popular fashion in hair colour has been to look as natural as possible. There are certain stages in life, however, when it is not acceptable to be silver (grey). A 20-year-old woman, for example, may want to cover silver hair because few people her age have silver hair. The same client at, say, 60, may look out of place without silver hair, when her other features are aging. The overall effect will not look natural and she realises that at some stage she must reveal her real colour by growing out the artificial colour.

Advice

'Growing out' the colour is not technically or strictly what the client wants, for the only advice in this case would be to simply to stop colouring the hair. This, of course, would leave an unsightly line of coloured hair growing out over a period of months. Once the regrowth is sufficiently long, the balance of the hair can be cut short.

The client, however, probably wishes to camouflage the regrowth during the growing-out phase. Growing the colour out can include lightening the hair to a silver (grey) colour, thereby making the regrowth less noticeable, but you may need to prepare the client psychologically to accept such a sudden drastic change.

The alternative is to grow out to a noticeable regrowth and then semipermanently rinse the regrowth. As the hair grows, cut it into a short style. This procedure will need to be done two or three times, rinsing, say, every six to eight weeks. This also has the advantage to you that you do not immediately losing a colour client. Eventually, the grey hair will come through and the rinsing can be discontinued. The rinsing will be a good camouflage during the growing-out period and should not damage the hair.

Streaking is also a possibility. This, again, will camouflage the growing-out period. Fine frostings can be woven or drawn through a cap and placed discreetly, especially in the front so that the growing silver hair mingles and merges with the fine frostings. Frostings will give a lighter overall effect and get the client used to the final lighter result.

Whatever advice is suggested, the process of growing out a colour requires patience on the client's part and sensitivity on the part of the hairdresser. The client will have given the procedure a lot of thought and will have discussed it with others who may be affected by the change.

Ultraviolet radiation in New Zealand

Waiting for summer to get those natural golden streaks? Are clients complaining that their colour rinses and tints fade or go brassy? Is the outdoor sportsperson tired of having harsh, dry hair in summer?

It is widely believed that sunshine in New Zealand has a particularly harsh ultraviolet element. In general, hairdressers and hairdressing manufacturers and suppliers are aware of New Zealand's solar radiation and the role it plays in hairdressing. Clients are also aware of the problem of colour fading, not only in artificial hair colourings, but also in the hair's own natural colour, melanin.

The intensity of the sun's radiation depends on:

1 the elevation of the sun in the sky, which in turn depends on the time of day, the season and the latitude (the distance from the equator);

2 the atmosphere and its haziness and cloudiness.

New Zealand has a fairly sunny climate. Our skies are much less hazy than those of most northern hemisphere countries, though the New Zealand Meteorological Service does not think this makes a huge difference. It does say, however, that many people forget that our latitudes are similar to sunny Spain and Italy, rather than the more northerly Britain and Germany.

Also, because New Zealand's climate is so pleasant, people probably spend much more time outdoors. It is wise to suggest that clients who spend time outdoors protect their hair from the sun's radiation. This is worse when the sun is high in the sky. As the top part of the head is more exposed, this area will be most affected. Men who are balding should wear some form of protection.

The ultraviolet levels in New Zealand should be little different from those of other places of similar latitude and cloudiness, such as coastal Victoria, but there are still some puzzles to be solved on this matter. In any case, it appears that hair will continue to bleach as a result of the sun's radiation. Tensile strength and flexibility are valued properties of hair. Exposure to a New Zealand summer sun reduces the strength of the hair, and the hair becomes weathered, harsh and can break rapidly. All you can do is advise customers to protect their hair during summer months. Manufacturers of hair colour will have to develop a product which will make artificial colour more 'light stable'.

Questions

1   How are tints formulated?

_____

_____

2   a   What are semipermanent colourants based on?

_____

_____

    b   Why might a semipermanent contain soapless detergents?

_____

3   In which products are the following chemicals to be found:
    a   magnesium carbonate?

_____

    b   sodium salts?

_____

    c   colour intermediates?

_____

    d   nitro-amino phenols?

_____

    e   lauryl sulphate?

_____

_____

4   How is permanent colour oxidised into stable colour pigment?

_____

5   Outline three causes and three remedies for a colour result which is too dark.

_____

_____

_____

_____

_____

6 What can cause the final colour result to be too drab?

_____

_____

_____

7 How may the hair become chemically damaged as a direct result of colouring or lightening?

_____

_____

8 A client complains that the beige toner which followed a lightener has lost its colour. Give one possible cause and the remedy to rectify the problem.

_____

_____

_____

9 How can you overcome brassy tones in the hair after it has been lightened?

_____

_____

_____

10 What advice would you give to a client who wishes to grow out his/her coloured hair and retain the natural silver look?

_____

_____

_____

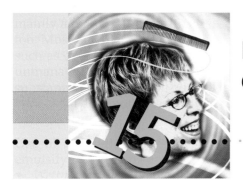

Boardwork and the making of postiche

In this chapter, you will learn about:

- wigs;
- making postiche;
- men's postiche;
- hair extensions.

Introduction

Boardwork involves the making of postiche. Postiche is any form of additional hair, such as wigs, wiglets, toupees, false moustaches, beards, and even eyelashes. There are skilled professionals who can knot, weave and sew up postiche. Boardwork is a trade very closely related to hairdressing. There are a variety of reasons why people need postiche:

1 to change their appearance;
2 where they may be losing their hair for medical reasons;
3 as an aid for theatrical plays;
4 just for fun.

Hairdressing salons are responsible for measuring, fitting and caring for postiche and some hospitals even advise patients with hair loss to visit such salons for consultation. Salons sometimes sell postiche pieces or have clients who bring in some form of added hair for cleaning, dressing and fitting. Hairdressers who work in television, film or theatre need to know how to work with postiche, especially for the dressing of period hairstyles. So, even though your salon may not handle postiche, you can see that there is good reason to learn about the way it is made, prepared, measured, cleaned, dressed and fitted. One day you could be working with postiche.

Boardwork – the making of postiche – involves the measuring, preparing, sewing and weaving or knotting of hair. Postiche is either made on a weaving frame or knotted by hand with a knotting needle. Postiche made on a three-string weaving frame are looped marteaux, stem switches, chignons and diamond meshes. Crêpe hair, Pompadour rolls, frizettes and doughnut buns/pads are made on a two-string weaving frame. Transformations, hand-made wigs and toupees can all be knotted by hand with a knotting needle (using a similar process to that of rug making).

Wigs

In the salon you will come across two types of wig – hand-made ones and machine-made ones.

The craft of wigmaking has become very commercialised as a result of new technology being developed, especially in Asia. Wig manufacturers now incorporate new ideas in each individual wig they design. This competition has led to the sale of machine-made wigs for as little as $20 in the United States, and even cheaper in Korea.

The craft of wigmaking by hand is very time-consuming and this is why a hand made postiche is expensive. Unless there is a special reason, clients will be reluctant to pay to have their postiche made by hand. As a senior stylist in the salon, you will encounter many machine-made wigs and hairpieces. Most men's toupees, however, are hand-made. You should know how conventional hand-made wigs are made.

The technology that was used in the production of machine-made wigs has now been incorporated, in part, into the making of hand-made wigs, so that these are now much lighter than they were, say, ten years ago.

Instead of the heavy nettings which were once used, light nylon lace is now knotted with hair. The heavier clock springs used for positioning are now replaced by light stainless steel springs which don't rust or corrode. Velcro straps are used as tension springs and fasteners and even the wider galloon has now been replaced by petersham. Polyurethane sheet is sewn in and used to attach double-sided tape. Polyester silks, similar to those used in silk screening, are used to line areas of the wig. These are more durable and better wearing. This new technology has made wigs better than ever; they are lighter, more comfortable and look more natural.

Because many of the materials required to make a wig are not readily obtainable, it is more difficult for the hairdresser to make one than it was in the past.

Hand-made wigs

These are made from a paper pattern based on the measurements that you have supplied to the wigmaker. The pattern is placed on a malleable block or a wooden mounting block. Galloon (a closely woven ribbon) is then sewn around the pattern perimeter (a parting, if required, is included on the pattern), positional springs are sewn in place and the netting is attached to the galloon. Notice, in the diagram of the wig mount, the different mesh sizes in the netting. The crown area is covered with a caul netting, while the paper pattern area is covered with foundation netting and the parting is knotted on silk netting.

The knotting of the hair onto this netting requires skill, practice and patience. Usually every other hole on every other line is knotted. Double knotting ensures that the hair is doubly secure. The wig mount is held in place with block pointing.

Machine-made or wefted wigs

Machine-made wigs are often referred to as wefted wigs. Their manufacture involves machine-wefting hair or synthetic fibre and sewing it by machine onto a capless base. Such wigs usually have a skin part. They are light and comfortable and the tension is usually adjusted by velcro straps or tension springs. Machine-made wigs are produced in quantity in various workshops throughout the world.

Types of hair used for wigs

Most wigs are usually made from two types of human hair: European and Asian.

European hair

This is by far the most sought-after type of hair, much in demand by hair merchants, because of its fine texture and natural shine. Most hairdressing services can be performed on European hair as long as the necessary precautions are taken – a test curl for permanent waving and a strand test for colouring. European hair may be artificially curled by hair merchants before it is made up. This is done by curling the hair on a bigode stick, boiling it and then drying it in a postiche oven. Although European hair is not easy to handle, it does have a natural look when finished.

Asian hair (Chinese, Nepalese, Indian)

Asian hair is more readily available and considerably cheaper than European hair, but it is much coarser in texture and does not have quite the finished look of the European hair. Usually, Asian hair is 'processed'. This '100% human processed hair' goes through a stretching and colouring or curling process, which increases the value of the hair when it is made up. Great care must be exercised when working with a wig which carries such a label, especially if a client requests it to be permanently waved or coloured. The hair may also have been 'vat dyed'. This involves using an acid bath to strip the cuticle, which makes the hair less coarse, and also lightens the fibre. Most of the human-hair wigs throughout the world are made of processed Asiatic hair.

Sources of hair

Human hair

The hair bought overseas by hair and wig merchants to be made into postiche comes from three main sources. Hair is bought from Italian nuns, from peasant women (in Nepal) who grow and sell their hair, and as hair cuttings from hairdressing salons. Hair combings – hair taken from brushes and combs – is not highly valued. All hair must be a minimum of 18 cm long; 18 cm of hair makes a hair piece approximately 15 cm long.

Whatever the source, all hair used for postiche must be correctly 'turned' or rooted and pointed. This means that all the roots must be at one end and all the points at the other. If this is not done, all the ends will run up the strand when the hairdresser washes the postiche and the wig hair could quite easily become matted, making it almost impossible to comb out. Hair is 'turned' or 'rooted and pointed' by swishing it in water. The need to prepare the hair in this way is the reason why hair combings are not commonly sought after. Indian and Nepalese hair is fairly good and is used mainly for practice block manikin heads for student training.

Synthetic fibre

The most common fibre used for making wigs is kanekalon, a very fine fibre which can readily be mistaken for human hair by the inexperienced hairdresser. Its curl is usually 'set in' by rolling on aluminium tubes and baking in a postiche oven at a temperature of around 60 °C. To maintain this curl, you should avoid extreme temperatures on curling tongs or hot dryers when working with kanekalon fibre. Otherwise you could spoil the curl or even melt the fibre. Nylon hair is not readily suited for wigmaking except perhaps for theatrical use, shop window mannequins or dolls.

Animal hair

Animal hair can be used as a substitute for human hair which is sometimes in short supply. Hair from the yak, a long-haired ox, has been used for its hair length, and mohair from the angora goat has been used, especially for dolls' hair. Judges' wigs are sometimes made from horse hair, although these wigs are not usually made within the hairdressing profession. Sometimes wigs have even been made using sheep's wool. Animal hair is not a good substitute for lost human hair.

Figure 15.1

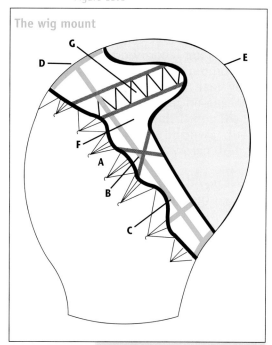

The wig mount

This shows:
A   Bracings
B   Positional springs
C   Bind
D   Galloon
E   Caul net
F   Foundation net
G   Silk netting on parting area

Figure 15.2

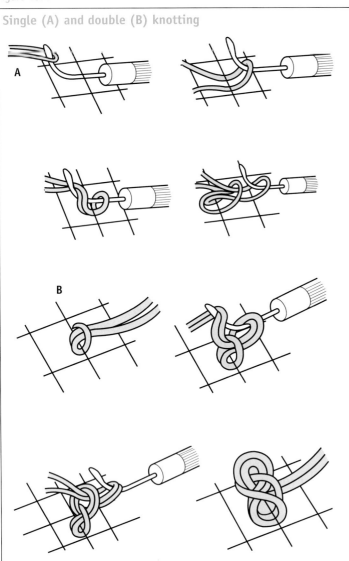

Single (A) and double (B) knotting

These exercises require skill, practice and patience. Double knotting ensures that the hair is firmly anchored to the netting.

 ## Making a postiche

Tools used in boardwork

A few simple tools are needed to make the different types of postiche. Ensure that you have adequate natural light when you are working.

- *The hackle.* Also called a carde, it is used for untangling the hair and mixing different shades of hair together. The hackle is also used for drawing the hair off in lengths. It is made of wood or metal and has large, sharp, upright or sloping teeth. Watch your knuckles when using this tool.

- *Weaving frame.* The English weaving frame has separate clamps and sticks. The right-hand stick has three grooves so that the weaving silks can be wound around it. The left-hand stick has a flat-headed nail to tie silks to. Wads of paper are used to tighten the silks individually. Wax the strings before use. Remember, it is the weaving frame that is used for making hair pieces.

- *Drawing brushes or mats.* These are used to hold prepared hair when weaving. Always ensure that the hair roots are facing you.

- *Jockey.* This is a useful tool which 'rides' the weaving silks to prevent the woven weft from becoming unravelled.

- *Knotting needle.* This small barbed hook comes in a variety of sizes; the size used depends on the size of the net being knotted.

- *Malleable block.* This is a head-shaped block filled with sawdust and covered with canvas.

- *Wooden mounting block.* This head-shaped block is made of solid wood.

Figure 15.3

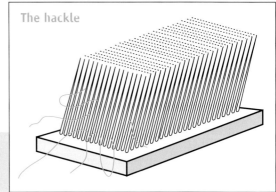

The hackle

This is a most useful tool in boardwork. It is used to untangle and draw off the hair lengths. Watch your knuckles on the sharp teeth.

Accessories used in boardwork

Silks for weaving	Silks wound on the weaving frame.
Nets: Caul	Used for crown area of a wig.
Foundation	Sewn around the pattern area.
Silk	Sewn along the parting only.
Galloon	A closely woven narrow ribbon, which comes in different colours according to the colour of hair used in the postiche.
Cache peigne	A hidden comb attached to a diamond mesh.
Postiche brush	Used to dress the added hair.
Wire	Used for positional springs, it is usually rust-resistant.

Figure 15.4

An English weaving frame

A The silks are all coming from the same direction.
B Note the paper wads for individual tensioning.
C Note the jockey which 'rides' the weaving silks to prevent the woven weft from becoming unravelled.
D Note the woven weft.

Different types of postiche

Postiche made on a three-string weaving frame should be made with at least 18 cm of hair length – 18 cm of hair will produce a postiche approximately 15 cm in length; a 25-cm hair length produces a 21-cm postiche (3–4 cm of the hair is used to produce the weft).

- *Marteau*. A marteau or fall is a wefted length of hair folded in three and sewn together. It may have loops attached to each end. It is covered and sewn with galloon and pinned into the hair with a scarf or ornament. It is used to add length and height to the hair.

- *Stem switch*. A weft of hair rolled up and shaped like a bell, the switch is usually wound around a cord with a loop at the top. Feel inside the postiche for a number of stems, either one, two or three.

- *Chignon*. A chignon is a postiche worn in the nape of the neck for ornamentation.

- *Diamond mesh*. Probably the most popular type of postiche seen in the hairdressing salon, the diamond mesh is a wefted length of hair with the middle silk replaced by wire. The weft is folded and sewn into a petal-shaped or diamond mesh base.

Figure 15.5

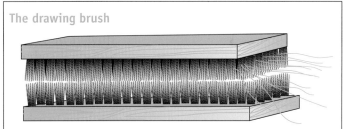

The drawing brush

This is used to draw off the hair when weaving.

Postiche made on a two-string weaving frame

Postiche made on a two-string weaving frame can be woven with hair 12 cm in length.

Crêpe hair. Having been woven in and out of the two strings, the hair is then boiled and baked in a postiche oven. Crêpe hair has been used for judges' wigs and is ideal for theatrical work to make beards, moustaches and sideburns. Crêpe hair is also used to make the following pieces.

- *Pompadour rolls*. These are used to gain height and fullness. The client's own hair is rolled around the Pompadour roll, either at the front or the side.
- *Frizettes*. Similar to a Pompadour roll. The narrow end of a frizette is placed in the nape area and the client's own hair is wrapped around it, as for a French plait or roll. It is used to pad out the hair.
- *Doughnut buns and pads*. These are popular pieces of postiche used for creating fullness in hairstyles. The hair is wrapped around the pad or bun and secured firmly in the nape area. Ballet dancers frequently wear a doughnut bun to hold their hair while they are dancing.

Cleaning postiche

How often a postiche needs to be cleaned depends on how much it is worn. In the case of a wig worn for medical reasons or a regularly used hairpiece, a weekly or fortnightly cleaning routine should be followed. Postiche used for special occasions or events will need cleaning less often.

Cleaning should always be done with great care and should not be confused with normal salon shampooing. The foundation of the wig can be stretched or shrunk if the correct procedure is not carried out. Be careful not to catch the teeth of the comb in the netting as this could cause rips and tears.

The most popular method of cleaning postiche is to use white spirit dry-cleaning fluids such as ether or trichlorethylene. If these white spirits are used, take care not to inhale the fumes as this can cause health problems, and wear gloves to protect your hands. These cleaners are ideal for removing grease, dirt and grime and can have an antistatic effect.

Procedure for cleaning wigs made from human hair (European and Asian)

1 Pour approximately 60 cc of white spirit into a glass bowl.
2 Hold the wig and gently immerse it in the white spirit, swabbing it through until the grease is lifted out. If the foundation needs cleaning, swab this area gently also. The white spirit will discolour when the dirt and grease is removed from the hair. One application should be enough, although two applications may be given if the piece is very dirty. Shake gently to remove excess white spirit.
3 The postiche can now be pinned onto a polystyrene block. (Covering the block with a plastic bag first will prevent deterioration.)
4 Comb through, being careful not to catch the netting or foundation.
5 The postiche may be given a gentle shampoo. Avoid any violent action or the normal sliding/rotating movement as this could tangle the hair. Rinse in tepid clear water. A conditioner may assist in the final combing. The postiche should now be clean.
6 Blow-dry or set in the desired style using a warm temperature. Dress to suit.

This is the most successful way to clean postiche. There should be no smell of white spirit.

Procedure for cleaning synthetic fibre wigs

Synthetic fibre should not need cleaning quite as often as human hair as it has no cuticle to collect the dirt and grime. Determine what fibre has been used in the wig and know what cleaning agents can be used on it. Some manufacturers do not recommend some dry-cleaning fluids, so read the instructions. Fibre wigs can be treated with an antistatic solution to prevent a fly-away condition and shampoo can remove this treatment, so ensure that this quality is replaced by applying a suitable fluid.

1 Pin the wig onto a polystyrene block and, with a sponge, swab through with warm soapy water. Ensure that the water is not too hot as this could relax the fibre curl.

2 Continue swabbing through with warm soapy water until all dirt has been removed.

3 Rinse in clear water.

4 If the foundation netting or galloon needs to be cleaned, do this also.

5 Set or blow dry in the desired style. Drying should be done with care or the fibre could melt or lose its curl.

Measuring for postiche

A number of different measurements can be taken to ensure that the client's wig is a comfortable fit. Your wig manufacturers will advise you of all the necessary measurements they require. Some men's toupee measurements are taken by wrapping clear plastic cellophane around the head and then drawing in the areas to be covered by the toupee. Plaster casts are also used to decide the fit of the toupee.

The ear peak is the area where most of the measurements are taken. Common measurements are:

- circumference – approximately 56 cm;
- ear peak to ear peak around the forehead;
- ear peak to ear peak over the crown;
- ear peak to ear peak around the back;
- ear peak to temple – approximately 5 cm;
- temple to temple around front hairline;
- temple to temple around the crown;
- forehead to nape;
- the nape area.

Figure 15.7

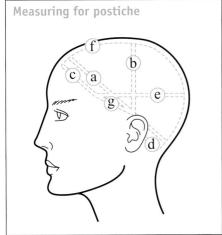

Measuring for postiche

Ask your wig manufacturers what measurements they require.
Common ones are:
a circumference;
b ear peak to ear peak over the crown;
c ear peak to ear peak around the front hairline;
d nape of neck;
e temple to temple around the back;
f front hairline to nape;
g ear peak to temple.

Figure 15.6 (a–e)

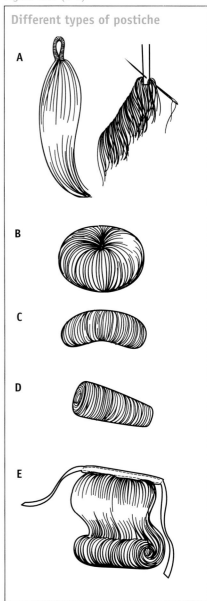

Different types of postiche

A A stem switch, showing a stem in the bell-shaped postiche.
B A doughnut bun, made from crépe hair, used for a chignon.
C A pompadour roll, made from crépe hair, used to give height in a final dressing.
D A frizette, made from crépe hair, used as a foundation over which to dress the hair.
E A two-looped marteau. A marteau is made with a flat sewn weft and a loop (sometimes two) at each end.

Figure 15.8 (a–d)

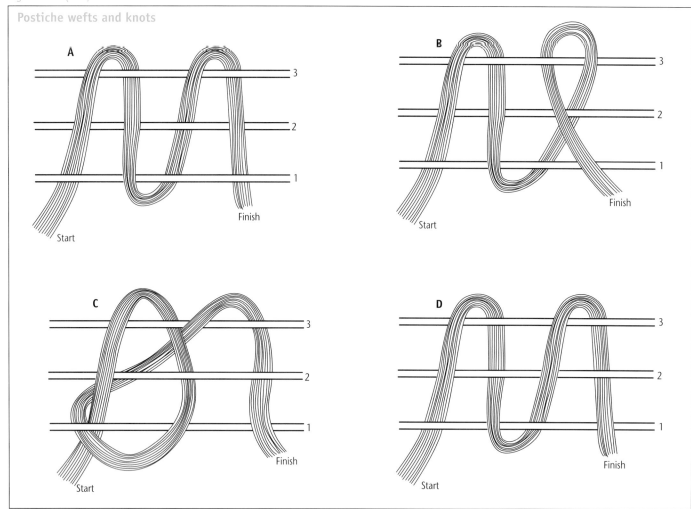

Postiche wefts and knots

A Flat weft – used for postiche sewn flat, such as a diamond mesh or marteau. When weaving the weft, use only the minimum length of hair to produce the weft. Slide the finished end of the weft to within between 1 and 3 cm of the no. 1 silk.

B Flat weft finishing knot.

C Starting knot.

D Fly weft – used for postiche that is rolled up, such as a one-, two- or three-stem switch.

Weaving

The most frequently used weft is the flat weft, used in any postiche that is sewn flat, such as a marteau or a diamond mesh. If the postiche is to be rolled up once it has been woven, the fly weft will produce a bell-shaped effect. To ensure the weft is secure, the wefts are started with the starting knot and completed with the finishing knot.

Practical boardwork exercises

1 Set up the weaving frame and weave 18 cm of weft, 5 cm of fly weft and the balance flat weft.

2 On a client or model, take five measurements necessary for the manufacturing of a wig.

3 Clean, set and dress a diamond mesh hairpiece.

4 Dress in a doughnut bun on a client with long hair.

Hairpieces

The making of a hairpiece is more of a possibility for a hairdresser as it does not involve using equipment, tools or materials which are hard to obtain.

The most popular piece of postiche is the diamond mesh. This involves weaving the hair on a three-string weaving frame and sewing it up into a diamond mesh pattern.

Circular- and square-based diamond mesh patterns

First, you need to draw a paper pattern to establish how much weaving is to be done. (This blueprint is actual size.) The base of the diamond mesh should be approximately 8 to 10 cm in diameter (64 to 100 cm²). The shape of the base can vary; it is usually round but it can be square or rectangular. You should decide this before the postiche is made. Once the shape has been decided, the weft of hair is folded into sections to form a diamond mesh. Generally, the weft should be slightly longer than the final length required since the folding and stitching tend to shorten it.

- *Equipment needed*: weaving frame, strong weaving silk drawing brushes, a pressing iron, a jockey, 30-amp fuse wire (stainless) or stainless floral wire and hair – a minimum 20 cm in length.
- *Accessories*: pencil, ruler, tape measure, needle and silk thread.
- *Preparation.* Set up the weaving frame by winding the silks two or three times around a small wad of paper around the groove of the right-hand weaving stick. The middle groove is prepared with the 30-amp fuse wire or floral wire in the same way as the top and bottom silks. The middle wire will give the base of the diamond mesh flexibility.
- *Preparing the hair.* Place the hair, which should be correctly rooted and pointed, in the drawing brushes. The last 5 cm of roots should be free of the end of the drawing brushes. The hair will need to be a minimum of 20 cm in length as this will make up a hair piece approximately 15 cm long.
- *Weaving.* Beginning with a starting knot, weave the hair in a flat weft. Maintain as much length in the hair as possible. Occasionally push the weft towards the left-hand stick; this will keep the weft tight and firm. As the weft is being woven, wrap the woven hair around the left-hand weaving stick. On completion of the weft, do a finishing knot and cut it down from the frame.

    Cut both ends of the no. 3 silk and tie it to the middle wire. Cut the middle wire and tie it to the no. 1 silk.

Finally, cut the no. 1 silk and tie it around the wire and the no. 3 silk. Do this at both ends of the woven weft. This will help to hold the weft secure. Trim any remaining silk or wire close to the woven weft.

At this stage, the weft can be covered with a cloth and pressed with a warm iron. Alternatively, it can be pressed with tongs while it is still on the weaving frame. The pressing of the weft makes the weaving firm and compact.

- *Sewing the circular-based diamond mesh.* Once the weft has been pressed, it is ready to be sewn up with strong silk thread. Using a pencil, bend the weft around and sew it firmly. The pencil's circumference is used to form a diamond formation. The hair can be finally shaped with the fingers; the pencil is merely used to keep the folds the same size.

    Sew the first four triangles to the first circle. Now form another circle around this first set. Make a second row of triangles and stitch to the circle. A four-, eight- and/or sixteen-pattern will keep the base symmetrical. The remaining hair should be long enough to encircle the base completely. The postiche can be moulded to fit the shape of the scalp.
- *Sewing the square-based diamond mesh.* When the weft has been woven and pressed, it should be moulded into the blueprint pattern shape. It is stitched at 1.5 cm or 2 cm intervals with a strong silk.

Once the weft has been finished it should be set and dressed, ready to be fitted.

Figure 15.9 (a–e)

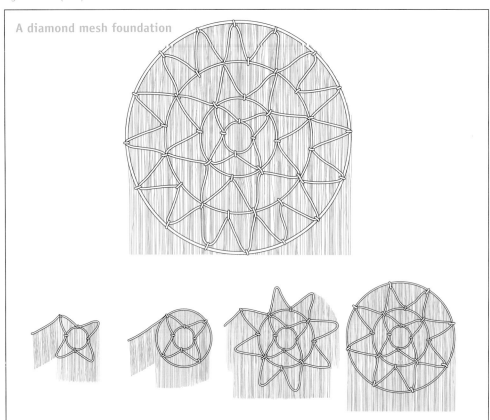

A diamond mesh foundation

This shows how the stitch holds are positioned. Wrap the weft around a pencil to achieve uniformity in the folds.

Figure 15.10

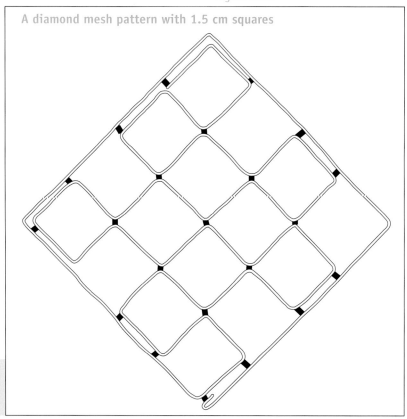

A diamond mesh pattern with 1.5 cm squares

Note how the meshes are folded and sewn to achieve the diamond foundation.

Men's postiche

How to measure for a toupee

The first stage is the preparation of a transparent shape. The manufacturer of the toupee needs this, along with samples of the client's own hair. The manufacturer will also want to know whether a parting is required, the direction of hair growth and any other information that will help to make the toupee look natural.

Discussion with the client is very important and thought must be given to the design and style of the hairpiece. Discuss the benefits of a natural skin part and the advantage of using grey at the temples to soften the look. If the client is married it can be a good idea to involve his wife to find out what she prefers. Show the client adhesive tape and explain where would be best to fit it in order to hold the hairpiece on.

Method

1 Cover the head with cling film. Ask the client to hold the sides of the film so that it fits tightly.
2 Cover the transparent film with five or six layers of overlapping strips of transparent adhesive tape. This will make a template.
3 Using a spirit felt pen, mark in the circumference on the base (approximately 1 cm inside the hairline to avoid a join line). Indent around the temple region for natural recession. Mark in the parting 1 cm into the natural hair to avoid a hard line effect and to allow for the knotting.
4 Mark the hair knotting direction and use the back of the parting for the crown. Mark the front and back of the template and label it with the client's name.
5 Attach clippings of hair, taken from the sides and back of the head.
6 Cut out the template outside the markings and check the fit, 1 cm inside the hairline.

When you send this template to the manufacturer, it is a good idea to include a couple of recent photographs of the client.

 ## Hair extensions

Hair extensions have now become a popular addition to hairdressing services. In addition to adding length, hair extensions can also add texture, a new colour or more density to fine hair. Both human hair and synthetic fibre (mono-fibres) can be used for hair extensions. Natural human hair will, obviously, look more natural and can be treated as the client's own hair. Hair extensions made from human hair will be more expensive than synthetic fibre.

Some disadvantages to hair extensions are that they do sometimes matt or tangle at the roots, especially if they have been secured with glue. They do take some time to position in the hair (and positioning them can involve two hairdressers, which can become expensive). The client should be advised to look after the extensions carefully. Advice should be given on shampooing; in particular, the client should be warned not to use a rotating movement during shampooing. Be careful with blow-driers and tongs if the extensions are made of synthetic fibre. Finally, extensions can start to look tatty after three or four months and should then be removed.

There are a number of ways in which hair extensions can be attached. Gluing, bonding and clamping involve either adhesives or heating to secure the hair

Figure 15.11 (a and b)

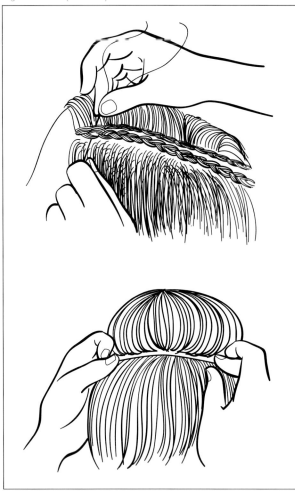

Practical exercise

Make a diamond mesh hair piece ... set, dress and present.

extensions to the client's own natural hair. A heat iron is used to assist the glueing and bonding.

Corn-rowing and sewing is another way of attaching hair extensions to the client's hair. The client's hair is tightly plaited and corn-rowed around the head; using a needle and thread, the hair extensions are then sewn on to the corn-row. The extensions are usually wefts of hair and are called tracks. The track is placed along the corn-row in the opposite direction to the natural fall of the hair. Using thread the same colour as the hair, the extension is sewn around the corn-row. The track is then folded down in the direction of the natural fall of the hair and the client's own hair is placed over this to cover the track.

Alternatively, the false hair and the client's own hair can be plaited together. This can be further secured by sewing with a needle and thread: take a 1 cm section of hair, divided into two, and lay the extension across it, then criss-cross the client's own hair with the extension. This creates a four-strand rope.

Clip-ons are also used to secure hair extensions.

Figure 15.12

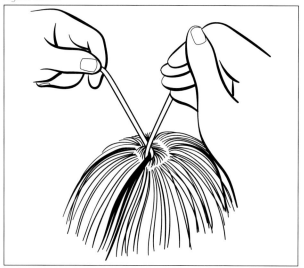

Figure 15.13

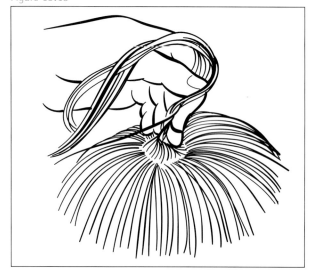

Questions

1 What do the terms *boardwork* and *postiche* mean?

_____

_____

_____

2 Name three pieces of postiche made on:

_____

a a three-string weaving frame;

_____

b a two-string weaving frame.

_____

3 Briefly describe how a hand-made wig is made.

_____

_____

_____

4 Describe the qualities of two types of human hair suitable for making postiche.

_____

_____

_____

5 What does the term '100% human processed' hair mean?

_____

6 a What are the three main sources of hair for wig merchants?

_____

_____

b What is the minimum length for hair which is to be made into a hairpiece?

_____

7 a Explain the term *turned* or *rooted and pointed* in the context of postiche.

_____

_____

_____

b Why is it important that the hair be correctly 'turned' before being made into a postiche?

_____

_____

8 **a** Name the fibre most commonly substituted for human hair in postiche.

_____

b What is the main precaution you should observe when working with this fibre?

_____

_____

9 Illustrate and describe three boardwork tools.

10 Using simple sketches, describe the following types of postiche:

_____

a marteau;

_____

b diamond mesh;

_____

c stem switch;

_____

d frizette;

_____

e doughnut bun.

_____

11 **a** Briefly outline the procedure for cleaning a human-hair wig.

_____

_____

b Name three cleaning fluids used in cleaning wigs.

_____

_____

c List two precautions which will need to be taken during the procedure.

_____

_____

12 a List six measurements required to make a full wig.

_____

_____

b What is the approximate average circumference of the adult head?

_____

c Name two common wefts which are used to make postiche.

_____

_____

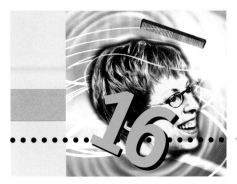

General business practice for the hairdressing salon

Now that you are approaching the final year of your hairdressing apprenticeship or training you will need to understand the more elementary aspects of the day-to-day running of a salon. This will give you a general appreciation of and introduction to the business principles and responsibilities you will require should you be the worker-in-charge or the senior stylist. If you are aiming for a managerial position or even to own your own salon one day, then the management section (Chapter 17) will explain the finer points of running a hairdressing business.

Even at this stage you may be given more responsibility for the salon's administration, so you will need a fundamental understanding of the aspects of general business principles covered in this chapter.

General business principles

The profit motive

A hairdressing salon is a very important part of the community. Hairdressing is a service industry but although the objective of a salon is to provide the public with a service, it also has to make a profit. This profit comes from giving clients the service they want and need. Generally, if this principle is followed, a sound business will produce profits and the clients will gain personal benefits. If the salon is to give the clients personal service and maintain profit, it must be well managed.

Assessing the salon overheads

Salon overheads are the costs and expenses involved in the day-to-day running of the salon: the bills which need to be paid for the salon to continue to run. If these overhead costs are not paid, people will refuse to supply you with the goods or services you need to keep your salon going.

A list of typical salon overheads includes:

- wages;
- salon stock;
- advertising;
- rent and rates;
- electricity and gas;
- insurance;
- telephone;
- laundry;
- accountancy and legal fees;
- repairs and general maintenance;
- interest on any loans;
- sundry items.

There will also be other costs, but these are the more obvious ones. This list comprises the bills which will arrive and must be paid out monthly or quarterly. Usually, goods and services bills need to be paid by a certain date; for example, stock, electricity and telephone bills will need to be paid promptly, or these services will be discontinued.

Generally, the salon owner will calculate the overheads as a percentage of the salon's turnover. Salon turnover is the total yearly income for the salon – the money taken for sales of services and retail products. As an apprentice, you may not be familiar with percentages. When we talk of percentages we talk in terms of units out of 100. For example, 10 per cent (%) equals 10 out of 100, or 1 out of 10. Forty per cent equals 40 out of a 100 or 4 out of 10. So, if your boss says that you have to sell retail products to 30 per cent of your clients, that would mean that 3 out of every 10 or 30 out of every 100 clients would have to buy retail products.

Wages are considered to be the biggest overhead. Stock, advertising and rent will probably come next. As an approximate percentage of the salon's turnover, wages should account for 35 to 40%. Stock should account for 8 to 15%, advertising for 5 to 11% and rent for 8 to 10%.

Most salons work on a 20% profit margin; that is, once all the overheads have been paid, the salon owner is left with 20% of the salon's turnover. This 20% is net profit *before* tax is paid. Once tax has been paid, it is net profit after tax. Salon owners do not pay tax as they earn but are assessed on an annual (yearly) basis and provision is made to pay tax twice a year. The less profit shown before tax, the less tax is paid. Profits can be put back into the business which, in turn, builds the business up.

 ## Taxation

As an apprentice, you will pay tax as you are paid, i.e. weekly. You are considered to be an employee and the salon owner is an employer. When you pay your tax every week, this is called *pay as you earn* (PAYE) taxation. You will see this abbreviation (PAYE) when you sign your wage book or receive your wage slip or if you are required to fill in a tax return at the end of the government's financial year (31 March). Your PAYE tax is calculated on the amount of money you earn. You will be paid a wage. A wage means you will be paid on an hourly basis for a 40-hour week; if you work a late night or on a Saturday, you will be paid extra or have time off in lieu. People who are salaried receive a fixed annual income regardless of the number of extra hours worked in a week. Most hairdressers are paid a wage and get extra pay for overtime worked.

The larger your wage, the more you pay in tax, so if you work any overtime during a week, your PAYE tax deductions for that week will be more than usual. What you earn before paying your tax is your *gross wage*. Once the PAYE tax has been deducted, this is your *net wage* or what you receive 'in your hand'. As an employee (apprentice) you may be able to claim the cost of certain items which are considered essential to improving your hairdressing ability. These deductions and expenses are added up at the end of the financial year (31 March) and claimed against your total income. At time of writing, these deductions are very few indeed. The policy concerning tax-deductible expenses relating to the betterment of your trade does change from time to time. Ask an expert what you can claim. Of course, you pay for all these yourself and must get into the habit of asking for and filing your receipts. If, however, *your* employer (the salon owner) pays these expenses, *he/she* can claim against his/her tax deductions.

In March 1999 changes were made to requirements for income and salary earners (applicable to the 2000 tax year). Employees are no longer required to complete IR 12 or IR 13 certificates. These have been replaced by a tax code declaration (IR 330). All new employees must complete an IR 330 tax code declaration when they start working. A new declaration must also be completed if an employee wishes to change his/her tax code. It is not necessary for employees to complete a new declaration every year, providing their tax code remains the same. All employees will need to read the notes on the IR 330 to work out their correct tax code. For the year commencing 1 April 1999, all existing employees will need to complete an IR 330.

Commissions, bonuses and incentives

If you receive an incentive payment, in the form of a commission or bonus, on top of your wage, this is added to the gross wage and then the tax is deducted. Commissions mean you are rewarded (possibly financially) for earning a certain amount for your employer for the week or month. As an example, let's say a commission of 20% is offered on any amount over $800 earned for the salon in any given week. Now, in week 4, say, you earn $1000 for the salon. So the commission payable to you is 20% of ($1000 – $800); i.e. 20% of $200, which equals $40. The commission you receive is added to your gross wage:

Gross wages	$ 300
Plus commission	$ 40
Total (gross)	**$ 340**

For that week (week 4), your PAYE tax is calculated on $340, not on your basic wage of $300.

The same principles apply for whatever financial incentive, bonus or commission is offered.

Economical use of time and materials

Profits must be maintained, especially during times of rising expenses such as increased stock prices or rent, and there may be times when raising the salon's prices is not the solution. Competition from other salons may stop you from doing this or there may be price control. Raising the prices continually is not the way to balance the books. An alternative – in addition to selling extra services and retail stock – is to look at the overheads and seek ways in which they can be reduced or used more effectively. If you can cut down on the overheads the salon carries, then profits can be maintained.

Electricity

This service is essential in the hairdressing salon. It is used for a variety of appliances but the biggest part of the electricity bill is the water heating (see Chapter 14 of *Hairdressing: A Professional Approach: Levels 1 and 2*), which can be as much as 60% of the cost. To ensure that hot water is not being wasted, switch the hot water tap off when you are massaging the client's hair during shampooing; otherwise you are literally pouring money down the drain. Some wash basins have a mixer control, with one lever for switching the water on and off. The temperature does not have to be regulated when it is turned on again. Others have a plunge-type attachment on the head of the spray which cuts off the water supply if it is pushed. These types of device help to save hot water (and electricity costs).

Any appliances not in use should be turned off. Heaters, dryers, curling tongs and heat brushes all use electricity at an alarming rate, especially if they are of a high wattage. The higher the wattage, the more it costs to run the appliance. Electricity is charged for by the kilowatt hour (1 000 watts or 1 kW for 1 hour equals 1 kWh). Thermostat-controlled plugs can help to reduce electricity costs where heaters are involved. These turn a heat appliance off once it reaches a certain temperature.

Materials

It is important to ensure that stock materials are not wasted in the salon. Junior apprentices should be taught at an early stage of their apprenticeship to mix and measure accurately, and to read instructions carefully, as these often advise how best to use the product and list the quantities and measurements which will ensure that the product is used economically.

Shampoos

Some bulk shampoos require diluting. If the information says '7 parts of water to 1 part of shampoo', don't guess; measure out seven parts of water and the one unit of shampoo, otherwise more shampoo than is necessary will be used and this will end up being washed down the sink. Use a shampoo container with a pump action measurer or look at the possibility of sachets (although you will need to keep scissors handy). Ensure that the apprentices know how to use the shampoo and don't pump it directly onto the client's hair. Pump the shampoo into the palm, rub the hands together and distribute the shampoo uniformly onto the client's hair. Don't spill any.

Setting lotions, mousse, gel and sprays

Setting lotions are bought either in bulk or in individual 15 ml units. If the hair is finely textured, the whole unit may not be required. If too much is applied, it will run off the hair and onto the towel or, worse, down the client's neck or onto his/her face. Don't use more mousse or gel than is required. Hairsprays will last longer if you pump the button instead of keeping your finger on it. Shake the can to ensure that the propellant is well distributed, else you will disperse only the propellant and be left with hairspray in the can.

Permanent wave solutions

Even though an individual unit of permanent waving lotion has been opened, it can be used again if it has been correctly capped. Don't open a new unit if a half-used one is available; you will end up with lots of opened half-used permanent wave units and that is wasteful. Read the instructions to check whether the lotion can be kept; some solutions cannot. Often, more neutraliser than is necessary is used. Junior apprentices should be taught that one unit is generally sufficient (unless the hair is extra long or a special winding technique has been employed). Ensure that the end of the container is snipped to create only a small hole, so that the neutraliser doesn't flow out uncontrollably.

Colours

Never mix more than is needed. Retouches need only half a tube of colour unless the regrowth is exceptionally long. A tube key on the end of the tube will ensure that its contents are fully exhausted; even rolling down against a hard surface will extract the last few grams. If you are putting a half-used tube back in the stockroom, ensure that you indicate clearly that there is half a tube left. Either hook the tube over a rail in numerical order or label the box or stack the half tube on top of the full box. In this way, the next hairdresser seeking the same colour will notice that there is a half-tube available and use that instead of opening up a new one. Semipermanent colours usually come in bottles; if the hair is fine, it may not be necessary to use a full bottle. Don't mix too much henna powder; it is always wiser to mix more if you run out.

Added up, all these small points become very important in saving money.

Sundry items

'Miscellaneous purchases' are a salon overhead which can add up quickly if some kind of budget is not provided and allowed for. You can lease a wide range of salon sundry items such as a cash register, plants and flowers and a coffee machine. Some firms offer a magazine hire service and you can even rent pictures. To save large cash outgoings, inquire about leasing to buy, hiring or renting some of these sundry items.

Stock control

Ordering stock

Your stock level should be sufficient to provide adequate customer service. The third-year apprentice is often given the responsibility of maintaining stock control. This is a responsible job and involves being frugal and economic to keep overheads within a budget. Manufacturers' sales representatives (reps) will call on your salon at regular intervals so that you can buy stock from them. Since these salespeople want to gain orders for their respective firms, it is best to make appointments to see them when:

a   you are not busy with clients;

b   you have completed the weekly stock check.

If you check the stock on a weekly basis, then you should have an idea of what products to order when you see the reps. Also, you will not run out of any essential stock items. This is bad stock control, and frustrating for you and your colleagues. Make a note in advance of what is needed and check the stockroom to make sure that all stock is in its appointed place.

Make your list of stock required in the stock control book. This should be a carbon-copy order book indicating the quantities, goods, price and date, plus the order number and a place for your signature. By doing this, you will know what products you have ordered. Some salons have a stock list in the staff room where stylists note what products they have used, including retail sales, during the day and the week. This will include setting lotion units, rinses, semipermanent colours, perm wave units and tints. This simple system can keep control of what stock is being used.

Never buy more from a rep than you know you need or can use within a certain time. Some manufacturers do offer goods on a sale-or-return basis, but don't rely on this. Ensure that supplies are fresh. Perm wave lotions and tints and hydrogen peroxides may have only a certain shelf life, so it is wiser to buy more often and have fresh supplies.

However, some products, such as shampoos, conditioners, setting lotions and hairsprays, will keep for a very long time.

Manufacturers often offer deals on these products; for example, if you buy three litre containers of shampoo you get one free, or buy twelve and get five free. This can be good buying, especially if you link up with other hairdressing salons in the area; you may find you get more free shampoo because the package deal is bigger, e.g. if you buy 25 two-litre containers, you get 15 free. You must remember, though, that you have to store these containers and space may be at a premium. You are also tying up more of the salon's capital, which may be required for other items later on. So make sure you can afford special deals. It is best to buy expensive items in small quantities and cheaper products in greater quantities.

Most hairdressing manufacturers operate on an accounts system for payment, i.e. they provide credit or payment is postponed. When the goods arrive in the parcel you will find a *packing slip*. This tells you only what is in the parcel – it is not a demand for payment. Check this packing slip against what you have ordered in your stock book – and against what you have actually received – and file the packing slip for your records.

The manufacturers may sometimes include the invoice in the parcel or they may send it out a week or so later. The invoice tells you what you have ordered, the individual costs of the goods and the charge for delivery freight, as well as the total amount due. If you wish, you can pay for the goods on receipt of the invoice or you may wish to wait for the *statement*.

The statement is the demand for payment and tells exactly what you owe the manufacturer for the goods you have bought in the previous three or four months. It will also include the date by which the goods must be paid for. Get into the habit of paying your cheque by the date due (usually the 20th of the month). Sometimes there may be a *credit notice*, which indicates that goods have not been received but have been paid for.

All these packing slips, invoices, credit notices and statements, mean, of course, extra paperwork and bookkeeping for the senior apprentice, manager, manageress or salon owner. Cash-and-carry warehouses are far more efficient. The salon owner or buyer will visit the warehouse once a week, say, and spend an hour or so choosing the salon's stock. The checkout will add up the total, supply a receipt and the buyer pays cash (cheque) and carries the goods away. This idea is similar to a supermarket concept. It gives the hairdresser the opportunity to viewing the stock, including all the new products, instructions, posters and booklets on display. Such systems, which operate overseas, may also save time on paperwork.

Laundry

There are a number of ways in which the laundry can be assessed as an overhead in the salon. Each way will need to be looked at and the best alternative will depend on your salon's needs. There may, too, be ideas which can save you money on your laundry bills. Disposable cloths, such as a dentist uses, can save your towels, especially when you're colouring. It is also a good idea to use black gowns and towels for your colouring work.

Laundry service

There are firms which wash, fold and deliver towels to your salon. You only lease the towels from them. The laundry charges by the single towel, so every towel that is put into the towel bin may cost 20 cents to launder. If you use approximately 250 towels a week, the laundry bill will be $50 a week. The service is usually good, with the towels being returned twice a week, clean and fresh-smelling. Colour is removed from the towels and the apprentice does not have to fold them before putting them away. Also remember that you didn't have the capital outlay of buying 250 towels in the first place.

Bag wash laundry

Towels are either collected or dropped off at the local laundry and the charges are usually calculated by the weight of the bag. Two or three bag washes may be done a week. At $10 a bag, the weekly bill will be around $30. Remember you have to buy the towels. They are considered semiconsumable, i.e. they will need to be replaced when they wear out, and this will happen sooner if you have bought poor-quality towels. Also, someone will have to fold the towels when they are returned, which wastes valuable time.

Laundering in the salon

If towels are going to be laundered in the salon, there is the initial outlay of buying a washing machine and dryer, at a cost of at least $1200. Extra space is needed to house these appliances and there will also be maintenance and repair bills and your electricity bills will increase, especially because the dryer uses a good deal of electricity. Also, someone must 'do the towels'. The urge can develop to put slightly soiled towels straight into the dryer. This is neither hygienic nor professional and any staff member caught doing this should be told so. In the long run, the laundry bill will be less but there is extra heat and noise in the salon and, again, you must buy your own towels. Some salon owners even take the towels home and launder them. Decide on what you consider the best way to launder your towels.

 # Simple account keeping

In an average-sized hairdressing salon, a number of different books must be kept. Being good at working with figures is a help, and a calculator is a great asset for adding, multiplying and working out percentages. Keeping a set of books is important for a number of reasons.

1   The Inland Revenue Department needs books in order to assess the salon's tax.
2   Annual accounts showing what the salon is worth, what its liabilities (what it owes) and assets (what it owns) are and where the money is are prepared using information in the books. This information is about how profitable the business is.
3   Sales figures and turnover figures can be compared with those of previous years to see if the salon is working efficiently.
4   The information is useful for the purpose of securing a loan.
5   The books will show who the salon's debtors and creditors are – what money is owed, to whom it is owed, and who owes the salon money.

6   Maintaining a complete, continuous and accurate record for the salon is essential if you decide to sell, so that you will be considered creditable and can justify your asking price for the salon.

In the average salon with, perhaps, two seniors and two apprentices, it takes approximately two hours a week to work on the books. Bookkeeping for a large salon will need a little more time. Accountants can help you do your books, but are not necessary in the day-to-day running of the business. You should expect to see your accountant two to four times a year. Accountants usually charge by the hour, so the more you use them, the more costly it is. Be prepared to do a certain amount of bookkeeping yourself if you are going to look after a salon.

All the appropriate books can be bought at a good stationery shop. They include:

- appointment book;
- petty cash book;
- day book;
- pay-in book (obtained from your bank);
- stock book;
- time and wages book;
- receipt book;
- chequebook (from your bank);
- dockets.

Some of these books are carbon-copy books.

Appointment book

Keep this as neat as possible: it could be shown to a prospective salon buyer as an indication of your clientele. The appointment book is usually drawn up in 15-minute intervals with a column used for each stylist. If 30-minute appointments are made, make sure you write only over that half-hour period. If you write over the next time slot, someone may make the next appointment at the wrong time. Don't space out the appointments unnecessarily as this wastes time. It is a good idea to record clients' telephone numbers to remind them of their appointments or to advise them if a staff member is unable to do their hair. Work in pencil so that appointment times can be changed easily.

Petty cash book

The petty cash book will record all the incidentals which are bought for the salon. Since these are tax deductible, they need to be accurately recorded. Petty cash incidentals will include light bulbs, cleaning materials, stamps, cheque clearance fees, sundry items for beverages (sugar and milk), cleaning agents and talcum powder. Usually the money for these items comes out of a petty cash tin or the till. Unless these purchases are recorded somewhere, the till will not balance, so enter the amount for purchases (paste or stick the receipt into the book) in the petty cash book and put the change back in the tin or till. Then when the till is balanced, i.e. when the till roll receipts are checked against the money in the till (the day's takings), the items entered in the petty cash book are noted and the till will balance.

Some tills now have a debit key. This means that when you press the receipt key and the debit key, the till opens and you take out the money needed to buy your petty item. This amount will be recorded on the till roll receipt. Once you have made your purchase, the receipt is placed in a compartment in the till. Alternatively, you can enter the item on the till roll and write down next to the amount what it was for. Keep your till rolls. This information will all help to balance the till takings.

Day book

The day's takings are recorded in the day book. Once the till has been balanced, the amounts are entered into a day book under various headings. The amount that each stylist has taken is recorded under a separate heading. The retail sales are recorded under 'retail sales'. Purchases from petty cash are also noted. All these figures are then added up to show what the total takings have been for that day. This is done every day and at the end of the week the takings are added up and the final week's total is noted. Usually a page is devoted to each week.

Pay-in book

This book may be used twice a day, depending on how frequently the salon banks the money from the till. It records what money is paid into the bank, either in cash, cheques or credit card vouchers. This book must be filled in accurately. The top part of the book is filled in with the date, your account number and name, the number of cheques and who is paying in the money. Make sure you have the carbon paper underneath and the correct way round.

You then write the details of cheques in the pay-in book. The name of the drawer – the person who gave you the cheque – is printed on the front of the cheque. If there is no name, just enter the account number.

You then record the bank that holds the drawer's account, the branch of the bank and finally the amount. These cheques are then totalled and the final amount entered in the column total at the bottom. If you have a lot of cheques, carry on to the next page and make a total there as well.

A smaller pay-in book is needed for cash. It is filled out in the same manner, although you will have to put in how the cash is made up:
- silver (5, 10, 20 and 50 cent pieces);
- notes (5 and 10 dollar notes, etc.),

and add up this amount.

The cheques and the cash now go to the bank. At the bank you will be asked for the cheque clearance fee – so many cents per cheque – so be sure you have this amount. Take it from the till and enter it in the petty cash book.

In addition to the cash and cheques entered in the pay-in book, you may also have to enter the total amount of credit card vouchers. At the end of the day, remove the merchant and bank copies of the vouchers from the till. Separate the different types of credit vouchers, for example, Visa and Bankcard.

Banking procedure for credit card vouchers

The details of the vouchers are entered onto a merchant's summary or sales summary. Make sure you have the correct one for the particular credit voucher. Run the form through the imprinter to record the salon's merchant name and number. Total all the voucher sales on this summary and write in the total. Date, sign and add the total number of vouchers – use a new summary if you run out of space. Retain the merchant's copy along with the merchant's sales voucher. Enter the total amount of each sales summary in the pay-in book. Put all the vouchers and summaries in the plastic bags supplied. These then go to the bank with the cheques and cash.

Stock book

This carbon-copy book duplicates the stock items that you have ordered from the sales representatives. This enable you to check what comes in against what you have ordered.

Time and wages book

Your employer must keep a record of all staff members who work in the hairdressing salon. This record is the time and wage book, in which the following information is written down:

1   the date each apprentice joined the salon and from then on a running total of the number of hours he/she has served in his/her hairdressing apprenticeship;

2   gross wages, PAYE deductions and net wages; dates of wage increases should also be noted;

3   any absences, the reason for these and the time of the absence;

4   holiday dates and pay.

You may have to sign this book every time you receive your weekly pay; a page is usually devoted to each staff member. The information in this book is confidential and the book should be kept in a safe place. Certain authorities, however, can have access to this book. Make sure it is filled in accurately. If you don't sign a wage book, you should receive a wage slip with your wages.

Ledger/debit/credit/receipt book

This book is usually alphabetically indexed down the side for easy reference. It records all stock, services or goods received and all cash or cheques given in payment. The book is divided into two parts. The left side is termed 'debit' (dr) and the right side 'credit' (cr).

If you receive anything from anyone, such as stock, goods or services, you debit them, i.e. you record the stock, goods or service and the amount on the left-hand side. For example, if the salon has bought stock from a wholesaler you debit them in the ledger; they are creditors – the salon owes them money.

Figure 16.1

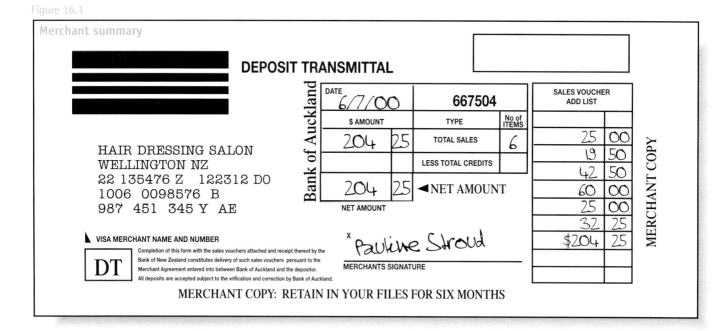

This is how the merchant summary for credit card vouchers should be filled in before you take all the sales vouchers to the bank.

Figure 16.2

DEPOSIT SUPPLEMENT

_____ 20

For credit of _____

the sum of _____

Lodged with _____ Branch _____

Paid in by (signature)	Account number	Teller
	/ 0				...		/	

	:
Total notes	:
Total coin	:
Total cash	:
Charges	:
No of cheques	:

With recourse on all documents, cheques, etc. included in this credit not to be available until collected.

	Drawer	Bank	Branch	Amount
1				
2				
3				
4				
5				
6				
7				
8				
9				
10				
11				
12				
13				
14				
15				
16				
17				
18				
19				
20				
21				
22				
23				
24				
25				
26				
27				
28				

Abbreviate names as follows

A– ANZ N– National
B– BNZ W– Westpac
R– Reserve

IMPORTANT: This schedule must be accompanied by a MICR ENCODED
DEPOSIT SLIP supplied by your Bank.

Total amount of cheques	
Total cash	
Total deposited	
Less charges	
Total	

This records how much money is paid into the bank.

The pay-in book

If you pay out any cash or cheques, you credit them, i.e. you enter the amount on the right-hand side of the book. So, when statements arrive, the salon pays them by cheque and credits the supplier with the amount.

This type of transaction is called an account. An account (A/C) requires a giver and a receiver. Two book entries or a double entry are involved, one for receiving the goods and one for paying for them. Usually, a page is devoted to each account and the book, as mentioned, is alphabetically indexed for easy reference.

Dockets

If your salon does not have an electronic, programmed cash register, then you could use a docket system. The client's name, service, total cost of the service and the name of the stylist are entered onto a docket and each docket is added and balanced with the till roll at the end of the day.

If the salon does have an electronic, programmed cash register, then learn how to use it, and press the correct buttons. Electronic cash registers can help tremendously with simple bookkeeping. They can add up the daily and weekly totals for each staff member, and indicate whether cash or a cheque was received. Such registers total retail sales and a final printout will add up the week's total takings. Some can be programmed to do far more than this and can become highly technical. There are firms which can advise you on the most suitable cash register for your business.

Chequebook

This important book should be kept somewhere safe. It is used to credit accounts and it is safer to write cheques than to use cash. Fill in the cheque carefully as follows.

Cross the cheque and write 'Not negotiable – account payee only' on it. This is the safest way of writing out a cheque, as it can then be banked only by the person to whom it is paid and is easy to trace should it be lost or stolen. If you don't cross your cheque, it can be cashed by anyone, especially if you write on the cheque 'pay cash'.

Always write a cheque out to a firm and never to an employee. Make sure no one can alter the sum to be paid in any way, for example by adding letters and altering figures. Once you have written the cheque, make sure you have dated and signed it; if you make a mistake and have to alter it, initial the alteration.

Now record the cheque details on the cheque butt. Enter the date, to whom it is paid, the reason for payment and the amount. The chequebook butt is one way to record your payments.

Pay accounts promptly on receipt of invoice or statement. This is a good habit to get into and builds up your creditworthiness. All the salon records involving the running of the business must be kept in a locked filing cabinet. They should be retained for a minimum of seven years. Keep the books accurately and set time aside solely for doing the books. Try to avoid interruptions and you will find that keeping the books can provide a pleasant two or three hours a week away from the hairdressing chair.

General salon retailing

Salon retailing means selling goods and products – the ones you use in the salon – to the client. Manufacturers make a range of products specifically to be sold in salons. They are usually special products not available elsewhere and some require professional instruction from the hairdresser before the client can use them at home. Such retailing is a quick and simple way to increase salon turnover and support your earnings during the low seasons. It also shows clients that you are interested in caring for their hair and are professional enough to offer advice. If your salon doesn't retail products, it does not provide the total salon service which the consumer should come to expect.

Figure 16.3

The time and wages book

RATES OF PAY

WEEKLY

HOURLY

TIME & HALF

DOUBLE

TEA MONEY

HOLIDAY RECORD

Holiday Entertainment	Total Days Taken
Date Commenced	
Date Terminated	
Date Commenced	
Date Terminated	

Total Gross Wage to Date		Paye ded. for Week		Total Paye ded. to Date						Net Wage in Week				Signature
$	c	$	c	$	c	$	c	$	c	$	c	$	c	

This records all details of the staff's wages, hours worked and so on.

Figure 16.4
Filling in a cheque

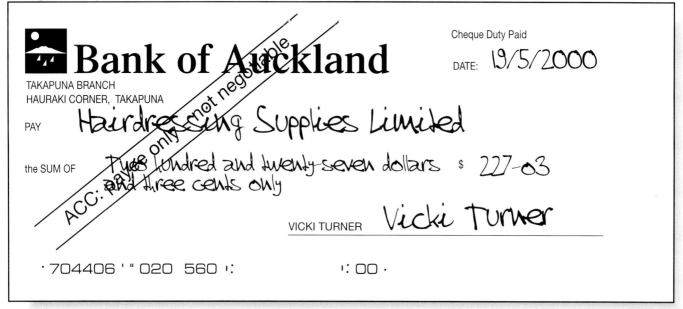

It is good for the salon's professional image if you offer shampoos and conditioners that you actually use in the salon. This also helps to strengthen your sales approach. Remember, you don't want to compete directly with pharmacies and supermarkets so there is no point in retailing non-professional products.

Make sure you're completely familiar with all the products that are for sale, so that you aren't hesitant about selling retail stock. If necessary, call in the local manufacturer's technician for an evening to explain all the benefits of the product.

Display

There are five important considerations in setting up a successful retail display.
- appeal and interest;
- lighting;
- area – floor space;
- ticketing and pricing;
- showcards and posters.

You should know not only how to use and sell retail products but also how to display them. Let the customer know you are serious about retailing by ensuring that the display area is always well stocked with products. Don't have small displays spread throughout the salon; concentrate on one area, around the reception and pack all your products into this area. Don't put retail stock away in cupboards or drawers. That stock costs money – if you were to substitute actual cash for this stock, you wouldn't keep it in the cupboard or drawer. So take the stock out and make the most of it: display it!

Make the display look significantly large; half a dozen cans of hairspray and twelve cans of mousse are not sufficient. Never run out of stock, as this is frustrating for clients who may choose not to return if they have been let down because of insufficient supplies.

Display is an area where you can look to the discount stores for ideas. They know how to display, and how to create the impression of 'come and get it while stocks last'. Some stock is hardly taken out of the boxes, which are piled up, easily accessible for the consumer to try. The area can even be untidy, but clean, giving the impression that stock is selling, that it's on the move, not just to be looked at, but to be picked up, tried and used. Stock will move faster when it is displayed at eye level.

Lighting is a prime consideration in retail selling. Make sure the selling area is well lit as this attracts attention. You should create a warm environment.

You need *floor space* for retail selling. Manufacturers sometimes supply retail stands, and these are fine as long as they don't take up too much room. The number of chairs in the waiting area can be reduced to accommodate a retail display. Unnecessary furniture such as lamps and tables can also be sacrificed to make room for retail stands. If such furnishings are already down to a minimum, consider the reception desk. This could be moved, put against a wall, made smaller or even taken away altogether!

For *ticketing*, plain, bold, black lettering on white is still the best. Showcards supplied by manufacturers are usually large, colourful and well thought out. Make sure that the price is always displayed. It is an excellent idea to have the salon's own ticket labelling system with the salon name and the product price. These labels can be bought at good stationers.

Promotional material such as showcards, manuals, leaflets, manufacturers' instructions and posters all make your retail area more attractive and noticeable, adding to the display and making it less likely to be ignored. Such material also gives your client more product information. An added bonus is to give your clients a salon bag in which to carry their purchases home; this is also good advertising.

Some salons operate a 'salon system'. This is where one make of product is used throughout the salon – shampoo, conditioner, permanent waving treatments, setting agents, sprays and fixatives are all under one label. This total package has a good, professional, uniform appearance, and it also streamlines your retail area. These are professional products designed and formulated for the client's individual needs. The fact that you use the same products throughout the salon is your seal of approval, encouraging the client to buy from the range.

Display checklist

1 Use professional products.
2 Know your products.
3 Display in bulk, concentrate displays and don't break your display up into smaller groups.
4 Never run short of supplies.
5 Keep the displays clean and free from dust.
6 Ensure the display area is well lit.
7 Place the display where customers can see, smell and handle the products.
8 Tickets should be clearly printed with the name, price and description of product and the salon name.
9 Brochures, posters and pamphlets add interest to the display.
10 Salon systems streamline your display.
11 Products used in the salon should also be available for retail; this is your seal of approval.
12 Give the client a bag with your salon name on it to carry the products home. This will also serve to advertise your salon.

The hairdresser who sells the product

Show skill in helping others to buy in the following ways.

1 Ensure you have a thorough knowledge of the product. This will give the client confidence in the goods being sold.

2 Understand what the client needs; never sell a client anything he/she doesn't need.

3 Have a general understanding of the selling principles.

  a You must recognise buying signals, such as: 'My hair is so limp', or 'I wish my hair was more controllable'. Your answer could be: 'Your hair would really benefit from a style support, so what I will do is …', or 'I'll give you a gel lotion especially formulated for your type of problem.'

  b You should arouse interest in the product.

  c You should get the client to listen.

  d Relay the benefits to the client.

  e Know how to answer objections such as: 'Why is it more expensive?', or 'Can anyone in my family use it?' Your answer might be: 'As you can see on the label, this quality product contains the ingredients best suited for your problem. Remember how little I had to use to get such good results.' or 'No, it's formulated just for your type of hair, as you can see on the instructions. We'd be happy to talk to the rest of your family and advise on a product suited for them.'

  f Close the sale correctly.

4 Be able to demonstrate products and talk to clients about them – and be able to listen to their point of view.

5 Have a knowledge of a broad range of products that are available, including any competing products.

6 Be sincere in your approach and your desire to give service to the customers. You can stimulate their interest in goods they need.

Insurance used in hairdressing salons

In most countries, insurance companies make it possible for the business community to protect itself against losses arising from unexpected events. With rapidly increasing risks, legal responsibilities and larger amounts to be insured, hairdressing salons are wise to safeguard themselves against unforeseen hazards which may, unfortunately, arise. In return for a premium (the cost of insuring), the insurance company will 'carry' the risk of such unforeseen events including fire, burglary, breakage and electrical fusion; these can be covered in an all-risks policy. Insurances should be reviewed annually and, following the advice of an insurance consultant, should be sufficient to cover your salon's needs.

Salons need to insure to cover:

- plant and equipment against theft, fire, burglary, breakage and damage;
- furniture and fittings;
- money and assets – both on and off the premises;
- public liability – damage to clients' or landlord's property;
- loss of profits (business interruption insurance).

Although the salon can be insured against most perils, you are expected to take all reasonable care in handling cash and in securing the salon against theft, burglary and fire. Police Crime Prevention Officers are available to advise businesses on salon security.

The types of cover offered by such insurance policies are more comprehensively explained in Chapter 17.

Accident compensation

From July 1999, as a result of the introduction of the new Accident Insurance Act, the delivery of accident compensation changed. The scheme itself will not change and it will remain 24-hour, no-fault, comprehensive and compulsory. As an employee you will be covered for all work-and non-work accidents. If you are an employee you need do nothing. You will continue to be covered for all injury resulting from accidents, 24 hours a day.

Accident injury insurance for employees will be split into two parts: work and non-work accident insurance.

- Insurance for work accidents will be provided by a registered workplace injury insurance company. Your employer will pay for this insurance.
- Insurance for all non-work accidents will continue to be provided by ACC. This also includes cover for any motor vehicle accidents.

Regulations affecting hairdressing salons

The Health (Hairdressers) Regulations

Although, as an apprentice, you are not ultimately responsible for ensuring that these regulations are complied with, you should be aware of why they exist and why they should be observed.

These regulations set down standards for the maintenance of healthy hairdressing practices, to ensure that the public is given the best possible protection against the spread of disease. The administration of these regulations is under the control of the Department of Health. The salon proprietor is responsible for meeting the necessary regulations. Health inspectors may periodically inspect the salon; they are responsible for enforcing the requirements. A copy of the regulations can be purchased at bookshops and an explanatory commentary can be obtained from the Department of Health.

The Employment Contracts Act

The Employment Contracts Act applies to every employee and employer in the hairdressing industry. If you have a job or if you are an employer, then you already have an employment contract. This may be written or unwritten. You also have rights and obligations under the Employment Contracts Act. Employees may choose whether or not to belong to an employees' organisation or union. They may also choose the organisation to which they wish to belong.

Employees and employers can authorise any person, group or organisation to be their bargaining agent or to represent them in negotiations for an employment contract.

Both employers and employees can bargain about the type of contract they want for the salon. They can also bargain about what goes into a contract.

Individual contracts

Individual employment contracts cover only one particular employee and his or her employer. Individual contracts do not have to be written, unless the employee asks for this. If the employee does ask for a written contract, this must be supplied. An individual contract can include anything that is lawful and on which employer and employee agree. However, there are some things that an individual contract must include:

- effective personal grievance and dispute procedures;
- a date on which the contract ends.

Contracts must also comply with minimum conditions set out in other Acts, such as:

- a minimum wage for employees 20 years of age and over;
- paid statutory holidays;
- paid annual holidays;
- special leave for sickness, domestic or bereavement reasons;
- equal pay;
- parental leave;
- job protection for defence force volunteers;
- protection against unlawful deductions from wages.

A typical individual contract will often cover matters such as:

- wages and allowances;
- hours of work and shift provisions;
- the type of work to be done;
- holidays and other leave;
- health and safety provisions.

Contracts may also deal with matters such as superannuation, bonus schemes or consultation arrangements.

Breach of contract

If an employer or employee has breached the employment contract by not doing what the contract says, the other party to the contract can apply to the Employment Tribunal for a remedy. The Employment Tribunal is the mediator and adjudicator which may suggest a compliance order to get the offending person to do what the contract says he/she must do.

Hairdressing training requirements

Most hairdressing industries set out requirements for the systematic training of apprentices or trainees. These are usually approved by the Industry Training Organisation. Apprenticeships that meet these requirements will receive national recognition by the hairdressing industry and a Certificate of Completion will be issued to trainees on the completion of the training requirements. Local training boards can sometimes assist or provide support for apprentices who meet specific training requirements.

Training requirement documents will cover such topics as:

- training agreement;
- training requirements;
- suitability for training;
- period of probation;
- prerequisites for apprenticeship;
- terms of apprenticeship;
- competency-based training;
- onjob training;
- offjob training;
- responsibilities of employer;
- responsibilities of apprentice;
- training record books;
- distance learning.

Accident compensation

All persons who suffer personal injury as a result of an accident are entitled to weekly earnings-related compensation under the Accident Compensation Act. Time lost during the first week as a result of an accident at work is usually payable by the employer at 80% of the employee's total lost time. That is, the employer must pay 80% of the full amount the employee would have earned in time lost from work on the day of the accident and the following six days. Earnings-related compensation after the first week is paid by the Accident Compensation Corporation (ACC) at the rate of 80% of the lost earnings.

The first week is not compensated for by either the employer or the ACC if the accident happens away from work. Sick leave, if outstanding, can be taken. After this, the ACC will take over responsibility.

Building up and maintaining clientele

The best way to build up a clientele is to provide first-class service in pleasant, hygienic surroundings. A new client should be impressed by the efficiency and cleanliness of a well-run salon. The stylist should be constantly alert to new developments and up-to-date methods of styling. Make a point of knowing the client's name and, if possible, keep a record of clients; this will help you to know more about them. Clients are always impressed with personal service and if you can remember details about them when they next call, this, too, can help. Take an interest in your clients and take pride in your trade. If your clients are satisfied, they will tell others that they enjoy visiting the salon. Do your best to please the customers.

Business cards

The client should always receive an appointment card with the stylist's name. It will also show the date and time of the next appointment, and the name, address and telephone number of the salon. These cards should be given to all clients who visit the salon, and should also be carried by the stylist to be given to any prospective clients or anyone who inquires about what hairdressing salon to visit. This promotes the salon.

Seminars, demonstrations, workshops, competitions

Stylists should take every opportunity to attend seminars, workshops, etc. so they can transmit the ideas they learn to their clients. Such occasions will also get you known on the local hairdressing scene as someone who is interested in improving his/her ability.

Window displays

Because it can affect the salon's identity, the window display should be attractive enough to impress upon prospective clients that the salon exists. The display should be changed regularly – at least once a month, but more frequently if possible. The front window is really free advertising space and so should be put to good use. The display should have a theme or advertise the salon's special services.

Display windows should be cleaned regularly both inside and out. The lighting should be arranged so that it lights up the display rather than the people looking in. Avoid overcluttering the display; keep it simple. If too much is put in the window, you may be tempted not to change the display frequently. Keep your display original and aim to attract the client's attention. Moving objects, flashing lights and bright posters draw clients to look at the window display.

Local hairdressing suppliers may help with advice and with dressing a window display, and they may supply the products if it means free advertising for them.

The stylist

Sometimes, because of the effort that goes into attracting new clients, the stylist can take regular clients for granted. Don't become too relaxed with such people; you still need to try just as hard to keep them. Show regulars that you value their custom by giving them continual good service. A small gift at Christmas or a card on their birthdays will show that you appreciate their loyalty.

The stylist's personality will influence the type of client he/she will attract. There should be someone in the salon who is able to handle and feel comfortable with clients' different personalities, they are quiet, shy, embarrassed or outgoing. Assess each client's personality and treat them accordingly. Remember, all salon clients are equally important.

Shows

You should be encouraged to give hair shows for local organisations, such as kindergartens and charitable associations, as these are good ways of attracting new custom to the salon and of making your salon well known. A show simply to promote hair styling and fashion is fun, exciting and a good promotion winner. Combine with a local clothing fashion house to show the community the latest hairstyles and clothes. Posters advertising the event should be well distributed.

These are just a few ways in which you can attract, build up and maintain clientele. Keep yourself popular with your clients and show that you genuinely enjoy doing their hair. The service you offer is also a psychological one and you should treat the client as an individual and not just as another head of hair. Most clients are not hard to please, but do expect the best that you can possibly give. Be friendly and show a desire to please; this will help you, and the salon, to succeed.

Questions

1 a What are salon overhead costs?

_____

_____

b What is considered to be the biggest overhead?

_____

_____

c Express the following as a likely percentage of salon turnover:

i wages;

_____

ii stock;

_____

iii advertising.

_____

2 What do these terms refer to:

_____

a salon turnover?

_____

_____

b net profit before tax?

_____

_____

c net profit after tax?

_____

_____

3 On which dates does the government's financial year begin and end?

_____

4 How can profits be maintained if competition prevents you from raising the salon prices?

_____

_____

5 Discuss three ways in which wastage of materials can be kept to a minimum.

_____

_____

6 If you are given the responsibility of ordering stock for the salon, what factors will you need to consider?

_____

_____

7 What are the following:

a an invoice?

_____

b a statement?

_____

c a packing slip?

_____

d a stock book?

_____

e a credit note?

_____

8 Discuss and elaborate on how the expense of some salon overheads can be minimised by effective use of materials.

_____

_____

_____

_____

_____

9 What is the purpose of maintaining an adequate system of financial accounting?

_____

_____

_____

10   Name five types of book which are necessary for simple account keeping.

_____

_____

_____

11   Outline how incidental items bought for the salon are recorded.

_____

_____

_____

12   To what do the terms '*dr*' and '*cr*' refer? Where would you expect to see these terms?

_____

_____

_____

13   How should a cheque be crossed and why is it important that this should be done?

_____

_____

_____

14   **a**   Name three types of policy cover for hairdressing salons, where an insurance company carries the risk.

_____

_____

     b   What is a premium?

_____

_____

15   What is the purpose of the Health (Hairdressers) Regulations?

_____

_____

_____

16   Briefly outline the Employment Contracts Act.

_____

_____

_____

17 How does accident compensation affect you as an employee?

_____

_____

_____

18 What steps can you take to build up and maintain your clientele?

_____

_____

_____

19 Elaborate on two ways to make a window display attractive.

_____

_____

_____

_____

20 What do the following abbreviations stand for:

a IRD?

_____

b ACC?

_____

c PAYE?

_____

d Not Neg.?

_____

e A/C?

_____

21 How should retail stock be displayed so that it is promoted to its best advantage?

_____

_____

_____

_____

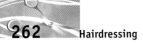

22 Name and discuss three ways in which retail stock can be promoted.

_____

_____

_____

_____

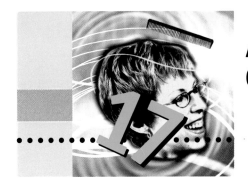

An introduction to the New Zealand Certificate in Hairdressing Management

In this chapter, you will learn about:

- starting a business;
- running the salon;
- taxation;
- goods and service tax (GST);
- costing a service;
- keeping the accounts (financial accounting);
- building up clientele;
- salon management;
- salon organisation;
- business legislation;
- salon design and decoration.

Introduction

Management means getting results through other people. This section on business management is aimed at those hairdressers who have just started out in their own salon or those who are toying with the idea of doing so. It is a guide for proprietors and managers who want to learn about the operation and day-to-day running of a hairdressing salon.

There are a number of factors to consider about the general administration of a small hairdressing salon. Usually, if you have been made responsible for the running of the salon or you are the owner, you will have to make your own decisions. There may be areas in which you have limited knowledge and in the early stages of business administration you will make mistakes through lack of experience. Unless your mistake is so costly that it puts you out of business, learn from it, avoid it next time and don't be put off.

You will need to know about:
- the fundamentals of establishing a business;
- buying the plant and equipment;
- ordering stock and materials;
- the products that you are using;
- the customers you serve;
- selling;
- how to handle finances;
- insurance;
- legal requirements;
- promotion, advertising and marketing;
- business management and business techniques.

In larger organisations, some of these jobs are done by specialists. Someone will be employed to promote and advertise the business, to buy stock or to advise on legal aspects. You will have to do all this yourself.

Starting a business

Location

Deciding where the salon should be situated is important. Renting in an area where there is a high pedestrian flow will cost more than in an area where the pedestrian 'foot count' is low. The extra money saved on rent, however, could be used to advertise and promote the salon.

Financing

A business needs starting-up capital – to purchase the lease, the plant, equipment and stock – and working capital to operate the salon on a day-to-day basis. Although an adequate amount of stock is necessary to ensure that the salon runs smoothly, overstocking should be avoided. Capital that is tied up in stock is unavailable for other purposes and there is a danger that the stock may deteriorate or become obsolete. The same rule applies for plant and equipment: don't tie up the working capital – use it to increase turnover.

Legal requirements

Local city councils are involved with business operation in three major areas:
1 general building requirements;
2 town planning;
3 health regulations.

Today the hairdressing business has become very competitive. For your business to do well and survive, you will have to keep up with changes in legislation. Be aware of your responsibilities toward your clients and your staff. These are further outlined in the Factories and Commercial Premises Act 1981, the Industrial Relations Act 1973, the Apprenticeship Act 1983, the Employment Contracts Act 1991, and the Health and Safety in Employment Act 1992. Your local I.T.O. will assist in giving you information.

What kind of business?

When you decide to start your business, you have three choices or alternatives. You can set up as a sole trader, as a partnership, or as a limited company.

Sole trader

You can establish the business in your own name – 'David's Hairdressing Salon', for example. Specialisation may be limited to the field of the owner's experience and expertise. There are no formal requirements for registration of the business name.

If you set up as a sole trader, you accept all responsibility for all work and any debts. All debts from the business must be made good out of the owner's personal assets, such as a house or car.

Advantages
1 No legal formalities need be completed to set up the business.
2 All profits are credited to the owner.
3 You have independence of action.

Disadvantages
1 It may be difficult to borrow money, especially in the early stages of developing the business – until your creditworthiness is established.
2 If the business does fail, you stand to lose the assets of your business and even your personal assets.
3 There are long working hours with little time off for holidays (or even for sickness).

Partnership

Although partnerships can increase the amount of capital available to set up the salon, they need to be well thought out before they are agreed to; in the experience of business counsellors, very few partnerships are successful. Planning, division of duties, responsibilities and wages or profit sharing are areas which can become problems and put a strain on the partnership. Communication is a key factor.

Points to be aware of regarding partnerships include the following.

1   Each partner is liable in full for the actions of all other partners, including borrowing by other partners.
2   It is desirable to have a partnership agreement, even if the partner is your best friend.
3   Interest in a partnership may not be transferable; partnerships can be wound up by agreement. Seek the advice of a solicitor.
4   All partners can be sued for the actions of each of them.
5   Profits as well as duties have to be shared.
6   Work and responsibilities can be shared.

Company

Companies are a common type of business organisation.

Company laws are governed by the Company Act 1993 and reading this Act will make you familiar with the provisions relating to the personal liability of the company. When a company is formed, it limits your liability for the debts of your business; it is the company which is liable for debts. Lenders such as banks, however, will usually hold you responsible for the amount they lend to the company, and this negates the limited liability concept. A company pays its own tax rate and shareholders are also taxed on dividends from the company. A lender will seldom risk lending more than the company's share capital.

Points to bear in mind about a company include the following.

1   The company's formation is defined by the Company Act 1993.
2   The Registrar of Companies must approve the trading name.
3   Annual returns must be lodged with the Registrar of Companies.
4   Directors are appointed by the shareholders.
5   Profits may be retained or paid to shareholders.
6   A large number of members can produce a larger initial capital outlay.

Franchising

Setting up a hairdressing business as a franchise is becoming more common. A franchise is where you pay a fee and the franchisors allow you to set up a salon under their brand name. You operate it as your own business, and it is very much like a business 'marriage'. Some of the benefits of a franchise include:

1   the business is likely to succeed because of the established name;
2   a lot of the problems of starting a business have already been 'ironed out' for you;
3   you will get a business package that will include promotion, training and advertising, and possibly benefits of buying products in bulk.

The cost of buying into a franchise will vary according to how established the name that you are buying is. The cost may also include payments according to turnover as a type of 'licence to trade'. For this initial cost you can expect a package that will include:

*   assistance with the location of the salon;
*   assistance with the design of the salon along with help with the fittings;
*   use of a well-known name;
*   help with management of the salon, including advice on how the salon system runs;
*   access to promotion, advertising and marketing facilities;
*   bulk buying privileges.

Questions should be asked of the franchisor. These should include the following.

- What is the company's track record; i.e. how long has the company been in business and how many franchises are running successfully? (You should also contact other franchises to see how well they are doing.)
- How many franchises does the franchisor intend to operate and will there be more than one in the same town?
- What are the implications of selling the franchise?
- Is the franchise for a set number of years?
- What is the true cost of buying the franchise?

If you are serious about picking up a franchise, it is obviously advisable to seek out a solicitor who is familiar with this type of business marriage. He/she will advise you and tell you the meaning of the small print in the contract.

Whatever structure you decide on, seek advice from your accountant and solicitor first.

Beginning your own business

Deciding

If you are deciding to venture into your own business, there are a few questions which you may like to ask yourself.

1 Do I have enough money to start?
2 Do I have enough money to support myself while the business becomes established?
3 Will I need a loan? If so, from where?
4 Do I have money to cover emergencies, such as illness, or the payment of provisional tax?
5 Have I thought about insurance?
6 Am I adept at keeping accounts?
7 What regulations do I need to be aware of which may govern my business?
8 How much will equipment cost? Can I hire, lease or buy good second-hand equipment?

Anyone who is interested in running a business can start a hairdressing salon. Running a salon is a risk but it can also be quite challenging. Decide whether you are the type of person who can handle the responsibilities involved. Are you:

- realistic?
- independent?
- optimistic?
- prepared to work hard?
- able to make decisions and plan?
- prepared to forgo holidays?
- able to deal with problems?

These are only some of the qualities necessary. You also have to decide whether you are going into business:

- to earn a better living?
- to be independent?
- for the challenge?
- for the financial gain (as an investment)?
- to do something different?

The reasons why you go into business will affect the way in which you run your salon and the rewards you will get for your efforts. It's up to you.

The success of most hairdressing businesses is very dependent on the skills and personalities of the owner/operator. The performance of this person needs to be assessed in relation to other factors, such as the salon's location, its staff, etc. Without that particular owner/operator, will the salon be able to produce the same results? Good ideas alone don't mean a viable business can be built up and sustained.

Legal requirements

There may be restrictions involved in operating a hairdressing business. The local council may have requirements about zoning, building, planning and health. Become familiar with these. Obtain copies of the Health (Hairdressers) Regulations 1980 and the Explanatory Commentary. These will tell you what requirements and standards the hairdressing salon has to meet in order to obtain a certificate of hygiene, which should be displayed in the salon. Check that you comply with the town planning zoning regulations set out by the local council.

Buying an existing salon

Is it better to buy an existing business or to start your own? Both alternatives have advantages. An existing salon is sold as a 'going concern' with an established clientele. The existence of this clientele is considered to be 'goodwill'. You need to find out why the salon is being sold and how old the equipment is. Watch out for any outstanding debts or hidden liabilities.

A typical advertisement may read:

'LADIES HAIRDRESSING SALON IN BUSY CITY CENTRE FOR SALE. GOOD LEASE, PLANT AND EQUIPMENT, TURNOVER $200 000 PER ANNUM – WALK IN WALK OUT – $45 000 + SAV.'

('SAV' stands for 'stock at valuation'.)

This salon is being sold as a going concern, but there is no indication as to why it is for sale, so you will need to find out:

1   why the salon is for sale;
2   about the lease, its length, the rent, when it will next be reviewed, how many years remain on the lease;
3   about the plumbing, electricity and hygiene and whether these meet council requirements;
4   how old the equipment is;
5   your accountant's assessment of the takings in relation to overheads (i.e. you will have to 'study the books');
6   what is incorporated in the asking price, i.e. how the figure is made up and how it was derived, e.g. how much is to be paid for goodwill;
7   about the stock at valuation (SAV). How old is the stock and how is it valued? You don't have to buy it; this may be a point of negotiation.

Never accept verbal information about the business; get it in writing.

Renting premises

A lease is an agreement between the owner of the building or premises and the occupier. Your solicitor will look over the lease and advise you on its provisions. This measure is protection for you and for the owner of the building. A lease will run for a number of years, perhaps from two to five years. It is advisable to ensure that the lease includes a right of retrieval clause. This means that, at the end of this period, you have a right to continue in business once the lease has expired. The end of a lease is also when the rent is revised. If a lease is for a long period, say seven years, the lease cost will be reviewed every three years, but generally, on short-term leases, the rent remains the same until the lease expires. Find out when a lease expires, whether there is a right of renewal, and by how much the rent will be increased.

A salon can be sold at any time during the lease period. The buyer of the salon buys the lease and continues to run the salon for the remaining years with a possible ROR.

Any structural problems are usually corrected and the building maintained by the owner, whereas maintenance of the interior is the occupier's responsibility.

The cost of a lease will depend:

1 on the size of the premises – some are calculated on a 'per square foot (psf)' (even though the country is 'metricated') per annum basis;
2 location – malls and arcades with a high pedestrian count or main street frontage are expensive. A salon away from the street frontage or on a mezzanine floor is cheaper.

Have the lease agreement inspected by your solicitor – it is a very important document and could make all the difference as you try to build your salon up into a successful business.

Goodwill

The hairdressing salon sold as a going concern will include goodwill in its price. Goodwill means the value of the salon's reputation (its name) and its popularity as a business. Time and money have been spent building up the business clientele and in training staff. These are intangible assets. Tangible assets are land, buildings, fixtures and equipment.

In hairdressing, paying excessively for goodwill can sometimes be dangerous, as clientele can often be built up by the owner's personality and style of hairdressing. In the hands of the new owner the goodwill may disappear very quickly, as will the profit.

Goodwill includes the salon telephone number, clientele, staff, and the value of any marketing, promotion and advertisement campaigns currently underway.

There are different ways of calculating goodwill, relating either to profits, turnover, or the length of time the business has been established. It's difficult to formulate a figure for goodwill but its cost should not be excessive and should be recovered in two or three years. You should also take into consideration whether the hairdresser who is selling the salon is likely to set up another business nearby. You would usually put a clause in the contract to prevent the vendor operating a business within a specified area for a specified number of years (this is called a radius or a restraint of trade clause). Goodwill is a negotiable factor, especially if you are not going to retain the salon's name.

Plant, equipment and stock (assets)

Evaluate the cost of the plumbing, electrical, carpentry and other work that will be necessary to get the salon operating – floor coverings, new paint etc. Ask what is leased or on hire purchase, e.g. the coffee machine, the plants, the cash register. Cost all the equipment and make sure you are getting value for your money.

You are not obliged to buy the stock if it is old, of poor quality or has been purchased by inexperienced buyers. It may not be a brand you enjoy working with, so if you don't want it, say so.

Accountants

Many hairdressers who are 'behind the chair' or 'on the floor' are busily involved in using their hairdressing skills and the artistic side of their craft. Many don't enjoy figure work, lack the time for it, or are 'not that good' with figures. Know your limitations: if you fall into this last category, you will obviously need the services of an accountant. Even if you are good with figures, you should still seek the help of an accountant (although maybe not as frequently).

It is important to remember, however, that accountants know nothing about hairdressing. They are employed by you to arrange finance, to prepare profit-and-loss accounts and balance sheets, to deal with government assistance programmes, and to prepare and submit tax returns. Accountants can assist in the financial running of your salon; they can save you time and money which will help increase your profits. Accountants' fees are scaled in accordance with the guidelines of the Society of Accountants. It is good policy to prepare yourself in advance before seeing your accountant.

Financing – getting a loan

Very few of us are lucky enough to have the ready cash to buy a salon outright, so part of the purchase price will have to come from somewhere else. Before you approach any of the lending institutions, you must know how much money you need and at what rate you can afford to pay it back.

The amount of money which you actually put into the business is called the 'capital outlay' or equity. This capital outlay is your contribution, consisting of money which you have accumulated from earnings or bequests and use to start the business. Hairdressing salons which start with a shortage of capital need to borrow more and must therefore make higher repayments, which come out of the profits. It is not regarded as sound policy to start a hairdressing salon with limited capital outlay.

Personal finance to capitalise a salon can be obtained from loans or mortgages. These involve paying interest on the amount borrowed; this interest is usually calculated weekly, monthly or quarterly. There are three main types of loan: long-term, medium-term and short-term loans.

- *Long-term loan* – 10 to 15 years plus capital mortgage. A long-term loan is usually for a freehold business which may include living accommodation or salon extensions/renovations. Such a loan is a 'table mortgage' where the interest and the principle (the money borrowed) are repaid monthly over the loan period. Banks, building societies, insurance companies and solicitors are good sources for this type of loan.

- *Medium-term loan*. This is a two- to five-year (approximately) loan or extended credit. You can arrange to pay either the interest only or the interest and the principle during the term of the loan. Trading banks, insurance policies and finance companies offer medium-term loans which are suitable for equipment, vehicles or to improve facilities.

- *Short-term loan*. This refers to an overdraft facility or bridging finance – a monthly arrangement where the interest and the principle may be paid at the end of the short term. Hire purchase agreements, banks and finance companies are the main source of this kind of loan. A short-term loan can be used as working capital, usually for stock purchases. The overdraft operates on the cheque account; the bank allows you to overdraw the balance.

The lender requires security so that he or she has sufficient confidence that the salon will be able to repay the loan in the event of a business failure. Security may be your life insurance policy or you may be able to get someone to guarantee a loan for you. Small business agencies may be able to help you and tell you more.

When presenting your case for a loan, you will have to prove or convince the lender that your income from the business will be sufficient for you to meet the repayments. Although banks are usually very cautious, they do make loans for businesses. You must present a good case. You will have to supply the lender with the following information:

- the purpose of the loan;
- proof that the loan can be repaid;
- what security you can offer;
- how the business is doing at present – profit-and-loss accounts and balance sheets.

Some lending institutions not only require security but are also interested in the salon's liquidity, i.e. the assets that can readily be converted to cash.

Government-assisted schemes

The government, from time to time, operates different employment subsidies or incentive schemes. These make provision for additional apprentices or for job creation, job opportunity, training assistance programmes or apprentice block course subsidies. Such schemes are intended to provide increased employment by supporting business expansion. They offer financial incentives for employers who create full-time jobs or take on additional apprentices. The assistance is given to offset wage costs during initial periods of employment and the less productive period of apprentice training. To find out more about these schemes, contact the Industry Training Organisation.

Banks

Trading banks

All salons will have a bank through which they operate the salon's finances. Cheques will be paid out, takings will be banked, loan finance can be arranged, term deposits will be opened and automatic payments can be made. Making use of these services will help you build up a bank case history. This is good as the bank gets to know you, you build up credibility and you are in a better position when you want to approach them for finance. The bank's job is, after all, to lend money. Let the bank manager know what is going on; get to know the manager before you need the bank's help. Establish a rapport, keep the bank abreast of developments and conduct your affairs professionally. Honour any undertakings which you give, be loyal and maintain your accounts.

Bank overdrafts

For a salon business, one of the first considerations when you require finance is to approach the bank for an overdraft. The salon must be in a position whereby it increases its borrowing potential. The bank's primary interest is in the security of any advances. For security purposes, a bank will consider the salon's assets:

- a mortgage over the building if owned (up to 80% of approved value);
- a guarantee (insurance policy or guarantor);
- plant and fittings – up to 33%;
- a debenture over the salon's assets (if a company);
- a motor vehicle.

Trading banks like to lend money to people who give them security. The biggest disadvantage of an overdraft is that the bank can demand the repayment immediately. This can suddenly change your cash flow and monetary situation.

Finance companies are a good source of short-term finance but loans from them are generally more expensive than a bank overdraft.

If you are turned down for a loan, don't give up. Try another source which may view your loan application in a different light.

Starting a business – a summary

- Reappraise and assess the reasons why you want to start business.
- Be prepared to work hard and accept the responsibilities that will come your way.
- Analyse your experience. Have you gained insight into the intricacies of managing a salon? If not, you will need to obtain knowledge in this area. Are you able to raise the finance to establish a new salon or buy an existing salon? Do you have enough capital for the initial outlay? Borrowing large amounts when you first start is daunting to say the least; the salon has got to work from day one.
- Visit your solicitor to sort out all the legal requirements, especially the lease.
- Make an appointment with your accountant and bank manager to get their advice on whether your plan is viable, and to ascertain whether they have a source of finance.
- Decide if you are going to operate as a sole trader, pull in a partner or set up a private company; each has advantages and disadvantages.
- Is the salon in the best location? Does it suit your needs and requirements? Consider the goodwill that the salon has built up.
- Finally, always take professional advice and never sign anything until it has been checked by your advisers. Ensure that all legal requirements are met.

 Running the salon

Once you are in charge of the salon you need to know more about the administration/management side of the business.

Hairdressing Associations and Organisations invariably have a Code of Business Ethics. These are a set of rules that members must adhere to so that business standards are met. As an example, the following would be a guide. Salon owners and their employees are expected:

- to uphold the dignity and honour of the profession and conduct business in a way that befits a professional hair salon;
- to stand by workmanship and correct any complaints which have occurred through faulty products or poor workmanship;
- to conduct themselves in such a way that a spirit of fair dealing, co-operation and courtesy shall govern relations between members of the profession;
- to refrain from directly or indirectly offering employment or hiring an employee of another salon except through advertising vacancies in the media (but this is not construed to inhibit an employee acting on his/her own initiative);
- to refrain from, and to ensure that employees refrain from, soliciting or approaching persons known to be clients of another salon;
- to realise that clients are deemed to be clients of the employer and not the employee;
- not to use the name of any other salon or a member in any advertising or public manner without written permission;
- to refrain from directly or indirectly, falsely or maliciously, injuring the good name or reputation of a fellow member, or discrediting that member's ability.

Insurance

A number of insurance proposals need to be looked at to ensure that the salon has adequate coverage. Most insurance companies now offer an insurance cover pack, i.e. all the insurance proposals come under the one policy which is especially formulated for the small business.

The policy will cover basic cover (all risks) insurance, business interruption or loss of profits insurance, public liability and personal disability.

Basic cover (all risks) insurance

This insures the salon building itself against loss or damage resulting from a very wide range of events. Usually, this policy is required only if the salon proprietor owns the building; in most cases the salon is rented. The items included under basic cover are assets such as furniture, fittings, plant and equipment.

Over the years a salon will accumulate valuable assets and these must be protected against loss or damage. Take care that you do not underinsure your salon assets. Inflation can quickly overtake the original insurance cover. Keep a close eye on the policy and review it regularly (yearly), increasing and updating when necessary.

You will need to insure your salon plant to cover a number of possible perils, such as:

- fire damage;
- flood, storm, water damage;
- earthquake;
- explosion;
- malicious damage – burglary;
- wind, hail, etc.

All risks insurance policies provide a wide range of cover but the premium (cost of insuring) is usually quite high because of the amount of cover offered. There is usually an excess to pay if a claim is made. This excess can vary according to what the claim is for, e.g. fire or water damage, and whether a deduction in premium cost has been calculated against a higher excess. Some insurance companies can, however, reduce the cost of a premium when the salon pays a larger excess called a deductible. This means that if a claim arises, the salon pays the first $100, $200 or $500 before the insurance company is liable. The higher the deductible, the lower the premium.

All risks policies may have some additional clauses which may mean an extra fee on the premium. These will include cover for damage to glass, electrical equipment and specified items.

Burglary

The stock, plant, fixtures and fittings are covered for specified amounts (as per the basic cover) against the risk of burglary. This also includes damage to the salon as a result of a forced entry. You'll need to enter the total sum insured. Tools of the trade can also be insured under this policy. There is usually an excess to pay, perhaps $100.

Keep an inventory (a list of salon assets – with serial numbers, if possible) in case of a salon burglary. This will assist the police and can help when establishing the amount of an insurance claim. There is a risk of underinsurance here, as the person insured tends to underestimate his/her susceptibility to burglary.

Money, including cheques, both on and off the premises is also covered by a clause attached to the policy. You need to specify the amount of cover required for both cash and cheques on and off the premises.

Glass

You will need this proposal as it includes breakage to mirrors, hand basins, display windows (including sign writing), glass doors and tiled areas. You are usually limited to one claim before an excess is considered. Insurance proposals may have their own maximum claim for glass.

Electrical equipment

This could be included in a policy package. Cover is the same as outlined in the section on basic cover but includes theft of, accidental damage to and electrical breakdowns of calculators, typewriters, electronic cash registers, air conditioning units, computers and word processors. The company may specify the maximum age of equipment which it will insure. You will need to itemise the equipment and add the total sum to be insured. An excess is usually implemented on claims of up to $100.

Special items

Items proved to have a value over a certain amount may include computers, cash registers, stereos, televisions or videos. Such items can also be covered against damage while they are being moved, say to a staff member's home or to a demonstration or seminar.

Business interruption or loss-of-profits insurance

This is an essential insurance for salons. If your salon suffers any of the events listed under basic cover insurance, loss of trade can be devastating and turnover can be completely lost. The policy provides cover subject to the provisions outlined in it. The period of the indemnity (cover) is determined by how long it would take to re-establish the salon turnover. The length of the indemnity depends on the premium you are prepared to pay. You state the sum you wish to insure for. There is generally no excess to pay on this policy if there is a claim. Various types of cover can be offered to suit individual needs.

Public liability

In 1974 the New Zealand Accident Compensation Act abolished the injured person's rights to sue for damages and the Accident Compensation Commission took over responsibility for Workers Compensation Insurance.

To cover legal liability for accidental damage to other people's property, including liability for goods sold or supplied and legal costs resulting therefrom, you select the sum insured, which is generally somewhere between $100 000 and $1 000 000. The reason for this is that the policy not only includes cover for damage to clients' property, such as clothing and jewellery, but also for liability arising from fire, flood or explosion. An excess is sometimes charged but you may be able to select a larger excess for a reduction of your premium.

Personal disability

For incapacity as a result of illness or accident, you fix the benefit required and the amount insured on a weekly basis. The benefit is payable for up to three years and the premium is calculated on the amount you state per week (e.g. $30 per year payable for every $100 per week coverage). The premium cost is also dependent on a comprehensive statement of your personal health and whether you partake in any dangerous or risk-inducing pastimes. You sign a declaration claim that all your statements are true. Many provisions and conditions are set out on the policy.

All these types of insurance proposal can be effective under the one-pack system. You will have to answer general questions on your previous insurance history. You must declare all the facts which may influence the insurance company's assessment of your proposal. The policies should be reviewed, updated and adjusted annually.

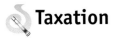

Taxation

Introduction (read IR 335 Employer's Guide)

As a salon owner you must deduct PAYE tax from the wages, commissions and bonuses that you pay your employees. These PAYE deductions are paid to the Inland Revenue Department (IRD). There are penalties for not fulfilling these obligations.

As soon as an employee starts work, he/she is required to fill in a tax code declaration (IR 330), to establish the rate at which PAYE tax is to be deducted. These deductions include the ACC earner premium which has been built into the PAYE tables and is deducted along with the tax. This form will also include the employee's IRD number and ask further questions of you. You are required to deduct the tax at the time of paying the wages – weekly, fortnightly, etc. Inland Revenue will send you an employer deductions (IR 345) form before the due date for each payment along with an employer monthly schedule each month. This tax is then paid to the IRD monthly. PAYE deducted in one month is due by the 20th of the following month. These deductions must be made and paid to the IRD to avoid serious penalties. The IRD supplies tax tables so that you can calculate the amount of tax to be deducted. You must keep the tax code declarations as part of your business records for seven years after the last wage payment has been made to the employee.

Once a month you must complete an employer monthly schedule (IR 348), which has details of your employees' gross wages and deductions made. This schedule will need to be completed at the same time as the Employer deductions (IR 345) form. This is due on the 20th of the month following deductions. Fill in the following details on the form for the period covered by the IR 345:

- PAYE deductions;
- child support deductions;
- student loan deductions;
- total deductions payable.

Payments can be made by posting a cheque with your payment slip in the reply-paid envelope provided, or you can pay electronically.

The employer's monthly schedule will include the following details for each employee:

- full name;
- IRD number;
- tax code;
- start/finish date;
- gross earnings;
- earnings not liable for ACC;
- lump sums taxed at lower rate;
- PAYE/withholding tax;
- child support;
- student loan.

Finally, at the bottom of each page, add up each column and put the total in the boxes provided. Sign and date the schedule.

Wages book

You must keep full and accurate records of wages. Cheque butts are not sufficient. The wages book should set out clearly details of wages, hours served in apprenticeship, commissions, tax, sick leave and holiday entitlement. The wages book should be kept for seven years after the making of the payments to which it refers.

How a salon owner's tax is calculated

Provisional tax

You should obtain the Inland Revenue booklets IR:240 *Taxpayer Obligations* or IR 335 *Employers Guide*. Unlike employees, who know what they earn each week, and are taxed accordingly (PAYE), the proprietor does not know what the salon's profit (taxable income after deductions) will be until after the end of the financial year. At the beginning of the tax year, the salon owner estimates income for the coming year. Most businesses end their tax year on 31 March. (If yours ends on a different date check with the IRD as to when your instalments are due.) This estimated figure is the one used to calculate the tax rate.

A salon owner becomes a provisional tax payer, i.e. enters a temporary tax arrangement, which is not finally settled. Salon owners pay their provisional tax in three instalments: one-third on each of the following dates: 7 July, 7 November and 7 March of every year.

Terminal tax

At the end of the tax year, actual income is calculated. Provisional tax that has been paid is subtracted from the tax to be paid on the amount earned, and if you have not paid enough you owe the balance, called terminal tax, which is due on 7 February of the following year. If your provisional tax payments were greater than the actual tax calculated, you will receive a refund. Most hairdressing salons base this year's estimated income on last year's performance. This is at least a guide. In the business's first year, because there is no basis for estimating income, provisional tax is not paid. Tax on the first year's profit is paid as terminal tax in the second year of business, due on 7 February. In the second year of business this tax is a heavy cash drain, as provisional tax is also due on 7 March.

The structure of the business will influence the rate at which you will be taxed. Company tax is 33 cents in the dollar (at the time of writing).

Tax allowable deductions

A hairdressing salon is entitled to claim the costs incurred by the business in the process of earning profits. A chartered accountant is the best person to advise on how to arrange the salon's expenses for maximum allowable deductions. Keep all receipts to support your claim.

Stock

Remember that stock is money tied up and will cost approximately 10% of your annual turnover. Keep your stock controlled so that you never run out. Keep stock levels low, never ordering more than you know you will use in a certain time. Holding excessive stocks means:

- losing interest on the money tied up in stock;
- extra work in maintaining records;
- using up extra space;

- encouraging wastage if staff think you have plenty of certain items;
- stock can become old or stale.

If stocks are small, you can readily see what is available and therefore know what is in short supply. If you have stock tucked away in cupboards, back rooms and drawers, it is difficult to keep track of what is being used. In major towns and cities, manufacturers' representatives come around frequently and you can order monthly. Two thousand dollars' worth of stock which is held continually on the stockroom shelves could be earning you 10% interest somewhere else!

Keep a watch on stock price rises; you may need to keep salon service prices in line with rising stock costs. Many hairdressing products are imported and are subject to numerous levies. Overseas oil prices can affect the cost of the preparations and cosmetics as this commodity is used in most hairdressing products.

Goods and services tax (GST)

The goods and services tax (GST) introduced on 1 October 1986 forms a part of sales tax. It brings within its scope the widest range of goods and services sold in New Zealand. Unlike a sales tax, which is collected at one stage in the distribution chain (when a commodity is sold), the goods and services tax is collected in instalments at each transaction in the production and distribution system. Every time a transaction is carried out by a hairdresser, the hairdresser must charge tax of $12^1/2\%$ (at the time of writing).

Taxable transactions

The goods and services tax operates on an invoice system The tax invoiced to a taxable trader is deducted from tax invoiced by the taxable trader to arrive at the net tax liability. This system is used in all countries which operate similar taxes. Taxable transactions include the following.

1. Supply of goods or rendering of services to any person in New Zealand by a taxable trader in the course of business.
2. Use of goods and certain services for private and certain business purposes by a taxable trader.
3. Importation of goods by any person, whether a taxable trader or not.

Goods and services tax is charged whenever a transaction is performed. Liability does not depend on the profitability of the outcome of the transaction.

Operation of the goods and services tax

Although the tax is a legal liability of traders, it is ultimately passed on to the consumer who is spending. This is because each time a trader invoices tax to a customer, the trader has claimed a credit of the tax previously invoiced to him/her. Thus, the tax paid earlier is netted out of the amount of tax charged and the trader is liable only for tax on the difference between sales (outputs) and purchases (inputs). The effect of this crediting mechanism is that the tax rolls forward at each intermediate transaction until the point of sale to the consumer. If the path of a commodity is followed through the distribution system and the amounts of tax paid are added up, the total of goods and services tax paid is equal to the revenue from a retail sales tax levied at the same rate.

The invoice system can be seen by tracing the path an item follows as it is built up from imports and raw materials, is manufactured and then passes from a wholesaler to a retailer for final sale. In this example, the goods and services tax is set at $12^1/2\%$.

	Transaction value $	Goods and services tax $	Tax payment to Inland Revenue $
• Producer of intermediate goods imports materials into New Zealand	2.00	0.25	0.25
• Producer makes intermediate product and sells it to a manufacturer	5.00	0.625	0.375
• Manufacturer makes final product and sells it to a wholesaler	10.00	1.25	0.625
• Wholesaler distributes product to retailer	12.50	1.56	0.31
• Retailer sells article to the final consumer	20.00	2.50	0.94
• Sales price	20.00		
			Tax collected
Goods and services tax		2.50	2.50
Total paid by the consumer	**$22.50**		

At each stage, tax is charged and credit is given for tax already paid. When the article reaches the consumer, the total tax paid by all the traders exactly equals the tax on the final product. This example illustrates that the goods and services tax is simply an alternative means of collecting tax. Most retailers include the tax in the price of goods and services sold to members of the public.

Costing a service

In a free market the right price is the one which the customer will pay; people will shop around only if your price is not good value.

There is sometimes confusion between the terms costing and pricing. Price is the amount of money customers are prepared to pay for your services. Cost is the amount of money you have to pay to provide what the customer wants. Thus, your net profit will be the price you get minus your costs.

Pricing a service is not easy because skill is difficult to measure. How much should you charge for the service in your salon? Many hairdressing salons take into account what their competitors are charging and fit somewhere in between. Some salons charge as much as they think they will get away with. Others try to undercut their competitors, especially if their overheads are low. These are accepted ways of pricing your service. There is a certain amount of strategy involved in calculating salon prices (as the client pays for the result); each salon will have a different philosophy.

It is generally accepted in the hairdressing trade that the price of service is lower in a suburban than a mid-city salon. This is because the cost of the service is less – the rent is usually lower. Because each salon has a different location, size, clientele, staff and general overheads, it is not sound policy to rely solely on the going rate to calculate your prices. You should know what your break-even point is on the services offered in your salon. This is an important part of running a business, as it allows you to ensure that services are correctly charged out.

Costing a service – wages

One way to assess the cost of services is to use a system based on consideration of the stylist's wage.

Let's imagine that wages (including the owner's/proprietor's wage) make up 40% of turnover. Working on a 20% profit margin, this would leave 40%

for all the other overheads. Most costing can be calculated according to the hours your staff work on the clients.

The cost of employing a senior hairstylist is, say, $400 per week gross, so:

$400 x 52 weeks = $20 800 per annum (not including Accident Compensation levies of $1.65 + GST or $1.85c per $100) (at time of writing).

This $400 per week figure is not, however, a true weekly rate because the stylist can have the following time off work every year:

3 weeks' holiday
11 days for statutory holidays
1 week sick leave
2 to 3 days on seminars, shows, etc.
totalling approximately seven weeks away from work annually. You are paying for this time off, so the stylist's 'year' is only 45 weeks:
$20 800 divided by 45 weeks = $462.22 per week.

Thus $462.22 is the actual cost per week for the senior hairstylist. If $462.22 is 40% of turnover, to be a viable operator this stylist should be taking approximately $1156 per week:

$$\frac{\$462.66}{4} \quad x \quad 10 \quad = \quad \$1155.55$$

Calculating an hourly rate

If the stylist is working 40 hours a week, we divide 40 into $462.22 to get the hourly rate which is $11.55. However, the stylist very seldom works 40 hours a week in giving the customer actual service. Time is spent on organising the day, tea breaks, personal needs, teaching the apprentices, answering the phone, supervising duties, attending to stock and so on. Let's say that 30 hours are productive hours. Remember, you are still paying the staff wages when they are physically earning nothing! Divide 30 hours into $462.22; this comes to approximately $15.40 per hour. This is the true hourly rate of the senior stylist who earns $20 800 per annum. If $15.40 is 40% of turnover, this hairstylist should be earning:

$$\frac{\$15.40}{4} \quad x \quad 10 \quad = \quad \$38.50 \text{ (approx.) per hour}$$
$$\text{for the salon}$$

Costing a service – labour and overheads

The salon can cost its services based on labour and overheads. This involves calculating the total overheads the salon carries and recovering costs in the number of working hours that are available. The labour cost will allow for holidays, statutory holidays, sick leave and so on. This second method is calculated on a per annum basis.

Labour cost

One senior operator employed 40 hours per week x 52 weeks	=	2 080 hours
minus 7 weeks (annual holidays, sick leave, statutory holidays, etc.)	=	280 hours
		1 800 hours
minus 10 unproductive hours per week (45 weeks @ 10 hours)		450 hours
		1 350 hours

This figure is the number of hours the senior will actually work on clients. Divide this by $20 800 per annum ($400 x 52 weeks) in total = $15.40 (approx.) per hour.

(This will not include Accident Compensation levies of $1.65 + GST $1.85c per $100.)

Calculating charge-out rates for the overheads

Overheads will be calculated at a rate per hour. Estimate the salon's overheads for the year. For a typical salon the overheads may be as set out below.

	$
Rent – $200 per week	10 400
Stock – $120 per week	6 240
Advertising	5 000
Electricity – $350 x 6 payments	2 100
Insurance	500
Gas – $50 x 6 payments	300
Interest (loans – 12% to 15%)	3 500
Depreciation (on plant 10%, on furniture and fittings 20%)	1 400
Telephone – $120 x 6 payments	720
Accountant/legal	1 500
Maintenance and repairs	500
Apprentices' wages	8 000
Miscellaneous (sundries)	2 000
Total	**$42 160**

Divide this by the number of actual working hours – 1350 – the salon has available to recover the cost:

$42 160 ÷ 1350	=	$31.23 (approx.)
plus labour	=	$15.40
		$46.63

This, then, is the minimum hourly rate that the salon can charge; *this does not include the 20% profit*. If you wish to calculate the hourly rate based on the 40 hours for which staff are employed, then add the total overheads to the wage bill:

$$
\begin{array}{r}
\$42\ 160 \\
+\quad \underline{\$20\ 800} \\
\underline{\$62\ 960}
\end{array}
$$

then divide by 52 weeks then by 40 hours; the hourly rate is $30.27.

To find the price of salon services, cost the charge according to the hourly rate of the senior stylist.

1 Wash, cut and blow-dry – medium length hair

	Time
Consultation and wash	10 minutes
Precision cut	20 minutes
Blow-dry and finish	15 minutes
Total	**45 minutes (approximately)**

Hourly rate
Senior   = $15.40
Apprentice   = $4.85
Total $\dfrac{\$20.25}{4}$ x 10 x 0.75 = $37.96 (approximately)

(As 45 minutes is not a full hour, this amount is multiplied by .75 to obtain the cost of the service.)

2 Permanent wave, blow-dry – short hair

	Time
Preparation, consultation, wash, cut	40 minutes
Winding	25 minutes
Process	15 minutes
Neutraliser	20 minutes
Blow-dry and finish	20 minutes
Total	**120 minutes (2 hours) (approximately)**

Hourly rate
Senior   = $15.40
Apprentice   = $4.85
Total $\dfrac{\$20.25}{4}$ x 10 x 2 hours = $101.25 for the service

Now establish what the profit margin would be in dollars and cents, working on the theory of a 20% profit expectancy.

1 The cut and blow-dry at a price of $37.96

Find the wage cost at 40% =

$$\frac{\$37.96}{10} \times 4 = \$15.18$$

Therefore

$15.18	wages (40%)
+ $15.18	all other overheads (40%)
$30.36	is the cost of the service

$37.96	price of service
– $30.36	cost of service (to break even – i.e. to make neither profit or loss)
$7.60	is the profit (20%) before tax.

2 The permanent wave at a price of $101.25

Find the wage cost at 40% =

$$\frac{\$101.25}{10} \times 4 = \$40.50$$

Therefore

$40.50	wages (40%)
+ $40.50	all other overheads (40%)
$81.00	is the cost of the service

$101.25	price of service
– $81.00	cost of service (to break even – to make neither profit or loss)
$20.25	is the profit (20%) before tax.

Similar calculations can be done to price all other salon services.

The 40% wage figure can, of course, vary from salon to salon. It may err on the conservative side, but it is nevertheless a realistic way of pricing and costing. Because hairdressing is a labour-intensive industry, wages are considered to be the biggest outgoing cost. Your wage bill may be higher or lower but the same principle still applies. To find your wage bill percentage, simply add up all the gross wages you pay (including bonuses, commissions, etc.) during a week, month or year. Total the turnover for the same period. Divide the wages into the turnover and multiply by 100 to obtain a percentage.

Although all overhead costs will vary, all salons will have the same overheads to consider. In most cases these include stock, rent, electricity, telephone rental, wages, advertising, insurance and laundry. The only real difference between a suburban and a city salon will be rent, a factor which can mean reduced prices in cheap rent areas. This, however, is often negated by spending more money on advertising. Naturally, the more staff, the higher the turnover, and the more expensive the overheads.

- *Variable* costs are the costs which are directly in proportion to the amount of business the salon does. For example, the cost of stock, material, electricity and employing part-time staff (casual workers) will increase as the salon becomes busier. These costs are items that need careful management and planning to keep them under control. The increase in overheads to meet demand should correspond to an increase in profit.

- Fixed costs are costs which do not vary with the level of business the salon does. These will include rent, telephone rental, insurance and loan repayments and depreciation.

Lack of profitability in a salon service usually arises from:

- too low a charge-out rate;
- insufficient business;
- spending an unnecessary amount of time on a friend at the expense of a client.

We have now examined the nature of profitability, looking at fixed and variable costs. Remember that turnover can vary between accounting periods. This variation will undoubtedly affect the cost percentage in relation to turnover. The figures in this chapter should be treated as a guide only because turnover will vary between different salons.

Break-even analysis

This form of calculation gives a salon owner the necessary information to determine whether or not the salon has made a profit. The calculations are reasonably simple, and can be summarised as follows:

1 To calculate break-even point (i.e. where no profit or loss is made), divide fixed costs by gross profit percentage (i.e. sales less variable costs expressed as a percentage).

Example: Variable expenses = 60% of sales
Fixed costs are $12 000 per year.

$$\text{Break-even point} = \frac{\$12\,000}{(1.0 - 0.6)}$$

$$= \frac{12\,000}{0.4}$$

$$= \frac{12\,000}{4} \times 10 = 30\,000$$

so $30 000 sales needed

Proof:
Sales = $30 000
Less variable costs (60%) = − $18 000
Gross profit $12 000
Less fixed costs − $12 000
Profit NIL

2 To calculate sales needed to obtain a predetermined profit figure for the owner:

Sales required = $\dfrac{\text{fixed costs + required profit}}{\text{gross profit percentage}}$

Example: As above, but owner requires profit of $20 000.

Calculation: $\dfrac{12\ 000 + 20\ 000}{(1.0 - 0.6)}$

= $\dfrac{32\ 000}{.4}$

= $32\ 000 \times \dfrac{10}{4} = 80\ 000$

so $80 000 sales needed

Proof:

Sales	$80 000
Less variable costs (60%)	– $48 000
Gross profit	$32 000
Less fixed costs	– $12 000
Profit for owner	$20 000

Figure 17.1

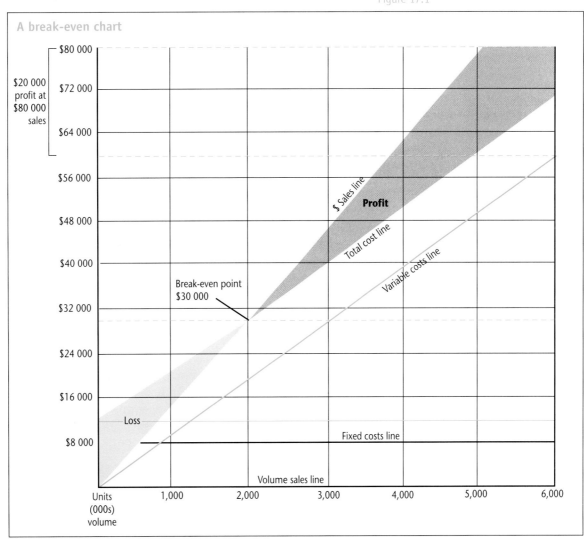

A break-even chart

Keeping the accounts (financial accounting)

Under the Income Tax Act 1976, everyone in business is required to keep proper records and books of accounts. Certain aspects of the salon's financial standing must be produced and recorded to support taxation returns. Fundamental records must exist to control the salon's financial standing and to maintain control of the cash. These records or accounts should be stored so that they are easily obtainable and can be referred to when necessary. Although some salons store this information on computers or word processors, filing cabinets with labelled suspended 'wallets' for easy identification are much more common. If the salon is large or more than one salon is involved, an index can be maintained for easy reference.

As each invoice or statement arrives, file it in alphabetical order. Check first:

- validity of the charge;
- the invoice against the statement;
- any credits.

The files and records will be quite numerous so it is important to work out a filing system which will prevent the documents from being misplaced or lost. The files will have labels such as:

- *Staff*: the wallet contains, in alphabetical order, manilla folders on each staff member.
- *Supplier's invoices*: the wallet contains, again in alphabetical order, the supplier's invoices from the various manufacturers.
- *Correspondence*: both incoming letters from trade associations, etc. and outgoing mail (copies of letters you have sent to people) should be kept.
- *Bank statements*: as manager or proprietor, you will also have to manage the salon's money and expenses.

Often the financial side of a hairdressing business consists of a quick glance at the bank statements; chequebook butts, bank deposit slips and any other receipts are handed to the accountant in order to prepare the necessary returns. The hairdresser then wipes his or her brow, heaves a sigh of relief and waits to see whether the business has been a success.

This, of course, is not the way 'the books' should be done. The owner of a hairdressing salon must know how well it is doing now, whether it is profitable, and must have a complete picture of probable trends in the future. It is assumed that a qualified accountant will be employed to complete the salon's accounts.

The situation to strive for is one where:

1 you know your cash situation – what has come in; what has gone out; whether it was a good week (i.e. you should have your finger on the pulse);

2 you should get your accountant to advise you on how to do little things to help reduce accounting costs. Providing a 'shoebox' full of old cheque butts, etc. at year end will cost you dearly in accounting fees. Many books on the subject will be of help and may be applied to hairdressing. The suggested minimum accounting records a salon owner should have are:

- a balance sheet;
- profit and loss – revenue statement;
- cash budget;
- reconciliation of bank statements;
- records of the handling of petty cash;
- wage records.

Balance sheet

A balance sheet is used for tax purposes and it can be produced quarterly, half-yearly or yearly (normally at the end of each financial year).

A balance sheet tells you what you own (assets) and what you owe (liabilities). Although it can be done at any time, your accountant usually puts it together at the end of the year. Its purpose is to show the salon's financial position. The worth of the business is determined by subtracting the liabilities (debts) from the assets.

Assets

- Liquid: usually convertible into cash within one month (bank term deposits, shares, fixed deposits).
- Current assets: usually convertible into cash within 12 months (stock and accounts receivable).
- Fixed assets: not convertible into cash within 12 months (lease, fittings and fixtures, equipment).

Liabilities

- *Current liabilities*: the amounts which you owe and will be expected to pay in the next 12 months; may include accounts payable and loans to be repaid.

Assets minus liabilities equals your equity (what you are worth). Your equity is increased if you make a profit or put more money into the business, and decreased if you make a loss or take drawings. Current assets minus current liabilities is working capital and this should be positive.

Balance sheet as at 31 March 20–

CURRENT LIABILITIES	$		CURRENT ASSETS	$	
(what you owe)			(what you own)		
PAYE owing	250		Stock – salon	750	
Telephone	75		Stock – retail	250	
Gas	50		Cash in bank	1 000	
Electricity	125		Cash in petty cash (float)	75	
Unpaid rent	200		Visa/bankings not yet received	100	
Creditors (for goods)	50				2 175
		750			
			FIXED ASSETS		
LONG-TERM LIABILITIES			Salon equipment	5 000	
Mortgage		100	*Less* depreciation (10%)	-500	
					4 500
Proprietorship			Fixtures and fittings	2 000	
Balance as at 1/4/–	6 000		*Less* depreciation (20%)	-400	
Retained profit after tax	4 150				1 600
Less drawings	-1 125		Furniture	2 000	
		9 025	*Less* depreciation (20%)	-400	
		9 875			1 600
					9 875

Profit-and-loss statement (or revenue or income statement)

All businesses have a standard profit-and-loss account (P and L account). It is normally prepared for a whole year (but can be done monthly) and shows income minus expenses. The purpose of the profit-and-loss account is to determine the profit from the salon's services for any given time; it shows the viability of the salon. The salon owner can take the drawings out of the profits. The profit-and-loss account is debited (dr) with purchases and expenses and credited (cr) with sales and income. To complete the statement, the accountant needs all the invoices and statements received, plus chequebooks, wages books, bank books and bank statements. The accountant also needs to know what stock is in hand (stocktaking) for salon and retail.

Profit-and-loss account
Year ending 31 March 20–

	$			$
Opening stock 1/4/–	750		Salon income	
			(including retail)	100 000
Plus stock purchases	3 000			
Less closing stock as at 31 March	– 500			
Less stock on shelf as at 31 March		3 250		
Retail opening stock	750			
Plus stock purchases	2 000			
Less stock on shelf as at 31 March	– 250			
		2 500		
TOTAL COST OF GOODS SOLD		5 750		
GROSS PROFIT		94 250		
		100 000		
Less EXPENSES (fixed and variable)				
Staff wages		30 000	GROSS PROFIT	100 000
Rent (fixed)		8 000		94 250
Rates (fixed)		1 000	Interest from bank	2 000
Advertising		5 000		
Interest (fixed)		3 000		
Electricity		1 500		
Gas		500		
Laundry		750		
Telephone (fixed)		600		
Insurance (fixed)		400		
Travel and entertainment		2 000		
Accident compensation levies (fixed)		150		
Allowances (meals) (fixed)		250		
Legal expenses		800		
Accountant (fixed)		800		
Petty cash expenses		1 000		
Depreciation (fixed):				
Equipment (10%)		500		
Fixtures and fittings (20%)		400		
Furniture (20%)		400		
Balance being net profit before tax		39 200		102 000
		102 000		

Using the profit-and-loss statement, you can look back over a period of months or years and compare figures. You can work out percentages on overheads and profit margins. The profit-and-loss account will show you which areas are becoming more expensive and which may need to be reduced. If there is more profit because of increased sales or advertising promotions, this is a pleasing reward if you know that competition prevented you from increasing your prices. You may have set goals or objectives in your budgeting and this is a good analysis for future budgets. Retail sales can be compared and appraised; the statement will serve as a guide and may indicate a need for a change in your selling approach.

Once you realise the statement's potential, you will want one drawn up far more frequently than you may have done in the past!

Cash budget (or cash flow forecast)

Your accountant will usually prepare this every six months. It's a projection of your cash income and expenses over the next six months (or whatever period you wish). This cash budget will make it easier for you to forecast funds which may be required for expansion or for improvements. It is also sound preparation for borrowing money; you will know whether the salon can afford a loan and what working capital will be available. In preparing the cash budget, the salon accountant, owner or manager estimates (using a safety margin) the salon's income on a weekly basis, referring to the salon's income history and past trading results.

If the estimated cash income is more than the expected outgoings, the difference is added to the cash balance at the beginning of the period. If the income is less than the outgoings, the difference is subtracted. The result at the end of the set period is the estimated cash balance. This type of information can also help in covering a salon's overdraft.

Example of a cash budget for the next six months

Income	Apr $	May $	Jun $	Jul $	Aug $	Sep $	
Cash sales: – salon	8 400	10 500	8 400	8 400	10 500	6 400	(bad month)
– retail	1 400	1 750	1 400	1 400	1 750	1 000	
TOTAL INCOME	9 800	12 250	9 800	9 800	12 250	7 400	
Cash payments							
Wages – net	3 200	4 000	3 200	3 200	4 000	3 200	
PAYE	800	1 000	800	800	1 000	800	
Stock purchases	1 000	1 250	1 000	1 000	1 250	1 000	
Rent	400	500	400	400	500	400	
Other expenses	400	500	400	400	500	400	
New equipment	–	–	500	–	–	–	
Term loan interest	100	100	100	100	100	100	
Tax – provisional	–	–	–	–	–	1 200	
Owner's drawings	1 200	1 500	1 200	1 200	1 500	800	(not enough $ could draw on funds)
TOTAL PAYMENTS	7 100	8 850	7 600	7 100	8 850	7 900	
Surplus (deficit)	2 700	3 400	2 200	2 700	3 400	(500)	
Opening balance at bank	10 000od	7 300od	3 900od	1 700od	1 000	4 400 in funds	
Closing balance at bank	7 300od	3 900od	1 700od	1 000 in funds	4 400 in funds	3 900 in funds	

In the example of the cash budget, salon sales were estimated at $2100 with retail $350 per week. The four-week months of April, June, July and September made the cash sales $8400 and retail $1400, making a total of $9800 for these months (except for September, which was not a good month ($7400 total)). May and August each had five weeks so salon sales were $10 500 and $1750 for retail, making a total of $12 250.

After paying out the estimated cash payments – some of which, such as rent, telephone rental, interest and insurance will be fixed – the total is added and compared with the income as either surplus or deficit.

Handling petty cash

Keep a petty cash tin or 'float' in a separate drawer or compartment in the cash register. The petty cash is required for small items and money is drawn out as required. Enter any spending money in the petty cash book. At the end of each week, add up the expenses in the book; expenses plus money left over should equal the float. Draw a cheque from the bank for the amount of money spent and put this cash back into the tin or drawer to bring the float back up to normal. This can be done daily or weekly. The normal float would be $40 or $50.

SET UP FLOAT 1/4/20– CHEQUE   **$50.00**

PETTY CASH BOOK WEEK ENDING 8/4/20–:

2/4	Postage stamps	12.00		
4/4	IOU Jenny	10.00		
	Milk Phil	2.00		
	Coffee	2.48		
	Tea	2.25		
5/4	IOU Jenny repaid		10.00	
6/4	Magazines	12.00		
7/4	Staff meals	18.00		
	TOTAL: Net spending	58.73	10.00	= $48.73
	Cash left			$1.27
				$50.00

Therefore draw cheque, 8/4/20– = $48.73.

Bank statement reconciliation

To assist in reconciling your account, follow the instructions as numbered.

1 Enter in your chequebook any debits or credits shown on the bank statement but not already recorded by you. Note: If account is overdrawn subtract deposits and add cheques. Watch for regular automatic payments for insurance, etc. These should be deducted from your chequebook.

2 List unpresented cheques:

Cheque no.   **Amount**

3 List deposits made before final date of the bank statement but credited after cut-off date:

Deposit no. (if any)	Amount

4 Final balance of bank statement   (A) $

    Total deposits   (B)

5 Add A and B   (C)

    Total cheques   (D)

6 Subtract D from C $

This should be your chequebook balance.

Banking procedure

Try and bank the salon's takings daily. This is a safe policy as large sums of money on the premises can be a risk.

1 Count the takings in the till and deduct the petty cash or float; this should balance.

2 Make a note of the cheques in the pay-in book (summary book) supplied by the bank, ensuring that the carbon copy is underneath. List the cheques, writing down the drawer (the person who originally wrote out the cheque), bank, branch and amount.

3 Fill in the deposit book, entering the total amount given in the pay-in book. Cheque fees or bank fees will need to be taken with you to the bank.

4 Remember, banks close at 4.30 pm.

Paying the wages

Obtain time sheets and a wage record book or use a system such as Kalamazoo.

1 Make a note of the total hours that each staff member has worked, noting any absences or overtime (extra late nights or Saturdays). The Hairdressing Award states the amounts which should be paid; keep up to date with any new awards and changes in rates of pay.

2 Make a total of the gross wages, including any overtime, commissions or bonuses.

3 Refer to the PAYE tables for the appropriate tax deductions. Tax is calculated on the weekly gross wage (PAYE). Once this has been deducted, the remainder becomes the staff member's net wage.

4 Add any non-taxable allowances to the net wage; this could include tea money for late nights (work after 6.30 pm). This total amount is paid to the employee.

5 Pay all PAYE deducted to the Inland Revenue Department by the 20th of the month following the month of payment. If you are a day late, you incur a 10% penalty.

6 A reconciliation of all wages and PAYE payments is required by the Inland Revenue Department by 31 May each year. Your accountant will normally do this.

Building up clientele

Sales promotion and advertising

All salons advertise in one form or another. Advertising can be anything from the simple business card to the advertisement on the television screen. Advertising is a salon overhead and approximately 10% of the salon's turnover should be budgeted for advertising. If you decide that you would like to promote your salon's services through advertising, it is best to plan the campaign with an advertising agent. Work out a budget and decide how much money you would like to spend. Then decide on the best way to advertise. You may decide to spend the entire year's budget on one or two very large advertising promotions or, as most salons do, spread the advertising budget over a longer period with a series of different ideas. Next you need to decide on what means of advertising you prefer; these are referred to as 'advertising media'. For salon purposes, advertising media fall into two categories:

- *That which the client can keep a copy of:*
    - newspaper advertising;
    - business cards;
    - circulars, brochures, pamphlets;
    - match books and other promotional material such as stickers, pens, combs, T-shirts, etc.
- *That which the prospective client cannot keep a copy of:*
    - cinema advertising;
    - radio announcements;
    - television coverage;
    - posters and billboards.

Some salons use all these forms of advertising. It is a good idea to advertise with a theme or to publicise a particular service at which the salon is expert. If you have been on an overseas trip to learn new techniques, this could play a part in the advertising promotion, although it is important to avoid promoting individuals in the salon; advertise the salon, not the stylist. Some hairdressing manufacturers sponsor advertising campaigns if their product is used in the advertisement. Ask the local manager whether the manufacturer is prepared to sponsor an advertisement in the local newspaper, for example, if its product is used to attract clients.

If your salon wants to advertise in a newspaper, it is important to decide whether the regional paper or the local suburban paper is best. The cost of advertising in the regional paper is greater than for advertising in the suburban paper. If your salon is in the central city, choose the regional paper because most of its readers travel to the city anyway. The suburban salon, however, may choose the local paper, as only 10% of regional paper readers may live in the salon's area, meaning that 90% of these readers may not visit the salon. The people who read the local paper are prospective clients so the catchment area is better.

The fundamentals of advertising promotion

A salon advertises to:
1. remind the public that the salon is still there;
2. promote the salon's services;
3. convince the client that the salon offers the best service.

Advertising aims to attract the client's attention and arouse interest. You must determine:

1   at what part of the public the advertisement should be aimed; for example, homemakers, young single people, pensioners;
2   who is going to advertise the salon services, and what advertising media to use (you may need to use different media, according to the service you want to advertise, and even the time of year may influence your choice of medium);
3   the salon's objective for advertising (do you want to stress retail or services such as permanent waving or colouring, or do you just want to build up an image and sell the salon's name?);
4   the main theme of the advertisement (is it to release a new style, to launch a new product, to let clients know that you are open at certain times?);
5   whether the salon is going to co-ordinate with a hairdressing manufacturer to promote a total package involving a particular product. In this case, who pays for what?

Deciding on an advertising campaign

There are many ways of advertising apart from the paid advertisement. These include demonstrations, public relations exercises, word-of-mouth, competitions, free gifts, special deals and samples.

Spread your campaign over a longer period of time and try to use more than one medium to present your message. Newspapers and radio are the prime media for hairdressing salons, with back-up advertising through business cards or promotional shows. Develop a theme for the type of client your salon attracts (once you are able to identify the salon's main clientele). Sometimes the clients themselves can give you ideas which can provide a refreshingly independent viewpoint.

Remember that you are constantly affected by other people's advertising campaigns, offering new products and brands which are always claimed to be better than anyone else's. We are exposed to advertising in the papers and magazines we read, and our letterboxes are full of promotional material. Radio, television, billboards and hoardings along the roadway, signs on buses, vans, cars, business cards, gifts and novelties in the cinema – we are surrounded by advertising!

Practical exercises

1   Do a survey at your salon to find out where most of your clients come from. Then decide whether the regional or the local paper is best for advertising.
2   Design a salon card using colour to illustrate your ideas.
3   In a 6 cm by 8 cm space, lay out an advertisement, using a theme offering a salon service. The advertisement is to be in a medium that the client can keep.

Salon management

Essentially, the manager's job is to show skill in achieving organisational goals through leadership. The manager is accountable and responsible for such matters as:

•   providing a service to the customer;
•   ordering stock;

- maintaining budgets;
- organising staff;
- training;
- making decisions.

To be successful at these tasks, the manager must be skilful in these areas:

- working with people;
- budgetary control;
- managing time;
- communication;
- training (giving instructions);
- solving problems;
- stimulating morale.

Managers are often appointed and given responsibility without having undergone training in any of these areas.

As a manager you must know what your responsibilities are, understand what has to be done and decide on how you are going to achieve it. Managers are paid to make decisions.

Unless the salon proprietor (owner) has given you a clear indication of the extent of your authority and responsibilities, you cannot be held accountable. You should, therefore, have a job description so that your performance can be fairly assessed.

Communicating

If you know what is expected of you, it is only right that the staff know what is expected of them. You must, therefore, know how to communicate. Staff must know what hours they are to work, their starting times, tea breaks and lunch times; what standards are required of them; what levels of productivity or efficiency they must meet. Good working relations will be maintained if both parties know where they stand. And if these good relations, in turn, mean efficiency in the salon, this is a credit to the manager. All this adds up to increased or maintained profitability, and the salon will survive.

Controlling budgets

As the manager's work is going to involve sales and figures, he or she must know the basics. These include such things as profits, simple accounting, bank balances, cash flow, payments, purchases, taxation, stock control and operating costs. The effective manager knows what resources are available; if he or she does not, there can be problems. Budget controls can be charted to assess progress, and appropriate plans and adjustments can be recorded. Having access to and using cost-saving information here may mean the difference between profit or loss. A computer can prove to be an excellent, time-saving tool for budgetary control.

Working with staff

The manager must take a broad view of the staff, using their minds as well as their hands. Most people have areas of capability which are often underdeveloped. Staff can frequently make significant contributions to increasing sales production and efficiency. Usually, if you give someone added responsibility, you will get a good response. Seek out any talents which may be untapped.

Managing time

Time is money in hairdressing so time must be controlled and managed efficiently. It is not the hours of work you put in, but what you put into the hours that is important. Rather than working harder or longer hours, aim to manage your time better. You can achieve this by:

- delegating more;
- handling each piece of paper only once;
- setting yourself bite-size targets.

Ask yourself, 'What would happen if I didn't do this?' Very often the answer may be, 'Nothing'.

Training

Training costs time and money and this must be allowed for when planning budgets. Training is designed to improve the performance of staff, and to teach apprentices so that they can become productive as quickly as possible. To check and evaluate the training programme, use an apprentice record training book to rate performance during the apprenticeship period. An effective training policy must become a positive commitment by the salon management to ensure that all staff members are competent in their sphere.

Keep all staff members up to date with technical and practical developments. They should be aware of the benefits they will derive from their involvement in training. The manager is responsible for ensuring that staff are properly trained, and properly trained staff take pride in the work they do. If trade qualifications are a prerequisite for advancement, all staff should know about this.

Time and money spent on training staff, paying wages and generally investing effort and exertion in the employment area will give a good return, and ensure that staff want to stay with the salon. For this reason, avoid transfers and terminations; productivity is dependent on the people employed.

It is also the manager's job to establish the factors which attract staff to the salon and keep them working there. They may have a variety of reasons for working in the salon, such as:

- the salon's location;
- security of employment;
- the salon's design and the type of work (fashion) it offers;
- the possibility of learning more;
- promotion within the salon;
- prestige;
- staff privileges;
- wages.

These factors determine staff members' attitude towards their jobs and can help to maintain morale. Factors such as job security or staff privileges may even help stimulate staff to make an extra effort and so increase productivity. Monetary reward is not, however, necessarily sufficient to stimulate staff to work.

Staff problems

These can be kept to a minimum if all employees know what is expected of them and understand their conditions of work. Again, communication is the key. Problems will be encountered if the manager:

- has favourites;
- does not recognise staff efforts;
- treats staff unfairly, either in terms of trust or of opportunity.

Any staff problems should be dealt with promptly and should not be allowed to get out of hand. Ensure that you have all the facts before giving either a verbal or written warning. If the problem occurs again, suspend or dismiss the offender, giving the correct notice. If you are an effective manager, however, it should not come to this.

Salon organisation

Managing and encouraging – the role of the manager

In general, there should be a hierarchy of employer and employees in a salon, a system that involves different areas of responsibilities, with each rank controlling the one below it. The owner of the salon (the employer) is ultimately responsible, legally, for what happens at the salon. If the salon is sued, taken to court, or does not meet hygiene or planning requirements, the proprietor must deal with the problem. The salon owner may, however, pass some responsibilities on to the manager who is in charge of the running of the salon. This person, then, should be recognised as the true manager. He or she will probably be very experienced, with many years of varied hairdressing experience. The manager should be approachable, so that staff can come to him/her with any problems or difficulties.

The manager should be supportive, showing an interest in staff as individuals, and a willingness to talk things over in a friendly way. Approve, encourage and recognise the staff's abilities and look after their interests. Always keep promises and don't bear grudges; staff will often have their failings, but don't keep on about them. Give credit and recognise good work – good bosses tell their staff when they have done a good job. The manager should delegate and not interfere, unless guidance is called for. This gives the staff an opportunity to show and develop their skills. It is surprising what some people achieve when you give them scope to extend themselves in areas such as window dressing or arranging demonstrations and small fashion shows. You can't motivate people; they have to motivate themselves.

The manager who is dedicated to the industry and to the salon will be successful and popular as a leader. Criticise if necessary (not in front of others) but don't make people feel silly, and help staff to overcome difficulties. Always inform employees of the salon's or the company's policies and keep them in touch with what is going on. This attitude makes staff feel as though they belong and are part of the organisation, especially if you take them into your confidence. Inform staff of the salon's objectives and aims. Rewards are necessary but they don't need to be financial ones – praise for a job well done, a good pat on the back and, 'You've worked really well today – thank you,' are often all that is needed.

The duties of the manager include:
- seeing that the salon runs smoothly;
- supervising the training of apprentices;
- being responsible for the daily cleaning and maintenance of tools and equipment;
- maintaining the appointment book;
- opening and closing the premises;
- cashing up the till;
- satisfying the customers' needs;
- ordering replacement stock;
- supervising the behaviour of staff;
- engaging and dismissing staff (at the request of the employer).

Salon staff

Worker-in-charge

This is a journeyperson who deputises for the manager when the latter is absent from the premises for periods not less than five consecutive working days and not more than 15 consecutive working days. Such a person is paid the allowance as provided.

Senior stylists

Staff will vary in age and range of experience, but everyone should be given individual responsibilities. Staff training nights should be rostered so that each stylist knows when he/she is expected to participate in workshops. Stylists can also be given the job of deciding what stock needs to be ordered, and they can be asked to suggest promotion ideas. Suggestions that will improve the salon's image or will create a better atmosphere will build confidence among the staff.

It is up to the employer or manager to keep the stylists busy with hairdressing work by bringing clients into the salon. It is up to the senior stylists to ensure that these clients come back because they are happy with what has been done to their hair.

Intermediates

These are hairdressers who are nearing the completion of their apprenticeship or who are sitting their final trade examinations or unit standards examinations. Their areas of responsibility can be: displaying stock (either at reception or in the front window); keeping an eye on any in-salon incentives or promotions; checking stock lists; adding till takings, and doing the banking.

Intermediate apprentices should do the shampooing of their clients' hair unless:

1 a junior apprentice is free and will remain so for the shampoo period;
2 the intermediate is busy with clients and has asked a senior stylist if a junior apprentice can help out. Animosity can develop if a more advanced apprentice with nothing else to do, asks a busy, less advanced apprentice to shampoo.

Junior apprentice

The junior apprentice is usually a busy hairdresser, as he/she must assist the senior stylists as well as maintaining the salon's tidiness and hygiene. Updating magazines, making and looking after style folders, checking new stock against invoices and packing slips and caring for plants are all areas that junior apprentices can be expected to attend to. They will also have to attend workshops, and learn from the stylists.

Job lists in the staffroom can be drawn up to allocate the various cleaning jobs that need to be done. Stick to the list so that the apprentices know exactly what jobs they need to do. The senior stylist (or manager) should oversee this task and should know whom to discipline if certain jobs have not been done.

Assistant

Employed to wash, shampoo and clean only, assistants may also be asked to answer the telephone and make appointments.

Receptionist

A well-trained receptionist can be the 'heart' of the salon and a valuable asset, if you can afford to employ one. The responsibilities of a receptionist are numerous, from organising the apprentices to doing simple book work. The worry that clients may be greeted inappropriately can be eliminated if you employ a well-trained receptionist. The business of answering telephones and control outgoing calls, booking appointments, distributing clients, answering inquiries, doing figure work, balancing the till, maintaining client records and arranging times for sales representatives to call can be left in his/her capable hands. The rest of the staff are free to get on with the job. Good receptionists are worth their weight in gold.

All staff should know the limit of their responsibilities and know where they stand.

Although hairdressing is one of the simplest of businesses – you could cut hair in your front lounge and call it a business – staff are the key factor; you must look after them. You may have a new, well-stocked salon, with all the latest equipment and even a clientele, but unless you have good staff (and can keep them), your business could be in trouble. So look after your staff.

Following these guidelines on staff encouragement will create a friendly atmosphere and certainly help the salon to retain staff:

- take an interest;
- recognise skills;
- be approachable;
- be fair;
- always keep your promises;
- give praise where necessary;
- listen;
- delegate – develop and extend the staff;
- criticise constructively;
- seek opinions;
- keep staff informed;
- trust your staff.

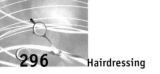

Dismissal

The employment of staff is deemed to be on a weekly basis, so one week's notice of termination of employment should be given by either employee or employer (except in cases of serious misconduct). In hairdressing it is worth considering letting the staff member leave immediately with pay (including accrued holiday pay owing) in lieu of notice. Some salons adopt this policy to avoid spreading discontent.

Business legislation

Accident compensation or disability compensation

Anyone in New Zealand who suffers personal injury by accident, and who is either an employee or self-employed at the time of the accident, is entitled to weekly earnings related compensation under the Accident Compensation Act. On 1 July 1999 several significant changes to the rules governing ACC came into effect; at the time of writing, following the November 1999 elections, several more are in the offing (see Chapter 16, p. 255). Consult your local office to find out more about these changes.

Employer

Employers must have a single, work-related injury insurance contract to cover all their employees. Employers must keep a permanent record of their employer accident insurance number and employer premium and claims history. An employer is required to deduct a levy based on the employee's gross earnings, including commissions and bonuses. This levy is paid by the employee at a given rate for the particular industrial activity classification – for hairdressers it is $1.40 including GST (at time of writing) for every $100 earned. Levies paid are tax deductible. The levy is calculated at the end of each tax year (31 March) and must be paid by 31 May. Even if you don't have employees, you must pay a levy to cover yourself.

The Inland Revenue Department (IRD) is responsible for collecting the levies, and can help you with the necessary forms, especially if you are a new employer, and it will explain what is required. If you are unsure of any procedure, ask.

Employee

If an accident or injury arises out of and in the course of employment (the ACC explains what constitutes an accident at work), the first week's compensation is paid by the employer who must pay 80% of the full amount the employee would have earned in any time lost from work, i.e. 80% of the gross wages, then deduct tax.

After the first week, Accident Compensation takes over responsibility and continues to pay 80% of the wages. All compensation is taxed and this is deducted from the 80%.

If an accident happens away from work or is not associated with work, then the employer is not liable for the first week's wages, nor is the Accident Compensation Corporation. Sick leave, if there is any outstanding, can be taken, but if not, the employee will not get paid. The ACC will take over responsibility after this first week.

Both the employer and employee must complete appropriate forms and send them to the Accident Compensation Corporation office without delay.

The corporation publishes numerous brochures and pamphlets dealing with the responsibilities of both employer and employee. Ask your local Accident Compensation Corporation office; they will gladly answer any queries.

The Hairdressers Award

Although the Employment Contracts Act was implemented in 1991, many apprenticeship contracts still include conditions under the Hairdressing Award.

A copy of the New Zealand Hairdressers (Male and Female) Award should be posted in a conspicuous place in the salon so that all workers can see it.

The award has been agreed to and settled on by negotiation between the Shop Employees Industrial Association and the workers' employers of the hairdressing industry.

Such negotiation between two parties is referred to as conciliation and is conducted before a conciliation council. The hairdressing industry employs an arbitrator to settle any disputes arising from the award.

The terms, conditions and provisions set out in the schedule are binding on both the parties. The schedule covers:

- industry to which agreement applies;
- definitions;
- hours of work;
- hours of work protection;
- meal and refreshment intervals;
- overtime and meal money;
- payment for customary late night;
- Saturday and Sunday work;
- wages – journeyperson;
- wages – assistants, shop assistants and receptionists;
- casual and part-time workers;
- uniforms;
- holidays;
- annual holidays;
- special holidays for long service;
- sick pay;
- compassionate leave;
- maternity leave;
- abandonment of employment;
- continuity of employment;
- weekly employment;
- payment of wages;
- tools;
- general;
- time and wages book;
- references;
- right of entry;
- union meetings;
- disputes;
- personal grievances;
- under-rate workers;
- unqualified preference;
- application of agreement;
- scope of agreement;
- term of agreement.

The Health and Safety in Employment Act

The object of this regulation is to prevent harm to employees while they are at work, and to ensure that actions at work do not result in harm to other people (including members of the public). The regulation sets out to promote excellence in health and safety management. It requires people in places of work to perform specific duties to ensure that people are not harmed as a result of work activities.

An employer must take all practical steps to ensure the safety of employees while at work. In particular, employers must:

- provide and maintain a safe working environment;
- provide and maintain facilities for the safety and health of employees while they are at work;
- ensure that equipment in the work place is maintained so that they are safe for employees to use;

- ensure that employees are not exposed to hazards in the course of their work;
- develop procedures for dealing with emergencies that may arise.

    Effective safety management requires the involvement of everyone in a place of work. Employees must look after themselves and must also ensure that their actions do not harm anyone else.

The Consumer Guarantees Act

The Consumer Guarantees Act came into effect on 1 April 1994. It states that services must meet four criteria:

a work must be carried out with reasonable care and skill;

b the work must be fit for any particular purpose the client has told you about;

c if a time for completing the work has not been agreed, it must be carried out within a reasonable time, and

d if the price for the work has not been agreed, it must be a reasonable price for the work done. For more information, see the Ministry of Consumer Affairs *Business Note no. 5.*

The use of computers in hairdressing

Computers are becoming commonplace in many small businesses today, and hairdressing salons can also make use of them. Computer consultants can assist you with information on the various options.

    The consultant or the hairdresser can set up the environment required by the salon, i.e. what data actually needs to be programmed. Although the consultant can advise on the various 'packages' that are available, the salon must decide on the system that bests suits its individual needs. This initial setting up takes only a matter of days. The effort involved in processing the data is not significant, but you must know what you want the computer to do.

The capabilities and components of a microcomputer

Computers can be used as an efficient tool for keeping hairdressing records. The equipment needed will depend on such factors as the size of the salon, the number of employees or how many salons are in a group.

Hardware

You will need *hardware – a visual display unit* (VDU), a *keyboard* and a *central processing unit* (CPU) where all the data is processed. All these pieces of equipment can quite easily sit on the reception desk.

    Disk storage is also necessary, and can take two forms, either:

1 a floppy disk – which is cheap but has less storage capacity, or

2 a fixed (hard) disk – which has more storage capacity but also costs more.

    Peripheral equipment can include a *printer*, which will give you a printed copy of report forms or documents. This need not be kept at reception, but can be stored in an office. A disk rack can be used for storing the disks.

The software

Computer software comes in packages – i.e. as prewritten programmes. The hairdressing salon can use these packages in the standard way. Packages can include the following.

1 **A stock recording or controlling system**. This can be used to keep an accurate control of stock; every purchase made or product used is 'keyed' into the system and will be automatically added or deducted. The keying

can be linked to an 'intelligent' cash register which can even calculate price increases on retail stock.

2 **Accounts payable and accounts receivable**. This type of package will tell you what you owe and what is owed to you – dates due, statements and invoice for costs.

3 **Payroll package.** The data will include details of pay, holidays, apprentices' hours, sick pay and anything else you may include in a time and wage book.

4 **Financial statistics package**. Annual statements, balances, salon takings, taxation, profit and loss can all be keyed into the system.

5 The salon can set up its own system for **client identification**, including all necessary data such as hair type, hair characteristics (texture, porosity), type of service – method, formula, and results – problems, treatments, new developments, etc.

Include anything else relevant to giving the client efficient service.

Many other packages are available and it is up to the salon owner to weigh up what each will do. At first, the facilities used will be basic. As the salon grows, you will use more packages which, if correctly selected, will all 'interface' (match up and complement each other).

Degree of usage

Apprentices can be given a password which will allow them to read only certain data on the computer, such as client information or stock files.

An identified password can also give access to the system in areas designated for the manager only.

The owner will have full access to information on salaries, profits, etc., information can be stored in such a way that it is inaccessible to other staff members.

If you and your staff can use a cash register, then you can use a microcomputer. Most are 'user friendly' – they prompt the user and ask for details should you forget to key things in.

Salon design and decoration

Introduction

Whether you are opening up a new or buying an existing salon, the chances are that it will need to be fitted out completely, redesigned or refitted. Although each salon proprietor will have his/her own ideas (and budget), certain principles need to be considered in creating the best possible environment for working in and for attracting clientele. You must comply with health regulations and you may need to consult local authorities about external alterations or additions, such as awnings, neon signs or advertising boards. Plumbing and electrical installations may also need inspection.

A salon need not be expensive to put together, but you should remember that furniture and fittings will need to last approximately ten years so buy quality products which should last longer and wear better. Although the salon should look attractive, the essential thing is that it should be functional. Remember, in hairdressing, the name of the game is beautiful people, not beautiful salons. The adage that kitchens should be designed by the people who are to work in them is also true of hairdressing salons. They should be designed by the hairdressers who have to work in them, with professional assistance.

There are pitfalls if you decide to design the salon without assistance. Interior planners or designers will be guided by the information you give them and they will ask how the salon operates, what services it offers and what furniture and fittings it needs. The salon should be designed for the quietest times as a large salon does not necessarily mean large profit. Nor does increasing the salon size necessarily increase the profit. It is better to concentrate on how well you do (your profitability) rather than how good you look. Use all available salon space; each part of the salon area should justify its share of the rent. There is no point in taking up salon space that does not contribute toward the profits.

To be effective and attractive, salon planning will need to take the following factors into account: lighting, client flow, reception area, furniture, washbasins, surfaces and flooring, placing of staff room, windows, colour, features, heating and ventilation and mirrors.

Lighting

Lights attract not only moths, but people! Lighting is one of the most important features of the salon. It is best, therefore, not to cut costs in getting the right lighting. Don't underestimate what correct lighting can do for the salon. Clients may even think that the hairdressing is better because of the atmosphere created by the lighting. Lighting requirements are outlined in the Health Regulations.

Both fluorescent and incandescent lighting will be needed in the salon. Fluorescent lighting is needed for lighting for the top of the hairstyle and incandescent lighting is needed to put light on the side of the head, at an angle. This enables the hairdresser to assess volume and movement.

Fluorescent lighting should be put continuously along the ceiling and in double strips on both sides of the salon.

Incandescent lights (spotlights) will need to be high at both ends of the salon, directed at the working area. The reception area will also need to be adequately lit, with both fluorescent and incandescent lighting; clients can be drawn to a salon with a well-lit reception area.

Keep all the lights on as, in part, the electricity bill is part of the advertising budget. Good lighting is an investment, not an expense.

Natural light through the salon windows is the best type of lighting for colour work. If natural light is not available, then suitable artificial light will need to be selected.

Fluorescent lighting

Fluorescent lamps produce light by converting ultraviolet rays from a phosphor powder coating. They give approximately four times more light than incandescent lights; that is, a 40-watt fluorescent tube will give the same light as a 150-watt lamp. Fluorescent lights last about seven times longer than incandescent lamps, generate less heat and distribute the light more evenly. If they grow dim, blacken or flicker, replace them, because they rarely fail like an incandescent light.

Get to know the range of colour that the tubes come in. A warm white delux is best for most colours. Similar to an incandescent light, it bathes the salon in a warm glow. If you put make-up on in this light it looks fine, as will the client's complexion. Some tubes, however, have a blue light which affects complexions and hair colour and can alter the client's appearance quite dramatically when they are in natural light. A fitting which diffuses the light will ensure that all horizontal and vertical surfaces are well lit. This diffuser produces glare-free light.

Incandescent lighting

The general lamp has a coil of tungsten wire in the centre of the glass bulb. It glows white-hot and is designed to last approximately 1000 hours. The bulbs are either clear, crystal or silicon-coated (these look white when unlit), but there is little difference in the light output through these finishes. Because it omits all the colour from the spectrum, the light from an incandescent bulb looks white. Incandescent light tends to give off warmish tones and blue colours appear darker. Bulb sizes are standardised and 40, 60, 75 and 100 watts are usual for hairdressing salons.

Incandescent lighting can be:

1 *refracted* – crystal glassware to 'sparkle' the light;
2 *shielded reflection* – part of the bulb coated to direct the light (usually down);
3 *diffused* – glare-free glow.

Client flow

Client flow refers to the movement of the client in and around the salon. The amount of walking the client does should be kept to a minimum. Walkways should be straight with clear movement and need to be at least 1.5 m wide. Otherwise muscle fatigue can result from continually twisting around objects.

Reception

The reception area is where the client first makes contact with the salon and it can be responsible for the image the salon projects. Make sure you create an environment in which the client feels comfortable, and not tense. Ensure that the reception area is clean, warm and attractive. Use lighting and keep the door open.

As space is usually at a premium in salons, the reception and waiting area should not be too large. Too many chairs, lamps, desks and magazine racks can give the client the initial impression that you are selling furniture instead of hairdressing! Keep furniture to the minimum. The reception desk, should, if possible, be placed against a wall, as it can otherwise seem like a barrier, especially with its chair. It should be big enough only to accommodate the appointment book, the till, the telephone, and, if necessary, the salon computer, and to allow space for the client to sign a cheque or credit voucher. Chairs in the waiting area can also be reduced to make way for retail stock, take-home hair care and stock display stands.

Furniture

Chairs must be comfortable, practical and suited to hairdressing services. Try to avoid a dining room or outdoor chair image. Although such chairs may look good, they are not always functional. Select one which is adjustable in height and which can swivel (so that you can check clients' profiles). A place at the back of the chair to keep the salon gown can be useful, although there should be nothing to impede the stylist's movements around the chair, and no edges which may protrude and injure the client. Furniture should look elegant but be practically designed and well made.

Chairs take up a lot of salon space. Do a chair-space exercise. Place a chair in front of a mirror as you would in the service area. Place a piece of paper where the stylist would stand. Place another piece of paper where the client's feet will be (the lower the chair, the more spread out the feet). Now draw an arc. You will see that plenty of space is needed, especially if a 1.5 m passageway is added behind the stylist.

Other salon furniture should be kept to a minimum as it is cheaper to use wall space than centre space, which may not work quite as well. The correct positioning of chairs is outlined in the Health Regulations.

Washbasins for shampooing

Avoid doing shampoo work, colouring and permanent waving near the window. It is also better to place shampoo areas out of view of the reception area as the sight of legs and feet can embarrass clients entering the salon. Side washbasins against the wall take up less room than centre-floor basins. A tilt-back or slant chair is most comfortable for the client. Requirements for washbasins are discussed in the Health Regulations.

Surfaces and coverings

Choose materials carefully so that they will look stylish, but still be hard-wearing. Vinyl surfaces are fine as they are easily kept clean by wiping. Tiled floors are hard to work on. A good quality vinyl resistant to staining is ideal. A light mottled colour effect can hide any stubborn staining and markings. Carpet in the reception areas creates a feeling of warmth. Requirements for surfaces and coverings are further outlined in the Health Regulations.

Mirrors can create the image of depth and light, and most customers like to see themselves after having had their hair styled. Salon decor should be changed every five years or so, to add interest. Wallpaper and paint is cheaper than permanent materials.

Staff room and office

This should be near the reception area so that you can keep a constant eye on the salon entrance. Having the staffroom here will also give the effect of movement and a busy environment around the waiting area.

If the staff room is made too large and comfortable, staff will want to spend too much time there. It should just be adequate for the staff's needs: having a staff room is a requirement of the Health Regulations.

If it is necessary to have an office, it should be small, with room for a desk, two chairs and a filing cabinet. It should be put in a place from where the whole salon can be observed.

Figure 17.2

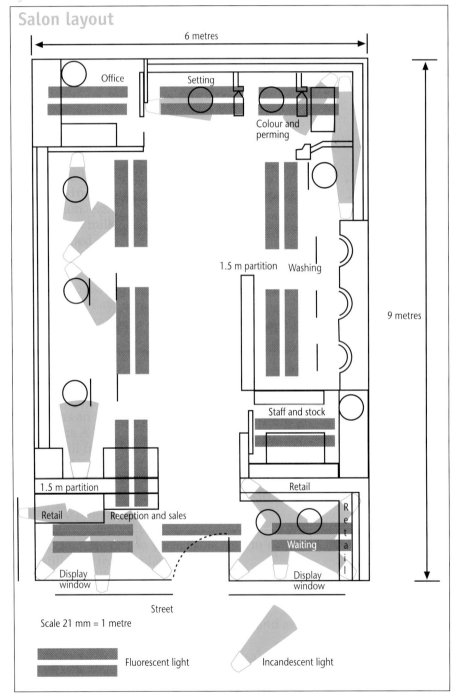

Salon layout

Windows

It is wise to have windows that allow a clear view of the inside of the salon from the outside. Although clients generally feel uncomfortable if they are seated in full public view, a side-on view is acceptable. A good view of the salon lets the passing public know what you are selling. Take care that the window is not cluttered with advertising material.

Colour

Colour choice tends to be personal but there are certain colours that will:
1 enhance the salon's image;
2 express a particular feeling.

Reds, for example, give the impression of a busy environment, while white is clean. Dark colours are solid while pastels are soft. Golds gives the impression of wealth.

Painting a wall or ceiling in the salon can bring it forward or make it appear deeper, depending on whether it is dark or light. Colours should attract and relax the client and for this purpose, warm colours are best, as they create an inviting atmosphere. Try and give your salon a feeling of warmth. Reds tend to draw the attention and say something about the salon.

Wallpapers should not have big patterns as these can dominate the salon. Select something more unobtrusive which is less noticeable. Art galleries cover their walls with a bland wall covering so that it will not detract from the displays.

You can include a special feature in your salon if you wish to do so.

Heating and ventilation

Salons do tend to get hot, especially in summer. If your salon is in an arcade or a new building, there may be air conditioning. A comfortable working temperature is around 17 °C in summer and 22 °C in winter. Bear in mind all the appliances that give off heat, including the steam from the hot water. This can make conditions uncomfortable for clients and extremely tiring for staff. Clients may wilt at the thought of a stuffy salon visit during summer, so ensure that the salon has a welcome cool and airy feeling (even though the colouring may be warm).

It may be difficult to supply adequate fresh air for the salon. You must consider a carefully balanced ventilation flow when laying out the salon. In arcades and malls there may, for aesthetic reasons, be restrictions on cutting into windows and shop fronts to install ventilating and extracting fans. Provisions for adequate ventilation are further outlined in the Health Regulations. A ceiling fan whirring around is effective and also has a psychologically cooling effect. In winter, a ceiling fan can also push warm air back down into the salon where warmth is needed.

Mirrors

Mirrors are essential fixtures in the hairdressing salon. They should be large enough for the client and stylist to see the total look of the hairstyle.

Mirrors are made of polished glass which is coated with a reflecting layer of silver metal or an amalgam of alloy mercury. Mirrors should be of good quality so that the surface won't flake off.

Mirrors can give an illusion of space in the salon, rather like the effect created when you use a light colour of paint on a wall. Two or more mirrors can be used to create a number of images. This type of arrangement can also be used to display articles at reception. It can also be used for wall mirrors to give the salon a feeling of depth.

It is a good idea to have mirrors which can tilt, especially in the colouring and perming area. These have the advantage that the clients cannot see themselves during the process. It is a good idea to have a large mirror at reception for the clients to arrange their hats, scarves or coats and to admire their new hairstyles.

The plan illustration on p. 302 is a good example of standard salon design.

Questions

1   Discuss the advantages and disadvantages of starting business as:
    a   a sole trader;

    b   a partnership; or

    c   a limited company.

2   If you saw a salon advertised for sale as a 'going concern' and 'walk-in walk-out', list and discuss what information you would require to establish if the business was a viable proposition.

3   **a**   Explain the conditions that are usually applicable when renting premises.

    b   How does goodwill affect the purchase of an existing salon?

4   **a**   Financing a salon can be done by borrowing money. Name three types of loan and explain the differences in their terms.

b If you required a loan, what steps should you take to present your case?

_____

_____

_____

5 Name three types of insurance cover suited to a salon and outline the type of cover each will offer.

_____

_____

6 Explain the procedure a salon owner would follow to pay the staff's PAYE deductions to the Inland Revenue Department:

a for the weekly wage; and

_____

_____

b for the annual deductions.

_____

_____

7 Explain the salon owner's responsibilities in paying provisional tax.

_____

_____

_____

8 **a** Discuss how the Employment Contracts Act affects you as a salon owner.

_____

_____

_____

b What is meant by personal grievance?

_____

_____

c What committee deals with complaints or breaches of employment contracts?

_____

_____

9 Outline the advantages of and some points to consider about franchising.

_____

_____

_____

10 If you pay a senior stylist $400 a week, calculate:

    a the true weekly cost of employing the stylist;

_____

_____

_____

    b the hourly rate of pay for

_____

       i 40 hours;

_____

      ii 30 productive hours;

_____

    c What weekly takings would this stylist have to earn to be a viable operator?

_____

_____

11 A client with long hair has had a permanent wave. The stylist has worked for approximately 2.5 hours with the client and the junior apprentice for 30 minutes, a total of 3 hours in all. The stylist's productive hourly rate is $12 and the apprentice's is $4. Working on the assumption that the wages make up 40% of the cost, and profit is 20% , calculate:

    a the final price that the client is to be charged for the permanent wave; and

_____

    b the net profit before tax.

_____

12 Calculate the total sales needed for a salon (with fixed costs of $15 000 per annum and variable costs at 60% of sales) to break even.

_____

_____

13 Explain the purpose of:

    a a balance sheet; and

_____

_____

b a profit-and-loss statement.

_____

_____

14 Outline the benefits of preparing a cash budget or cash flow forecast for the salon.

_____

_____

15 Using the following figures, prepare a cash budget for the next six weeks to establish the closing bank balance at the end of this period.

Cash sales: $1200 per week for 4 weeks; $2 000 for 2 weeks

Retail sales: $180 per week for 4 weeks; $300 for 2 weeks

	$
Wages	300
PAYE	80
Rent	120
Advertising	85
Interest	80
Stock	100
Other expenses	150
Owner's drawings	200
OPENING BALANCE AT BANK	**$3 000**

16 How should you reconcile your bank statement?

_____

_____

_____

17 In a 6 x 10 cm column, using colour, lay out an advertisement poster, offering a new salon service.

18 a Name two qualities of a good salon manager.

_____

_____

b List five areas for which a manager is responsible.

_____

_____

_____

c Who is accountable for meeting the salon's legal requirements?

_____

19 List and discuss five ways in which the salon manager can get the best possible results from staff.

_____

_____

_____

20 How does the ACC affect you as:

a an employee?

_____

_____

b an employer?

_____

21 a What are the advantages and disadvantages of using (i) fluorescent and (ii) incandescent lights?

_____

_____

_____

b Explain why lighting should be an important part of salon design.

_____

_____

_____

22 Describe how the colour of the salon decor can reflect the salon's image.

_____

_____

_____

23 a What is a comfortable working temperature in the salon during (i) summer and (ii) winter?

_____

b Name two ways in which the salon's temperature can be kept at a comfortable level.

_____

_____

24 Outline how a salon can be made to appear larger than it actually is.

_____

_____

_____

25 Draw a floor plan of a salon, incorporating:

a two washbasins; **b** five styling areas;
c a staff room and office; **d** a reception area;
e a retail stand; **f** lighting;
g a front window.

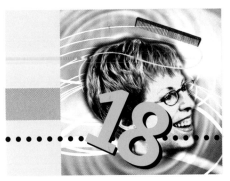

Final practical assessments

Guidelines for:

- applying hairdressing services under workplace conditions;
- performing hairdressing services in a commercial salon.

Apply hairdressing services under workplace conditions

The purpose of this practical assessment is to observe a demonstration of a variety of hairdressing skills/services in your salon. The duration of the assessment is two hours. The assessor will visit your salon to observe the way you handle the services. The services you will be assessed on include:

- client consultation;
- haircuts (scissor or razor);
- permanent wave or permanent colour;
- blow-dries/hair sets.

You will not be expected to complete these services in the two hours of the assessment, nor will you be assessed on how well you permanently wind the hair. The assessor will be observing from a distance how well you cope in the salon. Remember, you have passed all your units as a prerequisite to this assessment, so you are competent in your skills. The assessor will not check your work, but may ask you or your client questions relating to salon procedures. Key areas include:

- personal presentation;
- planning;
- professional approach and attitude;
- services meet consultation;
- telephone manner;
- reception duties;
- home hair-care recommendation;
- closing a sale;
- client comfort.

The assessor should make you feel relaxed during this assessment and will notify you of the outcome during the feedback at the end of the two hours.

Further, the assessment requires performing hairdressing services to meet the commercial requirements of a hairdressing salon. The purpose is to assess the candidate over at least a four-week period while he/she is performing hairdressing services in a commercial salon where he/she is currently employed.

The practical assessment consists of two parts: evidence is collected over four consecutive weeks and sent to the assessor for evaluation; and the second part is a two-hour visit to observe the candidate's performance in the salon.

The analysis of in-salon client services includes:

- the number of clients serviced per week.
- average number of clients per week;
- chemical services average;
- retail sales (if salon sells retail);
- corrective services.

Observation process covers:

- a pre-assessment meeting;
- assessment;
- post-assessment meeting (feedback).

During the assessment process, the assessor will want to observe two hairdressing services during a one hour session (it is not necessary that you complete these services in this time).

It is important to understand that the assessors are there to observe the way the services are handled – i.e. whether this is done in a professional manner – rather than the salon's operations. Assessors are there to assess how services are handled in the salon by the candidate. The assessors will not check the quality of the work itself but merely observe the services performed.

The assessors' observations will monitor:

- planning and time management;
- verbal communications;
- personal presentation;
- closing sales;
- client comfort;
- hair-care advice;
- service outcomes.

Guidelines which update requirements are available for this assessment. Ask you regional co-ordinator or employer for more information. As there is commercial sensitivity in an assessor coming into a salon to observe services on paying clients, managers, employers and the candidate can be assured of confidentiality and discretion during this assessment.

Perform hairdressing services in a commercial salon

At the end of your training you will sit a seven-hour practical assessment. It is important that you should be well prepared. The assessment consists of a series of exercises to test your competency in the following:

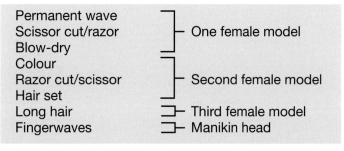

Permanent wave	
Scissor cut/razor	One female model
Blow-dry	
Colour	
Razor cut/scissor	Second female model
Hair set	
Long hair	Third female model
Fingerwaves	Manikin head

The permanent wave, scissor/razor cut and blow-wave exercises are of three-hour duration and you will be assessed on:

- consultation;
- perm service;
- fashion scissor cut or razor cut;
- fashion blow-wave;
- home hair-care advice;
- health regulations;
- service completed in time.

The colour, cut and set exercises are of three-and-a-half hours' duration and you will be assessed on:

- consultation;
- multi-shading;
- fashion cut – scissor cut or razor cut;
- fashion set;
- home hair-care advice;
- record of service;
- health regulations;
- service completed in time.

The long-hair exercise will be for one hour and will be assessed on:

- consultation;
- styling the long hair;
- home hair-care advice;
- record of service;
- timing.

The finger-waving exercise will be for 30 minutes and will be assessed on:

- finger waving;
- pincurls;
- timing.

You must demonstrate competency in all exercises. As the assessment day is yours, it is important that you have the final say as to what you do with your model's hair. Flair and artistry will be assessed. See that your models know where to go and won't get lost, and ask them to arrive well before the assessment begins.

The assessment: key points

Present yourself to your assessor in a smart, well-groomed and professional manner. Be polite. Make sure all your equipment is clean and well presented. You will need to bring all tools, materials and equipment with you. Make a comprehensive list during the preceding week so that you don't forget anything. Always comply with the Health Department Regulations.

Permanent wave

- Consultation.
- Fashion wave.
- Directional wind.
- 75% of hair to be permanently waved.
- Follow manufacturer's instructions.
- Home hair-care advice.

Scissor cut

- Correct cutting angles.
- Remove 3 cm minimum.
- Style suitability.
- Timing (30 minutes, at time of writing).
- Outcome.

Fashion blow-wave

- Correct use and control of brushes.
- Movement – volume (complex).
- Outcome.

Colour

- Allergy test.
- Correct selection.
- Multi-shading (roots to ends).
- Correct developer.
- Correct measuring.
- Developed according to instructions.
- Removal of colour.
- Outcome (result of colour).

Razor cut

- Cutting angles.
- Remove 3 cm minimum.
- Timing (30 minutes, at time of writing).
- Outcome.

Fashion hair set

- Directional pli (complex).
- Full head including pincurls.
- Movement and control.
- Fully dried.
- Outcome.

Long hair – an evening or wedding style

- Styling products and accessories.
- Control of hair.
- Firmly secured.
- 75% of hair up.
- Finish.
- Outcome.
- Timing (1 hour, at time of writing).

Finger waves (manikin)

- Evenness.
- Wave joining.
- Side parting.
- Pincurls (10).
- Full head required.
- Timing (30 minutes, at time of writing).

A solid, confident approach and well-executed exercises should bring you a good result. Your assessor will give feedback and notify you of the outcome at the end of the day.

Note

Requirements for these assessments may change periodically. The information given here is accurate at the time of writing and is to be used as a guide only. You will be fully informed of the latest, updated requirements prior to assessment. Contact your ITO Regional Co-ordinator who will give all the information necessary.

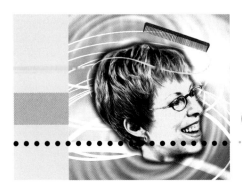

Glossary

A-helix A protein coil of outstanding strength and stability.

A-keratin The substance of human hair. *See* Alpha-keratin.

Accelerator That which increases the speed.

Accident Compensation Corporation A corporation set up by the government to give financial compensation after an accident.

Account Statement of money, reckoning of money paid and received, goods bought where payment is postponed.

Acetic acid Substance such as vinegar, diluted and used as a hair rinse.

Acid hair rinse Weak solution in water of either citric/acetic acid.

Acid mantle An acid covering on the skin formed from the secretion of oil and excretion of perspiration which form an emulsion.

Acid side chain An amino acid with an extra carboxyl group.

Acidic A corrosive substance with a sour taste and a pH of less than seven. A solution with more hydrogen ions than hydroxide ions.

Acne A skin problem.

Activated texture A rough surface texture where the hair ends are visible.

Adhere Stick.

Adornment Decoration.

Adsorb To take in a liquid by concentration on a surface.

Advertising Publicity, making known, public announcement.

After-rinse A preparation used as a rinse after hair treatment, the rinsing of the hair after treatment.

Aftershave A deodorised lotion used on the face after shaving.

Albino A person who has no colour pigment in their hair or skin.

Alcohol Class of organic compounds derived from the hydrocarbons.

Alkaline A substance which neutralises acids. Has pH of more than seven.

Allergy Sensitivity to a substance, e.g. metal, animal or hair product.

Alopecia Loss of hair.

Alopecia areata Loss of hair in areas or patches.

Alopecia post-partum Loss of hair by the mother soon after birth.

Alopecia senalis Loss of hair in old age.

Alopecia totalis Loss of hair on the scalp.

Alopecia universalis Loss of hair of the scalp and body.

Alpha-keratin The hair fibre in its natural unstretched state. *See* A-keratin.

Alum An astringent.

Amino acids Organic compounds in the breakdown of proteins – the body's building blocks.

Amino group The characteristic group to which nearly all acids belong.

Ammonia NH_3 – A pungent colourless alkaline gas, insoluble in water.

Ammonium hydroxide A colourless, pungent alkali liquid.

Ammonium thioglycollate A chemical used in permanent wave lotions and straighteners to open the cuticle and break the sulphur links.

Anagen The growing stage of the hair life cycle.

Analine derivative A colourless liquid obtained from coal tar.

Analyses To distinguish the main points, examine.

Androgen Male sex hormone.

Angle Measured in degrees, space between two intersecting lines.

Angora Long-haired (usually white) variety of rabbit or goat.

Animal protein Protein – amino acids – obtained from animals, e.g. chicken, beef, lamb, liver, dairy products.

Anionic Negatively charged ion.

Anodised To coat metal with its oxide by electrolysis.

Anterior Front end.

Anti-clockwise In the opposite direction to the hands of clock.

Antiperspirant A substance which acts against perspiration.

Antiseptic A substance that will prevent the growth of bacteria.

Antistatic Against static electricity in the hair.

Aponeurosis Attachment of muscle.

Apollo knot Hair looped, plaited or coiled on top of the head, fashionable in the early nineteenth century.

Appointment An agreement fixing the time and place.

Apprentice A person learning a trade who is bound to serve the employer for a set number of years in exchange for instruction.

Apprenticeship The state of being an apprentice.

Apprenticeship award Conditions of service and payment of wages.

Apprenticeship order List of provisions in employing apprentices, agreed upon by the industry and the Shop Employers Association.

Arrector-pili The involuntary muscle attached to the hair follicle.

Arteries Major blood vessels carrying oxygenated blood from the heart.

Arteriols Fine capillaries supplying arteries oxygenated blood.

Ash A matt, cendre colour reflect – green or blue. A shade that has no red or yellow tones.

Assets Valuable possessions which add value.

Astringent Having the effect of contracting skin tissue.

Atoms Smallest portion of an element which can take part in a chemical reaction; a minute particle.

Auricular Of the ear.

Azo dyes A type of temporary colour containing nothing organic.

B-helix The stretched form of the protein coil.

B-keratin The stretched form of the protein of human hair. *See* Beta-keratin.

Bacilli Rod-shaped bacteria which cause flu.

Back-combing Combing the short hairs of the strand toward the scalp to form a cushion of support.

Bacteria Microscopic organisms, germs.

Balance Equilibrium.

Balance sheet Statement showing financial position.

Bald Part or the whole scalp hairless.

Bandrowski base A possible formation resulting from the action of hydrogen peroxide and para phenylene diamine.

Barber/surgeon A term used in the fifteenth century (medieval times) when the barber also acted as minor surgeon and dentist.

Barrel curl A curl clipped in a stand-up position with a uniform depth around the curl.

Barrier cream A Vaseline-type cream used to prevent chemicals burning or harming the skin.

Basal A layer of cells at the base of the epidermis, closest to the dermis.

Base Foundation, anything acting as a support, a starting point.

Base *See* Basic.

Base part A parting taken against the scalp, especially when cutting.

Basic alkaline A pH of above seven. A solution with more hydroxide ions than hydrogen ions.

Basic side chain The amino acid with an extra amino group.

Beige Yellowish-grey colour.

Benzines Liquids distilled from crude petroleum.

Beta-keratin The stretched state of the molecular structure. *See* B-keratin.

Bigode (bigoudi) A carrot-shaped stick used for curling hair.

Bind The outer edge of a wig.

Blanching Sudden greying (whitening) of the hair.

Bland Mild.

Bleaching Removing the natural pigmentation.

Bleaching Lightening the hair.

Blemish A flaw of the skin.

Block A practice manikin.

Block points Thin, headless nails approximately 1 cm long used to tack galloon etc., in position on a wooden block.

Blunt cut Club cut, cutting the hair straight across.

Blusher A cosmetic which gives a pink or rosy colour.

Boardwork The making of postiche.

Bob A level haircut above the shoulders.

Bracing (1) Done to hold the foundation of the wig in place. (2) The position of the cotton or silk thread from the galloon at the point where the block point holds it to another block point.

Break-even point The point where no profit or loss is incurred.

Bridging finance A short-term loan.

Brochure Booklet or pamphlet.

Budget A provision for estimated costs.

Buffer A solution the acidity or alkalinity of which is practically unchanged by dilution.

Building blocks A phrase describing the amino acids which make up the protein molecule.

Bulbous Like a bulb.

Bulk Volume, body.

Business interruption Loss of profits.

Butane Gas propellant used in pressurised cans.

Cache peigne A hidden comb.

Calcium A chemical element, the metallic basis of lime, found in hard water.

Callus A hardening of the skin through friction.

Canities Loss of pigment in growing hair.

Capillaries Small blood vessels connecting the arteries and veins.

Capital Financial contribution to start a business.

Capitis Pertaining to the head.

Carbohydrate An organic compound composed of carbon, hydrogen and oxygen: starches, sugars and fibrous food.

Carbon Non-metallic element – the major element found in keratin.

Carboxyl The characteristic group to which nearly all acids belong.

Carotid The chief artery found in the neck.

Cash and carry Where cash is paid and the goods carried away.

Cash flow Ready money.

Casual client A client who does not have an appointment.

Catagen A state of the hair during its replacement cycle – clubbed hair in the follicle.

Cation Positively charged ion.

Caul net The net of a wig, usually on the crown, with a soft open weave.

Caustic potash Potassium hydroxide – used in the making of some soaps.

Caustic soda Sodium hydroxide – used in some hair straighteners.

Cellulose A raw material used in plastics and obtained from plant cells.

Cendre A matt, ash colour reflect – blue or green.

Character Distinguishing quality, distinctive colour.

Characteristics Distinguishing features, qualities pertaining to the hair.

Chemical damage Damage to the hair fibre through the overuse of chemicals such as permanent waves, colour, hydrogen peroxide, ammonia.

Cheque A written order directing a bank to pay money as stated.

Chequebook A book of blank cheques with counterfoils.

Chignon A large bunch or coil of hair worn at the back of the head or the nape of the neck, often dressed over a pad.

Chlorine Greenish-yellow chemical used in swimming pools, bleaching powder and disinfectants.

Chlorofluorocarbons Chlorinated propellant released from aerosols said to adversely effect ozone layer in the earth's atmosphere.

Cholesterol White waxy substance present in human tissue.

Circlet Circular band especially of gold, often bejewelled, worn on the head.

Circumference The distance around a circle.

Citric acid Diluted with water, citric acid such as lemon juice is used as an after-rinse.

Classical Pertaining to Greek or Roman in style.

Clientele Customers.

Clockwise In the same direction as the hands of a clock.

Club cutting Blunt cutting the hair straight across.

Coal tar A thick black oily liquid obtained in coal manufacture.

Cohesive A holding force between molecules.

Coiffure A hairstyle.

Cold wave Curling the hair by means of chemicals, without the application of heat.

Collodion A clear syrupy liquid of alcohol used to cover a patch test when testing the client's reaction to tint.

Colour bath A diluted permanent colour formula, e.g. half a tube of colour, 30 cc of H_2O_2 and shampoo.

Colour filler A formula, e.g. a rinse, used to prepigmentate light hair when colouring back to a darker colour.

Colour reduction The removal of tint by chemical strippers which reduce the molecule size.

Colour rinse A semipermanent or temporary rinse which stains the cuticle.

Colour stripping Removing artificial colour by bleaching or using chemical colour strippers.

Colour test A method of determining the action of a colour on a small strand of hair.

Column A list of clients in the appointment book for the stylist.

Comb-out Second pli – dressing the hair with brush or comb into desired style.

Combings Hair collected from the brush or comb and used in boardwork.

Commission A percentage taken in payment.

Communication The flow of information.

Competition Contest for a prize, test of skill.

Complementary colour Colours displaying maximum contrast, e.g. green and red (when mixed produce brown).

Complexion Natural colouring of the face.

Compound Chemically united element; something made of various parts.

Compound henna Egyptian henna with added metallic salts. *See* Henna.

Concave Hollowed, curved inwards.

Conciliation The settlement of labour disputes.

Concretion A knotted mass of hair.

Conditioners Creams, waxes and oils which help protect and maintain the health and condition of the hair.

Confidence Lack of fear, assurance, self-reliance.

Conical In the shape of a cone.

Consultation Seeking information, taking into consideration, asking advice.

Contagious Communicated by contact or indirect contact, capable of spreading disease.

Contour winding A loose wave, winding the perm rods to the contour of the head shape.

Convex Curved outward.

Corneum The top horny layer of the epidermis.

Corporis Of the body.

Cortex Forms the inner structure of the hair fibre.

Cortical fibrils Fibrous second layer of the hair shaft.

Cosmetic A preparation applied to enhance the skin.

Counter (colour) In opposition, e.g. red and green.

Cover note An insurance protection while details are finalised.

Cowlick A tuft of hair on the forehead which will not lie flat.

Cranium The skull.

Cream shampoo Any shampoo that has a creamy consistency.

Cream tint A tint which is of a creamy consistency and is presented in tubes.

Credit Right-hand side of an account – sum of money coming in.

Credit card A card which promises payment at a later date.

Credit note Acknowledgment of credit.

Creditor One to whom money is owed.

Crêpe hair Hair that has been permanently kinked by means of weaving on two strings and boiling.

Crest The top position of a wave.

Crest line The widest point of the head. A line that divides the interior from the exterior of the head.

Croquignole Winding the hair from ends to roots.

Current assets Transferable into cash within one month.

Cuticle The outer layer of the hair; the hard skin at the base of the fingernail.

Cylinder Rectangle rotating around one side as an axis.

Cysteic acid Formed when overoxidation (neutralising) occurs which affects rebonding.

Cysteine An amino acid found in the hair constituting less than 1% of the protein.

Cystine An amino acid found in the hair constituting approximately 17% of the protein.

Dandruff Excess accumulation of dead skin cells on the scalp.

Day book A book to record the day's takings and retail sales.

Debenture Certificate that a sum of money is owing to a specific person.

Debit Left-hand side of an account – sum of money owing; charge.

Debtor One who owes you money.

Decomposition Process of disintegration, breaking up. A test to establish if there is any metallic covering on the hairshaft – 1–20 test.

Degree A position or stage in a scale or series.

Demarcation A line caused by overlapping tint retouches.

Demonstration A practical lesson.

Denman Trade name.

Density The number of follicles per square centimetre.

Deodorant A substance which destroys or lessens offensive smells.

Depilatory Hair remover.

Deportment Salon behaviour, the way you conduct yourself in the salon.

Depreciation Reduction in value through wear and tear on property.

Depth Intensity, deepness, level.

Derivative Something originating from another.

Dermal papilla (1) The area concerned with the hairs' nourishment. (2) A collection of capillaries found in a cone-shaped elevation off the base of the hair root.

Dermatitis Inflammation of the skin.

Dermis A layer of skin found below the epidermis.

Design A plan or arrangement of a hairstyle.

Design element One of three components: shape; texture; structure, which make up a hair cut.

Design line The line which makes up the artistic shape.

Detergent A cleansing agent which, with the addition of water, removes grease, e.g. soap or soapless shampoo.

Di-sulphide The combination of two sulphur atoms.

Diameter A straight line passing through the centre of a circle.

Diamond mesh An arrangement of weft (including a fine wire) in a diamond-shaped pattern with a cache peigne.

Diet Prescribed course of food.

Diffuser An attachment on a blow-dryer that 'shatters' the flow of air so that the hair can be soft-styled.

Dilute Thin down a fluid by adding another fluid.

Direct winding Winding a permanent wave with solution.

Directional A point toward which movement goes.

Directional winding Winding the perm rods according to the finished style.

Disinfectant Destroys or renders germs harmless.

Distilled water Pure water containing no metallic salts, e.g. rain water.

Docket A document summarising sales details.

Double application Two applications in tinting to overcome resistance. The first application of tint is applied to the resistant areas without H_2O_2, then again with the H_2O_2.

Double crown A head of hair with two natural crowns.

Doughnut bun (donut) A small round chignon with a hole in the centre.

Doughnut pad A round pad.

Drab A colour with no red or yellow.

Drabbing A process whereby light coloured hair is toned down.

Draize test A test used on rabbits to determine whether shampoos irritate the eye.

Drawing brushes Brushes used to hold the hair when weaving.

Drawing mats Mats used to hold the hair when weaving.

Drawn-through parting On a hair-piece, wig or toupee, a parting constructed where the knotted hair is drawn through another piece of netting (silk) to give a natural appearance and hide the knotting.

Duct A tube in the skin for conveying fluid.

Dye To colour or stain the hair with tint.

Effilate To taper the hair.

Effleurage A stroking movement in massage.

Egyptian henna Egyptian privet. *See* Henna.

Elasticity The ability of the hair to stretch and return to its original form without breaking.

Element Substance consisting entirely of atoms of the same atomic number.

Elevating Level of point, act of raising, state of being raised.

Emphasise To bring out a particular idea, to heighten.

Emulsifying agent A substance used to form an emulsion, e.g. shampoo.

Emulsion A milky liquid with oily, insoluble particles suspended in it, e.g. oil in water.

End bonds *See* Peptide bonds.

End paper A small paper tissue used at the end of a strand of hair to assist with the winding of the perm rod.

Endocuticle Layer of individual cuticle cells of low sulphur keratin protein.

Endorsement Approval or confirmation.

Enhance To heighten or increase awareness.

Environment Surrounding, external condition in which a person or organism lives.

Enzymes Organic substances produced by living cells used as an aid in digestion.

Epicranius A large sheath of muscle covering the top of the skull from the occipital to the frontal.

Epidermal cyst A sac containing fluid (sebum) on the outer layer of skin.

Epidermis The top outside layer of the skin.

Epilate To pull out the hair.

Equity Capital invested in a business.

Essence A perfume in concentrated form obtained by distillation from a plant.

Essential oil Oil from plants, flowers, leaves, wood, etc., soluble in alcohol.

Ethanol Ethyl alcohol.

Ethics Rules of conduct toward the client and associates in accordance with moral code.

Ethmoid A bone forming part of the nasal cavity.

Etiquette Rules of polite behaviour.

Eugene A permanent wave system, named after its inventor, Eugene Suter.

Eumelanin One of two types of colour pigment found in the hair – blackish/brown.

Excess An extra charge, a sum of money which is paid if an insurance claim is made.

Excretion Waste matter from the body.

Exocuticle Individual cuticle cells with a high sulphur content.

Exothermic Self-heating chemical action.

Exterior The part of the head where the hair falls free from the head due to a gravitational pull below the crest line.

Fantasy colour A colour not found in natural hair, e.g. green, blue.

Fashion The prevailing mode, custom or taste, the latest style.

Fat Greasy substance in animal bodies.

Fibre A fine strand. A form of carbohydrate producing roughage.

Fibrils Small thread-like fibres.

Fillet A head bank or net used to hold the hair in place.

Fingerwaving Forming 'S' movement in the hair, using the fingers and comb.

Fish hook The double-backed point of a badly wound perm road.

Fixative A substance that fixes the hair in place, e.g. setting lotion, hairspray.

Fixed assets Assets transferable into cash within 12 months.

Florid Complexion with a pinkish cast, ruddy.

Fluorescent A lamp consisting of a cathode ray tube coated with fluorescent material.

Follicle A small well-like depression in the skin in which the hair root is to be found.

Fonz A soft-styler diffuser attachment for a blow-dryer.

Formaldehyde A good disinfectant and preservative.

Formula Prescription mixture.

Foundation net The net of a wig which forms the foundation around the pattern area.

Fractionated protein Protein broken down into small molecular units and effective as a hair conditioner.

Fragilistic crinium Brittle or broken hair.

Franchise Being given the privilege (to sell).

Freon Propellant used in pressurised cans.

Friction A rubbing movement in massage.

Frizette A pad of crêpe hair used as a foundation over which to dress hair.

Frontal In front.

Frosting Fine strands of hair over the entire head which have been lightened.

Fructose Fruit sugar.

Fundamentals Essentials, important foundations.

Fuse (1) To melt. (2) A small piece of wire in an electric circuit which melts when the current exceeds a certain strength.

Galloon A narrow closely woven ribbon, in different colours, used in the foundation of wigs and other postiche.

Gel A transparent, spirit-based jelly-like fixative used on dry or wet hair to sculpt or give a 'wet look'.

Germinal matrix The area of the root bulb where mitosis occurs.

Germinative The innermost layer of the epidermis adjoining the basal layer.

Glucose Granular sugar, purified grape sugar, sweet carbohydrate.

Glycerol Glycerine – a thick syrupy liquid obtained from fats and oils.

Glycerol mono thioglycollate A reducing chemical used in acid permanent waves.

Glycine An amino acid found in hair.

Glycol thioglycollate A reducing chemical used in acid permanent waves.

Goodwill Value of reputation and popularity of a business.

Graduation The grade at which the hair is cut by degrees.

Granulosum The granular layer of the skin.

Green soft soap Soft soap for which vegetable 'oil and alkali are boiled together, saponified.

Gross profit Excess of receipts over expenditure.

Growth pattern The shape that hair tends to grow in, especially at the nape.

GST Goods and services tax. A government tax on goods and services.

Guarantee A formal undertaking that conditions will be carried out; pledge.

Guideline A line to follow when shaping the balance of the hair.

Guidestrand A strand of hair cut to a predetermined length.

Gum tragacanth A gum from a plant used in making some setting lotions.

Hackle A block of wood or metal with closely set sloping teeth used to draw the hair off and disentangle it.

Hair bulb (1) The base of the hair root. (2) That portion of the hair found below the surface of the skin. (3) The root end of the hair which fits the dermal papilla.

Hair conditioner A treatment designed to improve the quality and condition of the hair; contains fats, oils and waxes.

Hair shaft That portion of the hair found above the surface of the skin.

Hair whorl A spiral effect of the hair's growth on the crown.

Hairdresser One whose business is to clean, cut, style, brush, colour, permanent wave, curl, lighten, arrange and dress the hair.

Hairline The outline of the growing hair on the head.

Hairspray A liquid fixative sprayed onto the hair.

Hairstylist A person who designs and dresses the hair.

Halo colouring Colouring the hair around the perimeter of the head.

Hard water A hardness in water caused by calcium and magnesium salts – soap will not lather readily in hard water, but soapless shampoos will.

Harmony A pleasing relationship of balance, proportion and rhythm.

Harsh Hard and rough to the touch.

Heat wave A method of curling the hair by applying heat to hair that has been dampened with a suitable chemical.

Height Elevation.

Henle's layer A layer of inner root sheath composed of clear cells.

Henna The powdered leaf of the *Lawsonia inemis* (Eygptian privet bush) which imparts red tones to the hair.

Henna shampoo A shampoo incorporating a small quantity of Egyptian henna.

Hereditary Of mental and physical characteristics transmitted from parent to offspring.

Herpes Cold sores.

High frequency A machine which causes the atoms and molecules of the skin to vibrate extremely rapidly.

Highlight To make prominent or emphasise with lightener or colour.

Hirsute An excessive unnatural growth of hair in unusual areas of the body, e.g. the backs of men or the faces of women.

Horizontal At right angles to the vertical.

Humidity Moisture in the air.

Huxley's layer A layer of the inner root sheath composed of coarse granular cells.

Hydrogen An element, positively charged atom.

Hydrogen bonds Unstable links or bonds formed between two molecules.

Hydrogen peroxide H_2O_2, a colourless, unstable liquid marketed as a solution in water in concentrations from 3% to 20%. A compound containing hydrogen and oxygen used as an oxidising agent tor tinting, lightening and neutralising.

Hydrolised protein Protein broken down into small molecular units and effective as a hair conditioner

Hydrophilic Having an affinity for water.

Hydrophobic Water repellent, having no affinity for water.

Hydroxometer An instrument for measuring the strength of hydrogen peroxide.

Hygiene Practice of maintaining health sanitation principles, cleanliness.

Hypersensitive Excessively sensitive.

Idiopathic Primary reason.

Imbrication Overlapping scales.

Impetigo A very contagious pustular disease of the skin.

Incandescent State of glowing at a high temperature, white light.

Income statement Profit-and-loss statement.

Incompatability Failure to agree, oppose.

Increasing layer Each layer becoming greater, longer.

Indemnity Insurance against loss, compensation for loss.

Indentation Dent, hollow.

Indirect winding Winding a permanent wave with water instead of solution.

Infection The act of infecting, communication or disease.

Inferior Below.

Infestation Infested, plagued.

Inflamed Swollen, sore, hot.

Inhibit Restrain, prevent from acting.

Intercellular Between cells.

Interior That part of the head where the hair lies that against the head, above the crest area.

Intermediates Artificial colour pigments found in tinting.

Invoice A detailed list, with costs of goods which have been dispatched.

Ion Electrically charged atom or group of atoms.

Jockey A clip to hold the woven weft on a weaving frame to stop it from unravelling.

Journeyperson A qualified hairdresser.

Jugular A large vein of the neck.1

Kanekalon A synthetic fibre used to replace human hair.

Keratin A tough fibrous protein forming hair and nails.

Kilowatt One thousand watts.

Knotting The tying of a small strand of hair to a net or gauze with a hooked needle, can be single or double.

Knotting needle A fine hook used to knot the hair onto netting during the making of postiche.

Lacquer A hard glossy varnish made of shellac.

Lactose Milk sugar.

Lanoline A waxy substance obtained from wool and used in shampoos, conditioners and cosmetics.

Lanugo Hair that is present before and sometimes at birth.

Lawsone The active colouring agent in henna.

Layer To cut hair in layers.

Legumes Seeds, pod fruit, e.g. beans, lentils, peas.

Liabilities Legally assurable sums which one is bound to pay.

Liberate Set free, release, allow gas to escape.

Lift Raise, position higher; upward movement.

Lightener A product used to lighten or brighten the hair.

Lightening Removing the natural pigment or artificial colour from the hair.

Liquid shampoo A shampoo in liquid form, usually clear.

Liquid tint A tint which is of a liquid consistency and presented in bottles.

Liquidity Assets that can readily be converted into cash.

Loading Add extra charge (insurance).

Louis style Any hairstyle worn by the French kings, Louis XIII to Louis XVI.

Loyalty Faithfulness.

Lucidum The less horny layer of skin beneath the corneum found only in the palms and soles of the feet.

Lymph A straw-coloured fluid which supplies the cells with nourishment.

Lysine An amino acid found in hair.

Machine-made wig A wefted wig sewn in spiral patterns.

Macrofibril Seven coiled microfibrils.

Magnesium A light silvery-white mineral found in hard water.

Magnesium carbonate A white powder used with straighteners.

Magnetic roller A roller with a smooth plastic surface.

Male pattern baldness The natural loss of hair by the male caused by genetic traits.

Malleable block A head-shaped block filled with sawdust and covered with canvas.

Maltose Malt sugar.

Manicure Shaping and polishing the nails of the hand.

Manikin A head form on which to practise hairdressing.

Marcel Grateau Inventor of the Marcel wave.

Marketing A planned system of pricing, promoting and distributing goods or services to meet customer needs.

Marteau A postiche made with flat sewn weft and having a loop (or two) at each end.

Mascara A cosmetic for covering the eyelashes.

Massage Treatment in which scalp or body are rubbed or kneaded, usually with the hands.

Masseter A muscle of the face, used for chewing and facial expression.

Matrix The area at the base of the hair root where the hair fibre forms and develops, part of the skin under the nail.

Matrix protein Hard fibrous keratin found in the cuticle.

Matt An ash colour reflect.

Maxilla The upper jawbone.

Maxillary Of the jaw.

McDonald An early discoverer of the permanent wave, especially cold waving.

Mechanical Physical action.

Medicated (of shampoos) Contains antibacterial qualities to help scalp conditions.

Medulla The hollow pith or core of the hair fibre.

Medullated Having a medulla.

Melanin The hair and skin pigment.

Melanocytes Cells producing the colour melanin.

Mentalis A muscle found in the chin, concerned with facial expression.

Merchant's copy The trader's copy (of a credit card voucher).

Merchant summary Details of credit vouchers which are to be banked.

Mesh Small section.

Meta-toluene diamine A chemical used in hair colouring.

Metabolism Rate of energy expenditure at rest.

Metallic dye A dye which incorporates a metallic salt, e.g. silver nitrate.

Method A systematic way of doing a service, an orderly procedure.

Methodical Done systematically, in an ordered way.

Microcomputer A small computer designed for a single user.

Microfibril Coiled protofibrils.

Micrometer An instrument for the accurate measurement of small distances.

Mineral Natural inorganic substance found in the earth, a substance containing metal which is mined.

Mineral oils Liquid hydrocarbons obtained from petroleum.

Mitosis Process by which cells reproduce.

Mohair Hair from the angora goat.

Moisturiser That which replaces water.

Molecule Smallest portion of a substance capable of existing independently.

Mortgage Using property as security for money lent until the loan is repaid.

Motor nerve A nerve that stimulates a muscle, moving part of the body.

Mounting block A head-shaped block made of wood.

Mousse A spirit-based aerosol foam used as a fixative on dry or wet hair.

Movement Moving, motion.

Mulch Spread around using the fingers.

Multi-shading Colouring the hair using two or more colours.

Muscle Tissue through which movement is effected.

Nail bed Part of the skin beneath the visible part of the nail on which it is bedded.

Nail matrix The part of the nail root from which the nail grows.

Nasal Of the nose.

Natural fall The natural fall of the hair due to gravitational pull.

Natural parting The area of scalp where the hair divides naturally.

Natural projection The hair projected at a 90° angle from the curve of the head.

Natural tendency The inclination or development of hair in a certain way, e.g. cowlick, parting, etc.

Naturalising Colouring the hair using the same depth of colour but with different reflects.

Nerves Bundle of fibres transmitting sensory or motor impulses between the brain and the body.

Nessler, Charles The inventor of the permanent wave.

Net profit Excess of receipts when all deductions have been made.

Neutralise To render neutral.

Nevus A mole.

Nevus-pilosus A mole with hair growth.

Niacin Part of the vitamin B complex.

Nitro-amino phenols Chemicals used in semipermanent colour.

Nitrodyes Semipermanent colours with some of the qualities of permanent colour.

Nitrogen Element; main constituent in air.

Non-taxable allowance Allowances not liable to be taxed, e.g. tea money.

Not negotiable That which cannot be transferred.

Nourishment Food.

Nutrient That which nourishes.

Occipital Back part of the head.

Oil lightener An oil preparation using sulphonated oils and mixing these with H_2O_2 and ammonia.

Olive oil Oil processed from olives, used in treatments for the hair.

Opacifiers Chemicals which make a preparation opaque.

Optic Of the eye.

Optical Of the eye.

Orbital Of the eye.

Order form A direction for goods.

Organic Having bodily organs; substances derived from living organisms.

Organic acids Chemical compounds containing carbon.

Organisms Bacteria capable of growth and reproduction.

Osmosis Flow of liquid through a semipermeable membrane.

Outline The outer edge.

Overdirected A roller sitting above its base.

Overdraft Overdrawing an account.

Overlap Overrunning with tint or lightener the area of hair already coloured or lightened.

Oxidation Combining with oxygen.

Oxidation dye A tint that needs oxygen to develop.

Oxygen Element, essential to life.

PAYE 'Pay as you earn' – as applied to taxation.

PVP Polyvinylpyrrolidone.

Packing slip A detailed list of goods or stock.

Pamphlet Short printed booklet.

Pancreas Large intestinal gland secreting digestive enzymes.

Pancreatic juices Juices of the pancreas which aid in digestion.

Papilla A cone-shaped elevation at the base of the follicle, concerned with hair nourishment.

Papillary The outer layer of the dermis.

Para Abbreviated term for para phenylene diamine or para toluene diamine (some people may be allergic to it).

Para phenylene diamine An analine derivative dye producing colour ranging from black to lightest brown, a tint dependent on oxidation.

Para toluene diamine An analine derivative dye used to provide red and black tones; it is dependent on oxidation.

Para-amino-phenol A chemical used in hair colouring.

Paraffin wax Derived from petroleum, a hydrocarbon used in cosmetics, which retards water evaporation from the skin.

Parallel Equivalent to, comparative line, similar.

Parallel graduation Graduation between two parallel lines.

Parasite An animal that lives on the resources of another.

Parietal Bones covering the upper surface of the scalp.

Parting A line along which the hair is divided.

Partnership A sharer in an enterprise, someone who shares in the profits or losses of a business and owns part of the capital.

Pastel shade Soft, delicate pale tone, e.g. beige, silver, champagne, platinum.

Patch test A test on the skin to determine the individual's reaction to chemical preparations such as hair tints.

Pathogenic Causing disease.

Pay-in book A book supplied by the bank which accompanies cheques and cash which are to be paid into the bank.

Pediculosis Head lice.

Pedicure Shaping and painting the nails of the feet.

Peptide bonds (end bonds) The chemical bonds that join the amino acids together to form a chain called a polypeptide.

Percentage Rate per hundred.

Perm Abbreviation for 'permanent wave'.

Permanent Long lasting.

Peroxometer An instrument for measuring the strength of hydrogen peroxide.

Perpendicular At right angles to any plane or line (90° angle).

Personalised Given personal, individual attention.

Perspiration The act of sweating.

Petersham Strong ribbon.

Petrissage A kneading movement in massage.

Petty cash book A book for recording incidental items, small items of expenditure.

pH scale A scale of measuring the hydrogen potential concentration of liquids – i.e. their degree of acidity and alkalinity.

Phaeomelanin One of two types of colour pigment found in the hair – reddish-yellow.

Phosphate Salt of phosphoric acid, used in hydrogen peroxide as a stabilising agent.

Physical damage Damage to the hair fibre through physical actions such as brushing, overheating or stretching.

Physical properties Qualities of the hair perceived by the senses.

Physiology Study of the working function of the body.

Pilar Epidermal cyst.

Pincurl (1) Moulding the hair with fingers and comb into a flat curl secured with a clip or pin. (2) The name given to this flat curl.

Pityriasis Dandruff.

Pityriasis steatoide Greasy dandruff.

Plant Complete set of equipment.

Plasma The fluid part of the blood, rich in nutrients.

Plasticiser A substance used to give a plastic composition.

Platelets Blood cells which assist in clotting the blood.

Platinum Silver-white, the lightest of all blondes.

Pli The setting and dressing of the hair – first pli: setting rollers and pincurls; second pli: dressing out.

Policy Document outlining an undertaking.

Polymer A complex molecule built up from a number of simple molecules of the same kind.

Polypeptide A chain of amino acids linked together.

Polystyrene A plastic material with good insulation.

Pomatum Apple grease – an early hair fixative.

Pompadour roll A large sausage pad of crêpe hair to give height.

Pore A minute opening in the skin.

Porosity The ability of the hair to adsorb moisture or chemicals.

Porosity filler A substance that slows down the adsorption of moisture or chemical into the hair fibre, e.g. conditioner.

Positional springs Flat springs used in a wig or other hairpiece to hold the edge firmly in position against the scalp.

Posterior Behind.

Postiche Added hair.

Post-partum alopecia Loss of hair by the mother at or soon after giving birth.

Potassium hydroxide Caustic potash – a base used in the making of soap.

Precise Exact.

Predisposition Susceptibility.

Preliminary First steps in any preparation.

Premium Annual renewal cost of sum and policy.

Preparation Making someone ready for a service.

Prepigmentation Prior colouring, usually red.

Presoftener A solution or preparation that will make the hair more receptive by softening the cuticle.

Primary (colour) Colours that cannot be produced by mixing others – red, yellow and blue.

Principle General law as a guide to action.

Private limited company A company whose obligations to meet any losses are limited.

Processing Continuous chemical action, especially colouring and permanent waving.

Professional Someone who earns a living by practising a specified art with expert skill.

Profile The side view of the face.

Profit Financial gain.

Profit-and-loss account Statement of performance over a year.

Projection The position the hair is held in relation to the curve of the head.

Promotion Publicising.

Propellant To drive forward by force.

Proportion A comparative relationship in size, relationship of parts.

Proprietor Owner.

Protection Shelter and safeguard.

Protein Complex organic compound of numerous amino acids, such as hair and nails.

Protofibril Three coiled helix chains.

Provisional tax The payment of tax which is not finally settled; payable on 7 September and 7 March of each year.

Psoriasis A skin condition characterised by a reddening of the skin, or silver/yellow crusty scales.

Psychological In or of the mind.

Pull burn Scalp inflammation resulting from excessive tension during winding of a permanent wave.

Quinone diamine Polymer of para diamine.

Reagent Substance used to produce a chemical reaction.

Rebonding Rejoining the lines and bonds on the keratin chains – neutralising.

Receipt Fact of being received.

Receipt book A book which shows written acknowledgement of money or goods received.

Reconciliation The act of settling and adjusting, making compatible.

Record card A card which records details about the client's hair type and service, e.g. the timing of permanent waves and colour formulas – acts as a guide for future reference.

Red corpuscles Blood cells containing haemoglobin which carries oxygen from the lungs to the cells (used for energy production).

Reducing agent A chemical that deprives another of oxygen.

Reduction Reducing, state of being reduced, e.g. the sulphur atoms during permanent waving.

Reflect To throw back light.

Reflection Throwing back light and colour.

Rep Abbreviation for a manufacturer's representative.

Resistant Opposing or withstanding; unaffected by chemical especially a colour; how hard it is for moisture or a chemical to be adsorbed into the hair fibre.

Retail To sell goods in small quantities to the customer.

Reticular The inner layer of the dermis.

Retouch To recolour the regrowth.

Revenue statement Profit-and-loss statement.

Reverse Position in the opposite direction to the present one.

Revitalise Bring back to vitality or durability.

Rhythm Movement in regular occurrences, pattern and distribution of lines.

Riboflavin Part of vitamin B complex.

Ridge line A line that divides surface texture.

Ringworm A vegetable parasite infestation – tinea.

Root and pointing Arranging a bunch of hair so that all the roots are at one end and the points at another.

'S' wave A wave alternating from clockwise to anti-clockwise movement.

Salary Fixed payment for work.

Sales summary A voucher showing details of credit card payments.

Sanitation Public hygiene, prevention of infection through dirt and contagion.

Saturated Containing as much substance as can be adsorbed.

Saw cut Where the teeth of a comb have been cut with a saw rather than press cut.

Scabies A skin disease caused by an animal parasite and characterised by intense itching.

Scrunch Crush.

Sculpture To build up a form.

Scurf Flakes of dead skin, dandruff.

Sebaceous Oil glands of the skin and hair.

Seborrhoea An oily condition caused by an active sebaceous gland producing excess sebun.

Seborrhoea dermatitis A reddened, greasy, scurfy scalp.

Seborrhoea oleosa Greasy surface – especially face and scalp.

Sebum The oily secretion of the sebaceous gland.

Secondary (colours) Colours that are produced by mixing two primaries, e.g. green (blue and yellow); second in order.

Secretion A product produced by the body for the use of the body.

Section Portion, subdivision.

Security Guarantee, pledge for payment of a loan.

Seminar A group or class for advancement of learning, working together under guidance.

Semipermanent Partly permanent; temporarily long lasting.

Senior (hairdresser) One who has completed an apprenticeship, a journeyperson.

Sensation Power of feeling through the senses.

Serrated Having a saw-like edge.

Setting lotion A liquid used to facilitate setting, retaining the holding power of the set (or blow-dry) by coating the hair fibre and thereby resisting the adsorbtion of moisture.

Shade Degree of difference in colour.

Shampoo Fluid for washing the hair.

Shellac A colourless resin produced on tree bark by insects (India). Soluble in alcohol but not in water, it is used in hair lacquers.

Shingle Hair cut gradually longer toward the crown, without showing a definite line.

Side chain Groups of atoms which, when connected to other amino acids, become known as bridges or bonds.

Silicone Compounds of silicon used in lubricants, polishers, lacquers.

Silk net Strong silk net usually of the colour of hair being woven and used in the parting area of a wig.

Slither A cutting motion used in thinning the hair with the regular scissors.

Soap Solid or liquid cleaners formed by the combination of particular fats and oils with alkaline bases.

Soapless shampoo A shampoo containing no soap, synthetic detergent manufactured from lauryl sulphates and sulphonated animal and vegetable fats and oils.

Sodium bromate A chemical used in neutralisers, an oxidising agent.

Sodium hydroxide A powerful alkaline produced in some chemical hair straighteners or hair relaxers.

Sodium perborate A chemical used in neutralisers, an oxidising agent similar to hydrogen peroxide.

Sodium salt A positive sodium ion combined with a negative ion, e.g. sodium chloride (common salt).

Soft styler An attachment on a blow-dryer to diffuse the airflow.

Sole trader Someone who operates a business as a single person.

Soluble Ability of a substance to dissolve in water.

Specified item An item which is specifically mentioned in an insurance policy.

Sphenoid A bone in the cranium.

Spinosum The prickle/spiny cell layer of the epidermis.

Spiral winding Winding the hair from roots to points.

Stabilise To keep steady, to make not liable to change.

Stable Not easily broken down or upset.

Stack winding A method of permanent waving whereby the perm rods are built up on top of one another, in a pile.

Stand-up pincurl A curl clipped in a stand-up position but which narrows towards the curl's end, used to give fullness.

Staphylococci Bacteria which are grouped in clusters and are found in pimples, boils and pustules.

Starch Carbohydrates stored in plants as granules.

Stem The part of the pincurl that produces the movement.

Sterilise To destroy bacteria and render them incapable of reproduction.

Stock control book A carbon copy book used to order stock and to control its use.

Straightening Making straight.

Stratum Layer.

Streaking Layers or strands of hair with a contrasting colour, usually placed so as to enhance the appearance.

Streptococci Bacteria which are grouped in lines and are found in blood poisoning.

Strop A length of leather (horse hide) on which the razor's edge is set.

Structure A design element: the length arrangement of the hair across the curve of the head.

Style support A permanent wave which will support the style between services.

Subcutaneous/subcutis A layer of fatty tissue which is found below the dermis and covers the muscles.

Sucrose Cane sugar.

Sudoriferous Sweat glands of the skin.

Sugar Sucrose, sweet substance, sweet carbohydrate.

Sulphonated oil Oil used in soapless shampoos.

Sulphur Element.

Sulphur bonds Cross-bonds in the hair fibre which hold the chain of amino acids together.

Sulphur side chain The sulphur amino acid cystine and cysteine representing 17% and 0.7% of the hair's total amino acid content.

Sulphydral group Reduced di-sulphide molecules – (SH) + (SH).

Sundry items Varied unspecified items, petty articles.

Superior Higher.

Surface tension A film or skin on the surface of a liquid.

Surface texture The surface appearance of a haircut – unactivated or activated, or a combination of these.

Surfactant A soapless detergent (a soapless agent).

Switch A postiche consisting of a long bunch of hair.

Symmetrical Hair equally distributed on both sides of the head.

Symptomatic As a symptom, indicating a disease or disorder, abnormality.

Synthetic fibre Fibre produced by chemical, e.g. nylon, a substitute for a natural product.

Systematic Done according to plan.

Table mortgage Using property as a security for money and repaying the ultimate source of the loan plus interest.

Tallow Animal fat.

Taper To diminish a strand of hair gradually toward the points by cutting. Removing bulk from the ends of the hair.

Tax Compulsory monetary contribution for the benefit of the state.

Tax deductible Item allowance against tax deduction.

Taxation Imposing a tax.

Technique Method of performance, showing skill in an art.

Telogen The resting stage of the hair's life cycle.

Temporal Of the temples.

Temporary For a limited time only.

Tension spring An elastic or Velcro strap at the nape of the neck on a wig.

Tepid Lukewarm.

Terminal hair Longer hair that replaces lanugo hair; hair of the scalp, eyebrows, eyelashes and beard.

Terminal tax The balance of tax owed after provisional tax has been paid, payable on 7 February of each year.

Tertiary (colour) Colours that are produced by mixing a primary and secondary colour, e.g. gold (yellow and orange); third in order.

Texture The degree of fineness or coarseness of the hair.

Thiamin(e) Vitamin B complex.

Thinning Removing bulk from the hair.

Thioglycollamides Reducing chemicals used in acid permanent waves.

Thioglycollic A colourless liquid chemical used to break the di-sulphide links on the keratin chain.

Thiolatic acid A reducing chemical used in acid permanent waves.

Time and wage book A book that shows the gross and net pay, sick pay, holidays and time served.

Tinea Ringworm – a vegetable parasite infestation.

Tipping Applying colour or lightener to the ends of the hair.

Toners The colours applied to hair which has been lightened – delicate pastel shades, e.g. champagne, beige, silver.

Toning The colouring process of blonde toners after the hair has been extensively lightened.

Tonsorial Of the barber.

Tortoise shell The shell of the tortoise, used for manufacturing combs.

Touch colouring Applying colour with the finger to various areas throughout the hair.

Toupee A small wig for a man which covers the front and top of the head.

Toupette A small piece of postiche for a woman.

Traction alopecia Loss of hair by the pulling or movement of hair at the roots – caused by tight braids or plaits.

Tragacanth A gum mucilage used as a thickening in setting lotions.

Transformation An artificial covering of the hair. Postiche.

Trapezius A muscle found in the neck.

Trichlorethylene A white spirit used for dry cleaning.

Trichologist A person trained in the science of caring for the hair.

Trichology The study of the structure and functions of the hair.

Trichoptilosis Splitting of the hair due to its swelling.

Trichorrhexis nodosa The breaking or beading of the hair.

Trichotillomania A mania for pulling out one's own hair.

Trough The lower part of a wave between two crests.

Ultraviolet radiation Invisible rays of the spectrum which are beyond violet.

Unactivated texture A smooth surface appearance where the ends of the hair are not visible.

Underdirected A roller sitting below its base.

Uniform layer Each layer exactly alike, without variation, consistent.

Unsaturated Able to dissolve more substance, not saturated.

User friendly A computer term meaning that a computer displays a prompt, so that you know which key to press next.

Van der Waal forces Weak attraction between molecules.

Variable Liable to change.

Variation Something different from another form, an alternative.

Vegetable oils Oils obtained from plants or vegetables.

Vegetable proteins Proteins (amino acids) obtained from vegetables, e.g. soya beans, nuts, beans, legumes.

Veins Blood vessels which convey blood back to the heart.

Vellus hair Fine, unpigmented hair covering most of the body that replaces lanugo hair.

Vent brush A brush with widely spaced plastic bristles designed to be used while blow-drying.

Venule Fine capillaries supplying veins with de-oxygenated blood.

Vertical Upright.

Vibrant Resounding.

Visual poise Correct impression – behaviour. Deportment in the hairdressing salon.

Vitamins Vital amino acids – organic substances found in food and essential for protection against disease.

Volt Electromotive force needed to carry 1 ampere of current against a resistance of 1 ohm.

Volume Height, bulk, (large) amount.

Voucher A document confirming some fact.

Vulcanite Hard rubber.

Wage Rate of pay at regular intervals for work, not including overtime.

Water winding Winding a permanent wave with water instead of solution.

Wattage Power of an electrical appliance expressed in watts.

Weft A length of hair woven on silks.

Weight Heaviness, bulk.

Wen Epidermal cyst.

Wetting agent A substance that facilitates wetting by reducing surface tension, e.g. detergent.

White corpuscles Blood cells which fight invading bacteria.

White henna An alternative term for a bleaching agent, containing hydrogen peroxide and magnesium carbonate or sodium perborate.

White spirit A mixture of petroleum and fractions (hydrocarbons).

Whorl A coil or spiral of hair on the crown.

Widow's peak Growth of hair into a point at the centre forehead.

Wig An artificial head of hair.

Wiglet A small wig which will cover part of the head.

Witch-hazel Astringent used to close the skin pores.

Workshop Practical lesson.

Yak A long-haired ox, the hair of which is sometimes used as a substitute for human hair when making postiche.

Zygomatic Of the cheekbone.

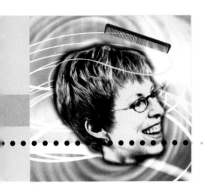

Bibliography

Accident Compensation Corporation. (1983) *Compensation at Work – A Guide to the Employer's Accident Compensation Liability*. Wellington, Accident Compensation Corporation.

– *Levies on Employees*. (1984) Wellington, Accident Compensation Corporation.

Airola, Paavo. (1965) *Stop Hair Loss*. Arizona, Health Plus.

Angelglow, Maggie. (1970) *A History of Make-Up*. London, Studio Vista.

Ashley, Ruth. (1976) *Human Anatomy*. New York, John Wiley and Son.

Asser, Joyce. (1966) *Historic Hairdressing*. London, Pitman.

Begg, Colin. (1983) *Setting Prices. Small Business Guide* (24). Wellington, Development Finance Corporation.

Biological Research Laboratory. (1980) *Through the Microscope*. California, U.S.A, Redken Laboratories.

Botham, Mary and Sharrad, L. (1964) *Manual of Wig Making*. London, Heinemann.

Brake, John. (1979) *Art of the Pacific*. Wellington, Oxford University Press and Queen Elizabeth 11 Arts Council of New Zealand.

Ceres. (1977) *Herbs for Healthy Hair*. Wellingborough, Thorson.

Clegg, Robert. (1981) *Practical Application of Adaptability*. California, Robert Clegg.

Collins, Sarah. (1979) *Beauty*. London, Artus Publishers.

Consumers Institute of New Zealand. (1977) *Cosmetic Care for your Skin*. Wellington, Consumers Institute of New Zealand.

Cooley, Arnold. (1866, 1970) *The Toilet and Cosmetic Arts in Ancient and Modern Times*. New York, Burt Franklin.

Cooper, Wendy, (1971) *Hair – Sex, Society and Symbolism*. London, Aldus Books.

Corson, Richard. (1965) *Fashions in Hair*. London, Peter Owen.

Cozens, Browyn. (1988) *Colour Crazy – The Complete Colour Guide for Hairdressers*. Melbourne, Clarity Publications.

Davies, David. (1976) *I've had a Transplant*. London, D. Davies.

De Courtais, Georgine. (1973) *Women's Headdress and Hairstyles*. London, B.T. Batsford.

Department of Health (New Zealand) (1983) *You – A Guide to Healthy Living for Young People*. Wellington, Government Printer.

Department of Industry and Commerce (Australia). (1982) *Cash Flow – Cash Management. The Small Business Series No. 23*. Canberra, Australian Government Publishing Service.

– (1982) *Retailing. Small Business Guide Series No. 3*. Canberra, Australian Government Publishing Service.

Di Salva, Ronald M. (1976) *Science and Men's Hairstyles*. California, Redken Laboratories.

Drake, Heaton. (1973) *Run Your Own Business*. Wellington, A.H. and A.W. Reed.

Factories and Commercial Premises Order. (1981) Wellington, Government Printer.

Factories and Commercial Premises Regulations. (1981) Wellington, Government Printer.

Fahy, J.L. (1983) *Accident Compensation Coverage*. Wellington, Accident Compensation Corporation.

Fletcher, Grace E., (1965) *Management for Hairdressers*. London, Chapman and Hall.

Foan, G. (1936) *Art and Craft of Hairdressing*. London, New Era Publishing.

Frieda, John. (1983) *Hair Care*. New York, Artus Publishers.

Galvin, Daniel. (1977) *The World of Hair Colour*. London, MacMillan.

Gambrill, Jill. (1980) *Cutting*. Australia, New South Wales University Press.

Grove Day, A. (1964) *They Peopled the Pacific*. New York, Duell, Sloane and Pearce.

Hair and Beauty. (1974) *Student Pic Strip*. London, Hair and Beauty, Consumer Industries Press.

Harrold, Robert and Legg, Phyllida. (1978) *Folk Costumes of the World*. Poole, Dorset Blandford Press.

Health (Hairdressers) Regulations. (1980) Wellington, Government Printer.

Helene Curtis. (1977) *The Salon Owner's Step by Step Guide to Salon Merchandizing*. USA, Helene Curtis.

Hibbott, H.W. (1963) *Handbook of Cosmetic Science*. New York, Pergamon Press.

Hix, Charles. (1979) *Looking Good: A Guide For Men.* London, Angus and Robertson.

Howells, William. (1973) T*he Pacific Islanders.* Wellington, A H and A W Reed

Hubbard, J., Thomas, C. and Varnham, S. (1989) *Principles of Law for New Zealand Business.* Auckland, Addison Wesley Longman.

Huggett, Renee. (1982) *Hairstyles and Head Dresses.* London, Batsford.

– *Main Styles and Head Dresses.* (1982) London, Batsford.

Jeremiah, Rosemary. (1982) *How To Make Money in the Hairdressing Business.* Cheltenham, Stanley Thornes.

Kassenbeck, Paul. (1984) *The Hair and its Structure.* West Germany, Wella.

Keyes, Jean. (1967) *A History of Women's Hairstyles.* London, Methuen.

Kibbe, Constance. (1981) *Standard Text Book of Cosmetology,* rev. ed. New York, Milady.

Kilgour, O.F.G. and McGarry, M. (1964) *An Introduction to Science and Hygiene for Hairdressers.* London, Heinemann.

Kilgour, O.F.G. and McGarry, M. (1984) *Complete Hairdressing Science.* Heinemann.

Kingsley, Philip. (1982) *The Complete Hair Book.* New York, Grove Pro.

Labour Market Information Division, Department of Labour. (1984) *An employer's guide to the department of labour's employment and training incentives and services.* Wellington, Department of Labour.

Law, D. (1968) *How to keep your Hair On.* Saffron Walden, Essex, Health Science Press.

Lee, Mary and Perelman, Susanne. (1973) *Natural Hair Care.* San Francisco, Straight Arrow Books.

Lindrop Tony. (1982) *Running A Small Business.* Wellington, Small Business Agency.

MacCoy, Susan. (1980) *Down the Shampoo Bowl.* USA, M.K. Press.

McCulloch, Menzies. (1983) *Survival Kit for Small Businesses.* Small Business Agency, Development Finance Corporation.

Masters, T.W. (1971) *Hairdressing in Theory and Practice,* 3rd ed. London, Technical Press.

Masters. T.W. (1974) *The Complete Hair Colourist.* London, Heinemann.

Meredith, Bronwyn. (1978) *Vogue Body and Beauty Book.* Book Club Associates.

Miller, Casey and Swift, Kate. (1982) *The Handbook of Non-Sexist Writing.* London, The Women's Press.

Moore, Angus. (1964) *Haircolouring and Bleaching.* London, Hairdressing Registration Council.

Mossman, Roxanne. (1979) *Schema.* Los Angeles, Sebastian International.

New Zealand Hairdressers (Male and Female) Award, 27 July 1982. Wellington, Government Printer.

New Zealand Ladies Hairdressing Industry Apprenticeship Order 14 December 1973. Wellington, Government Printer.

Openshaw, Florence. (1978) *Hairdressing Science.* London, Longman.

Pain, Alister. (1979) *Marketing Focus on Tomorrow.* Otaki, New Zealand, A.S. Pain.

Palladino, Leo. (1983) *Principles and Practices of Hairdressing,* 2nd ed. Macmillan.

Perry, John. (1982) *Hairdressing Management.* Cheltenham, Stanley Thornes.

Pivot Point International. Pivot Point Continuous Education Programme. *Leo Passage Aura Hair and Beauty Course.* Chicago, Leo Passage.

Powitt, A.H. (1980) *Hair Structure and Chemistry Simplified.* New York, Milady.

Price, Vic. (1983) *How to use Your Accountant.* Small Business Guide (17). Wellington, Development Finance Corporation.

Rabey, Gordon, P. (1979) *Manager.* Wellington, Paige Productions.

Redken Laboratories. (1981) *Hair Science and Beauty 1.* California, Redken Laboratories.

– (1976) *Dictionary of Cosmetic Ingredients and Technical Terms.* California, Redken Laboratories.

– (1976) *Acid or Alkaline.* California, Redken Laboratories.

– (1976) *Redken Science and Beauty II.* California, Redken Laboratories.

– (1977) *The pH of Hair.* California, Redken Laboratories.

Roddick, Anita. (1985) *The Body Shop Book.* London, McDonald.

Roe, Derek. (1982) *The Perfect Permanent Wave.* USA, Derek Roe.

Rose, Paul. (1983) *Marketing for Retailers.* Small Business Guide (13). Wellington, Development Finance Corporation.

Rowett, H.G.Q. (1959) *Basic Anatomy and Physiology.* London, John Murray.

Rudman, Richard. (1983) *People – Training Your Staff.* Small Business Guide (23). Wellington, Development Finance Corporation.

Sagay, Esi. (1983) *African Hairstyles.* London, Heinemann.

Salinger, David. (1982) I.A.T. *Guide to Hair Loss,* 3rd ed. International Association of Trichologists.

Salinger, David and Williams Jon. (1986) *Simplified Hairdressing Science.* Narrabeen, Australia, Saliam Books.

Salter, Mary. (1981) *Health for Hairdressers.* Oxford, Technical Press.

Sassoon, Vidal. (1978) *Cutting the Vidal Sassoon Way.* London, Vidal Sassoon (New Concepts) Ltd.

Shaw, Jo Kinross Sylvie. (1981) *Minding Your Own Business.* Australia, Cassell.

Small Business Agency. (1983) *Buying and Valuing a Business*. Small Business Guide (7). Wellington, Development Finance Corporation.

– (1983) *Buying Your First Computer. Small Business Guide* (12). Wellington, Development Finance Corporation.

– (1983) *Costing Your Service, Small Business Guide* (9). Wellington Development Finance Corporation.

– (1983) *Getting a Loan. Small Business Guide* (3). Wellington. Development Finance Corporation.

– (1983) *Starting Your Own Business. Small Business Guide* (20). Wellington, Development Finance Corporation.

– (1983) *Structures of Business. Small Business Guide* (2). Wellington, Development Finance Corporation.

– (1983) *You and Your Bank Manager. Small Business Guide* (15). Wellington, Development Finance Corporation.

Sneddon, J. Russell. (1974) *Natural Hair Care*. England, Thorsons.

Snowden, James. (1979) *The Folk Dress of Europe*. London, Mills and Boon.

Stevens Cox, J. (1979) *Shampoo and Shampooing*. Guernsey, The Toucan Press.

– (1971) *Hair and Beauty Secrets of the 17th Century*. Guernsey, Toucan Press.

– (1966) *Dictionary of Hairdressing and Wig Making*. London, The Hairdressers Technical Council.

Symonds N.G. (1965) *Modern Boardwork*. London, The Hairdressing Registration Council.

Thomson, James C. and Thomson, C.L. (1967) *Healthy Hair*. England, Thorsons.

Tortora, Gerard J. and Anagnostakos, Nicholas P. (?1982) *Principles of Anatomy and Physiology*, 4th ed. New York, Harper Row.

Wella Darmstadt. (1979) *Skills and Drills*. Germany, Wella Darmstadt.

– (1979) *Style Form System Technique Manual*. Germany, Wella.

Wilcox, R. (1965) *Folk and Festival Costume of the World*. New York, Charles Scribner's Sons.

Wilkinson, J.B. and Moore, R.J. (eds). (1982) *Harry's Cosmeticology*. London, George Goodwin.

Williams, Peter L. and Warwick, R. (1980) *Gray's Anatomy – 36th Edition*. Edinburgh, Churchill Livingstone.

Articles and Periodicals

Ayer R.P. and Thompson, J.A. (1972) Scanning electron microscopy and other new approaches to hairspray evaluation. *Journal of Society of Cosmetic Chemists*, 23: 617.

Badwan, A.A. et al. (1980) Preparation and characterisation of the C10 to C18 even-number triethanolamine alkyl sulplates. *International Journal of Cosmetic Science, 2*(1): 39–44.

Bauer, D. et al. (1983) Contribution to the quantification of the conditioning effects of hair dyes. *International Journal of Cosmetic Science, 5*(4): 113–129.

Bell, M. et al. (1979) Evaluating the potential eye irritancy of shampoos. *International Journal of Cosmetic Science, I*(2): 123.

Bjornberg, A, et al. (1983) Refatting rate of human hair lipids after exposure to selenium di-sulphide detergents. *International Journal of Cosmetic Science, 5*(1): 1–5.

Blakeway, J.M. and Seu-Salerno, M. (1983) Substantivity of perfume material to hair. *International Journal of Cosmetic Science, 5*(1): 15–23.

Bottoms, E., Wyatt, E. and Comaish, F. (1972) Progressive changes in cuticular patterns along the shafts of human hair. *British Journal of Dermatology, 86;* April: 379–384.

Brown, A.C. and Swift, J.A. (1975) Hair breakage: the scanning electron microscope as a diagnostic tool. *Journal of Society of Cosmetic Chemists*, 26: 289.

Clement, M.J.L. (1982) The specificity of the ultra structure of human hair medulla. *Journal of Forensic Science Society*, 22(4): 396–398.

– (1982) Mensuration of scanning micrographs. *Journal of Forensic Science Society*, 22(1): 86.

Di Bianca, S.P. (1973) Innovative scanning electron microscope techniques for evaluating hair care products. *Journal of Cosmetic Chemists*, 24: 609.

Donaldson, B.R. and Messenger, E.T. (1979) Performance characteristics and solution properties of surfactants in shampoos. *International Journal of Cosmetic Science, 1*(2): 71.

Dupre. A. et al. (1981) Assay of elements contained in human hair shafts. *Archives for Dermatological Research, 271*(2):233–236.

Estetica, E.S.A.V. Via Cavour 50, 10123, Turin, Italy, Published bi-monthly, (1946–).

Fair, N. and Gupta, B.S. (1982) Effects of chlorine on friction. *Journal of the Society of Cosmetic Chemists, 33*(5): 229–242.

Forestier, J.P. (1982) Henne, absorption de la lausone par le cheveu. *International Journal of Cosmetic Science, 4*(4): 153.

Garcia, Mario et al. (1977) Normal cuticle wear patterns in human hair. *Journal of Cosmetic Chemistry, 29*: 155–175

Hair and Beauty. (1866–) London, Consumer Industries Press, Vol 1.

Hairdressers Journal. (1882–) London, Consumer Industries Press, Vol 1.

Inland Revenue Te Tari Taake. (March 1999) *Employer's Guide* IR 335.

Kelly, S.E. and Robinson, V. (1982) *The effect of grooming on the hair cuticle.* Journal 4: 203–216.

Kirkland, D.J. (1983) The mutagenicity and carcinogenicity of hair dyes. *International Journal of Cosmetic Science,* 5(2): 51.

Knott, E.E. et al. In vivo procedures tor assessment of hair greasiness. *International Journal of Cosmetic Science,* 5(3): 77.

Maes, D.A. et al. (1979) Some aspects of hair degreasing. *International Journal of Cosmetic Science,* 1(3): 169.

Muto, H. (1981) et al. Electron microscopic fine structure. *Okajimas Folia Anatomica Japonica,* 58(2): 81–98.

– (1981) Fine structure of the fully keratinized. *Acta Dermatological Hifuka Kiyo (English ed.)* 76(101–106).

Patel, C.U. (1983) Antistatic properties of some cationic polymers used in hair care products. *International Journal of Cosmetic Science,* 5(5): 181.

Puri, A.K. (1979) Recent trends in the formation of permanent waving products for hair. *International Journal of Cosmetic Science,* 1(1): 59.

Riggott, J.N. and Wyatt, E.H. (1983) A possible means of hair identification. *Journal of Forensic Science Society,* 23(2): 155–160.

– (1980) SEM hairs of different parts of the body. *Journal of Anatomy,* 140(1): 121.

Robins, C. (1966) Weathering in human hair. *Textile Research Journal,* 37: 337.

Robinson, V. (1975) Split ends, a scientific study of a hair. *Australian Society of Cosmetic Science,* 90.

Ryder, Michael, L. (1981) *Hair – The Institute of Biology's Studies in Biology No. 41.* Edward Arnold.

Scandal, J. et al. (1983) Shampoos and their aesthetic effects. *International Journal of Cosmetic Science,* 5(5): 157.

– (1979) Studies on the cosmetic criteria of the hair after shampoo. *International Journal of Cosmetic Science,* 1(2): 111.

Shaw, D.A. (1979) Hair lipid and surfactants. *International Journal of Cosmetic Science,* 1(6): 317.

Van Abbe et al. (1981) The effect of hair care products on dandruff. *International Journal of Cosmetic Science,* 13(5): 233.

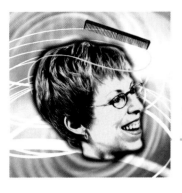

Index